Treatment Compliance
and the Therapeutic Alliance

Chronic Mental Illness

Series Editor
John A. Talbott, University of Maryland School of Medicine, Baltimore, USA

Advisory Board
Leona Bachrach • James T. Barter • Carol Caton • David L. Cutler • Jeffrey L. Geller • William M. Glazer • Stephen M. Goldfinger • Howard H. Goldman • H. Richard Lamb • Harriet P. Lefley • Anthony F. Lehman • Robert P. Lieberman • W. Walter Menninger • Arthur T. Meyerson

This book is part of a series. The publisher will accept continuation orders which may be cancelled at any time and which provide for automatic billing and shipping of each title in the series upon publication. Please write for details.

Treatment Compliance and the Therapeutic Alliance

Edited by

Barry Blackwell, MD

CNR Health, Inc.

and

University of Wisconsin School of Medicine
Milwaukee, Wisconsin

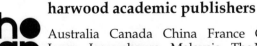

harwood academic publishers

Australia Canada China France Germany India
Japan Luxembourg Malaysia The Netherlands Russia
Singapore Switzerland Thailand United Kingdom

Amsteldijk 166
1st Floor
1079 LH Amsterdam
The Netherlands

British Library Cataloguing in Publication Data

Treatment compliance and the therapeutic alliance. —
    (Chronic mental illness ; v. 5)
    1. Mentally ill — Care   2. Mentally ill — Rehabilitation
    3. Patient compliance   4. Physician and patient
    I. Blackwell, Barry
    616.8'9'1

ISBN 90-5702-546-9

CONTENTS

INTRODUCTION TO THE SERIES

This series on chronic mental illness is a result of both the success and failure of our efforts over the past thirty years to provide better treatment, rehabilitation and care for persons suffering from severe and persistent mental illnesses. The failure is obvious to all who walk our cities' streets, use our libraries or pass through our transportation terminals. The success is found in the enormous boost of interest in service to, research on and teaching about treatment, rehabilitation and care of those persons who, in Leona Bachrach's definition, "are, have been, or might have been, but for the deinstitutionalization movement, on the rolls of long-term mental institutions, especially state hospitals."

The first book in our modern era devoted to the subject was that by Richard Lamb in 1976, *Community Survival for Long-Term Patients*. Shortly thereafter, Leona Bachrach's unique study "Deinstitutionalization: An Analytical Review and Sociological Perspective" was published. In 1978, the American Psychiatric Association hosted a meeting on the problem that resulted in the publication *The Chronic Mental Patient*. This effort in turn spawned several texts dealing with increasingly specialized areas: *The Chronic Mentally Ill: Treatment, Programs, Systems* and *Chronic Mental Illness in Children and Adolescents*, both by John Looney; and *The Chronic Mental Patient/II* by Walter Menninger and Gerald Hannah.

Now, however, there are a host of publications devoted to various portions of the problem, e.g., the homeless mentally ill, rehabilitation of the mentally ill, families of the mentally ill and so on. The amount of research and experience now that can be conveyed to a wide population of caregivers is exponentially greater than it was in 1955, the year that deinstitutionalization began.

This series will cover:

— types of intervention, e.g., psychopharmacology, psychotherapy, case management, social and vocational rehabilitation and mobile and home treatment;
— settings, e.g., hospitals, ambulatory settings, nursing homes, correctional facilities and shelters;
— specific populations, e.g., alcohol and drug abusers, the homeless and those dually diagnosed;

— special issues, e.g., family intervention, psychoeducation, policy/
  financing, non-compliance, forensic, cross-cultural and systems
  issues.

I am indebted to our hard-working editorial board as well as to our
editors and authors, many of whom are involved in both activities.

This fifth volume is typical of what we will publish; it covers a
specific portion of the field, although overlapping with other books
in the series; and it deals with experience, research, delivery system strategies and broader social issues. Its editor is a leader in the
area of the treatment alliance between provider and consumer and
has the unique ability to bridge the academic and practical worlds.

Future books in this series will cover inpatient care, psychiatric
rehabilitation, psychopharmacology, the homeless mentally ill and
the mentally ill in the correctional system. I hope you will look forward to them as eagerly as I do.

John A. Talbott, MD

INTRODUCTION

The purpose of this introduction is to familiarize readers with the volume and its contributors.

When Dr. John Talbott invited me to edit a text about compliance for the series on Chronic Mental Illness, I was delighted. After a quarter century of research and writing on the topic, I thought I knew something about it. Now that the task is complete, I recognize how much I still have to learn. An additional bonus has been the development of a new gestalt at a moment in history when the shift from paternalism to consumerism has accelerated dramatically. I hope that readers will share these twin benefits of new knowledge and a fresh perspective. These are best expressed by our early decision to modify the title to *Treatment Compliance and the Therapeutic Alliance*. I believe that every chapter reflects, to a greater or lesser degree, the profound semantic, practical, and philosophical gulf between the two words "compliance" and "alliance."

When psychiatrist Jay Katz wrote *The Silent World of Doctor and Patient* in 1984, he spoke about the long history of Aesculapian authority that stifled dialogue between providers and consumers. Interestingly, the word "compliance" did not appear in the index, and his book, although a classic, is seldom cited in compliance literature. What has happened since may well be considered a paradigm shift — one in which events have placed mental health professionals in a leading role. From the mid-eighties on, a rising tide of homeless individuals with severe and persistent mental illness forced us to consider the problems of providing access and services to an often-reluctant population. The words "outreach" and "engagement" extended our responsibility; it became "our" problem not just "theirs." What we have learned exposed the inadequacy of the concept "compliance" and invited us to become far more active in creating an alliance. That is what I believe this book captures.

A volume with thirty-four contributors presents its own problems; not the least of which being the compliance of authors to editorial requests. In order that conformity not constrain creativity, the requirements were kept simple. Person-first language, real-life examples, and reasonably concise writing were requested.

The volume is divided into three parts, reflecting a desire to capture the science, the art, and some special problems of the field.

For better or worse, there is a vast scientific literature codified in various data bases under the keyword "compliance." The first section of the book reports on the results of this research and debates some theoretical, philosophical, and policy issues reflected within this scholarly body of knowledge. The second section covers the spectrum of individual experience portrayed by many different participants in the treatment alliance. The third and final section dwells on the problems found among populations of people with special needs.

My first paper about compliance was published approximately twenty-five years ago. I became interested in the topic because it epitomized the nuances of a biopsychosocial perspective and it has remained a theme throughout my professional career at the interface between medicine and psychiatry. Over the years, collaboration and research with medical students, pharmacists, psychologists, internists, and ophthalmologists have shaped my thinking and writing. My opening chapter is a reflection of this general interest — it is an overview of the major conclusions derived from a quarter century of research in the entire compliance field. This creates a backdrop against which the special problems of people who treat or suffer from severe and persistent mental illness can be compared and contrasted.

Advance in any field is facilitated by theory development and conceptual clarity. This is particularly true for a topic as diverse and multiply determined as compliance. Howard Leventhal is professor of health psychology at Rutgers University, New Brunswick, New Jersey. For over two decades, he and his collaborators have reviewed and developed models for understanding the interaction between patients and providers in the entire arena of compliance. Their model of common-sense illness representations is particularly well-suited to the contemporary shift toward a more consumer-oriented approach. In chapter 2, for the first time, they apply their model to people with mental illness.

In today's climate, economic forces are beginning more and more to shape social policy and clinical care. Dr. Peter Weiden's NIMH (National Institute of Mental Health)-funded research on compliance in patients suffering from schizophrenia (chapter 3) forms the springboard for considering the clinical, economic, and social policy implications of this problem. As individual states place more and more people with severe and long-term illness into managed care, the economic consequences of both good and poor compliance will become increasingly apparent and influential.

Insight (or lack of it) is often the most commonly used (or misused) concept in our attempts to understand why people with severe mental illness do or do not follow treatment suggestions. Dr. Anthony David's research on this topic from England (chapter 4) stems from the intellectual challenge of integrating philosophy, neuropsychology, and the social sciences.

"Insight" is not only the clinical concept most often invoked to explain poor compliance, it frequently forms the basis for questioning a person's decision-making capacity and his or her ability to give informed consent. This ushers in the thorny problem of coerced treatment in patients who are involuntarily committed. This topic is addressed in a collaboration between Dr. Ansar Haroun, a forensic psychiatrist, and Grant Morris, a law professor (chapter 5). Both authors write from their practical experience in the California legal system, where they have worked to find a balance between the legal and ethical dilemmas posed by the patient's right to refuse treatment.

Coercion comes in many different degrees, some of which are far less obvious when they occur outside the legal arena and within what is often assumed to be a benevolent clinical context. These subtle forms of coercion are dealt with in chapter 6 by Ron Diamond, a psychiatrist with extensive experience in community care, and Laurie Curtis, an internationally known mental health consultant with the Center for Community Change, Trinity College of Vermont, Burlington.

The United States is a diverse society and in many ways it remains a melting pot. Often the two people attempting to form an alliance are from different cultures. Although seldom dealt with directly, cultural dissonance is a major contributor to faulty alliances. James Mason, who is completing his doctorate in urban studies, has taken his considerable experience as a service provider to culturally diverse populations of children and families, and has applied it to teaching and training individuals and organizations about how to improve their cultural competence in meeting the needs of clients (chapter 7).

The opening chapter in the second section of this book is literally "on the cusp" between the social policies that ushered in the first wave of deinstitutionalization and the practical problems of a program administrator faced with the contemporary task of completing the shift to community care. Dr. Mary Alice Brown, whose degree is in counseling psychology, has almost twenty years' experience as executive director of Laurel Hill Center, Eugene, Oregon, a large rehabilitation center responsible for designing programs to meet the needs of people with severe limitations and long histories of hospitalization. Her story carries the hopeful message that the lessons of the past have been learned so that those who need our services today do not have to express their dissatisfaction by staying away.

Having created the context in which our alliances can occur, it becomes time to introduce its most important participant — the patient or consumer of services. Dan Fisher is a psychiatrist, consumer, survivor, and teacher. Formerly the medical director of a community mental health center, he now serves as executive director of the National Empowerment Center, Lawrence, Massachusetts, a consumer-run, federally funded training and information center. Nobody can speak more knowledgeably and eloquently of the ingredients necessary for a satisfying alliance or of the shortcomings that can express themselves in compliance problems (chapter 9).

Next and closest to the person seeking services are the family members. Dale Johnson, the author of chapter 10, is the father of a son with schizophrenia and also a clinical psychologist who has played a leadership role in the National Alliance for the Mentally Ill. He therefore speaks from personal experience and the experiences of many other family members.

A variety of health care professionals enter into alliances with patients who have severe and persistent mental illness. Thomas Kuhlman is a clinical psychologist whose work among the homeless was the subject of his book *Psychology on the Streets*. In chapter 11 he discusses both the practical and theoretical considerations involved in forming a successful therapeutic alliance and in dealing with the novel concept of "reactance."

Next comes my own chapter on the physician role in medication management. It is based on personal experience working in a multidisciplinary health care clinic for the homeless. The much-maligned "med check" is an important part of everyday treatment. In addition to a knowledge of medications, an awareness of the interpersonal dynamics involved in prescribing and taking medications is essential.

Jayme Trott has a doctorate in pharmacy and experience working in both a state hospital and a private outpatient psychopharmacology clinic. She describes the important role that a pharmacist can play (chapter 13) in a multidisciplinary team helping to educate consumers and caregivers about barriers to medication compliance.

The concluding chapter in the second section of the book deals with the coordinating and integrating role of the case manager. An educator by training, Martha Hodge has been a pioneer in our field since the early years of deinstitutionalization. Her experience in community support projects and psychosocial rehabilitation facilities has made her an advocate in promoting ethical and supportive techniques that help people with mental illness enjoy enriched lives in the community.

The third section of the book describes the special problems encountered by individuals who are coping with particular problems. Its chapters span the life cycle and include each of the major psychiatric disorders.

Although familiar with the compliance literature, I knew of nothing that described the problems I felt sure must occur in the lives of children, adolescents, and adults with developmental disabilities. Tatiana Dierwechter is a social worker and director of services for a disability advocacy organization. Her insights and experience provide a unique description (chapter 15) of the ways in which choice and autonomy can be fostered in the interests of selective compliance by people of all ages who have intellectual disabilities.

Neal Cohen is a psychiatrist whose research in psychotherapy and psychopharmacology; leadership positions in public sector institutions; and outreach work among the homeless have equipped him to provide an informative chapter 16 on the difficulties encountered by people with schizophrenia and those who treat them.

Kay Jamison (chapter 17) is a psychologist with a unique perspective on bipolar disorder. She is both a nationally recognized author and researcher on the illness as well as someone who has described her own personal experiences with the condition in a recent book *An Unquiet Mind.*

No disorder poses greater problems with compliance than dependence on and abuse of alcohol, both by itself and in conjunction with other major illnesses. Dr. Allen Zweben holds a doctoral degree in social work and is a distinguished researcher in the addictions field. His fellow contributor David Barrett is a therapist and together they are investigators in a collaborative national research project exploring an innovative approach to individualized treatment (project MATCH). Chapter 18 describes practical steps that encourage commitment to a constructive treatment alliance. This approach differs markedly from the rigid and at times coercive traditional treatment model often unsuited to the needs of individuals struggling with their own sense of powerlessness.

The penultimate chapter in this section (chapter 19) is a collaboration among a team of six clinicians involved in caring for the elderly who have mental illness. The first author, Dr. Donald Hay, is a geriatric psychiatrist who describes a multidisciplinary integrated model that encourages compliance and provides continuity across different levels of care.

A particular problem affecting an increasing segment of our aging population is memory impairment. In the final chapter this neglected topic is discussed by Dr. Robert Hirschman, a neuropsychologist and educator with specific interests in rehabilitation medicine and geropsychology.

Altogether the thirty-four contributors of these twenty chapters provide a mosaic of information and advice from a variety of different perspectives. As people, they speak for consumers, educators, family members, administrators, and practitioners — who in turn include the disciplines of psychiatry, psychology, social work, counseling, pharmacy, and law. Some authors speak from both a personal and professional viewpoint. Out of this rich diversity emerges a clear consensus — compliance is no longer an adequate concept to convey the mutuality of a true therapeutic alliance.

CONTRIBUTORS

David Barrett, MS, CADC III, Southeastern Wisconsin Medical and Social Services, Inc.

Barry Blackwell, MD, Medical Director, CNR Health, Inc.; Clinical Professor of Psychiatry, University of Wisconsin School of Medicine, Milwaukee.

Sheila R. Botts, PharmD, Clinical Sciences Research Fellow, University of Texas Health Science Center at San Antonio.

Mary Alice Brown, PhD, Executive Director, Laurel Hill Center, Inc., Eugene, Oregon.

Neal Cohen, MD, Vice-Chairman and Clinical Director, Department of Psychiatry, Mount Sinai Medical Center, New York, New York.

Laurie C. Curtis, MA, Center for Community Change through Housing and Support, Trinity College of Vermont, Burlington.

Anthony David, FRCP.MRCPsych, MD, Reader in Cognitive Neuropsychiatry, Department of Psychological Medicine, King's College Hospital and Institute of Psychiatry, London, England.

Ronald J. Diamond, MD, Professor, Department of Psychiatry, University of Wisconsin Medical School, Madison; Medical Director, Mental Health Center of Dane County, Wisconsin.

Michael Diefenbach, PhD, Institute for Health and Department of Psychology, Rutgers University.

Tatiana Dierwechter, MSW, Services Director, ARC Milwaukee, Wisconsin.

Susan Essock, PhD, Director of Psychological Services, Department of Mental Health and Addiction Services, State of Connecticut; Associate Clinical Professor, Department of Psychiatry, Yale University School of Medicine, New Haven, Connecticut.

Daniel Fisher, MD, PhD, Executive Director, National Empowerment Center, Lawrence, Massachusetts.

Kari Franson, PharmD, Assistant Professor, Division of Geriatric Psychiatry, Department of Psychiatry and Human Behavior, Saint Louis University School of Medicine, Missouri.

Ansar M. Haroun, MD, Supervising Forensic Psychiatrist, Superior Court of California in San Diego; Assistant Clinical Professor of Psychiatry and Pediatrics, School of Medicine, University of California San Diego; Adjunct Professor, University of San Diego School of Law.

Rakhshanda Hassan, MD, Assistant Clinical Professor, Division of Geriatric Psychiatry, Department of Psychiatry and Human Behavior, Saint Louis University School of Medicine, Missouri.

Donald P. Hay, MD, Associate Professor, Vice-Chair of Clinical Programs, Division of Geriatric Psychiatry, Department of Psychiatry and Human Behavior, Saint Louis University School of Medicine, Missouri.

Linda K. Hay, PhD, RN, Assistant Professor, Director of Clinical Trials Unit, Division of Geriatric Psychiatry, Department of Psychiatry and Human Behavior, Saint Louis University School of Medicine, Missouri.

Robert S. Hirschman, PhD, Professor, Director of Clinical Training, Wisconsin School of Professional Psychology, Milwaukee, Wisconsin.

Martha C. Hodge, MS, Community Support Consultants, St. George Island, Florida.

Kay Redfield Jamison, PhD, Professor of Psychiatry, Johns Hopkins University School of Medicine, Baltimore, Maryland.

Dale L. Johnson, PhD, Professor, Department of Psychology, University of Houston, Texas.

Roisin Kemp, FRANZCPsych, Research Worker, Department of Psychological Medicine, King's College Hospital and Institute of Psychiatry, London, England.

Thomas L. Kuhlman, PhD, Licensed Psychologist, Minneapolis-St. Paul, Minnesota.

Jennifer Falconer Lambert, MS, Institute for Health and Department of Psychology, Rutgers University.

Elaine A. Leventhal, MD, PhD, Department of Medicine, Robert Wood Johnson School of Medicine, University of Medicine and Dentistry of New Jersey, Piscataway, New Jersey.

Howard Leventhal, PhD, Board of Governors Professor of Health Psychology, Institute for Health and Department of Psychology, Rutgers University, New Brunswick, New Jersey.

James Mason, PhD, (ABD), Director of Training, Research and Training Center on Family Support and Children's Mental Health, Portland, Oregon.

Grant H. Morris, JD, LLM, Professor of Law, University of San Diego; Clinical Professor, Department of Psychiatry, University of California, San Diego, School of Medicine.

Mark Olfson, MD, MPH, Associate Professor of Clinical Psychiatry, Columbia University School of Medicine, New York, New York.

Julie Renner, MD, Assistant Professor, Division of Geriatric Psychiatry, Department of Psychiatry and Human Behavior, Saint Louis University School of Medicine, Missouri.

Peggy Szwabo, PhD, ACSW, RN, C-CS, Assistant Professor, Director, Department of Psychiatry and Human Behavior Education Center, Saint Louis University School of Medicine, Missouri.

Jayme C. Trott, PharmD, Assistant Clinical Professor of Pharmacy, Clinical Pharmacy Programs at San Antonio, Department of Pharmacology, University of Texas Health Science Center at San Antonio.

Peter Weiden, MD, Associate Professor of Clinical Psychiatry, Columbia University, New York, New York.

Allen Zweben, DSW, Director, Center for Addiction and Behavioral Health Research, Associate Professor, School of Social Welfare, University of Wisconsin, Milwaukee.

SECTION ONE

Research, Theory and Social Context

1

From Compliance to Alliance: A Quarter Century of Research

BARRY BLACKWELL

Individuals with severe mental illness are people first; they experience many of the same problems in following treatment recommendations as anyone else. During this quarter century a vast literature has accumulated, mostly catalogued (for better or worse) under the term "compliance". This chapter summarizes its major conclusions. The goal is to provide a perspective that will help create the foundation for a fruitful alliance between health care providers and those who bear the burden of severe mental illness.

THE EBB AND FLOW OF INTEREST

Attitudes toward and interest in the therapeutic alliance between providers and patients have ebbed and flowed throughout the history of health care. This is testified to by the metaphors, myths, and language used to describe the relationship as well as by the volume and content of research and writing devoted to the topic.

Ever since Eve ate the forbidden fruit in the Garden of Eden, it has been metaphorically clear that people sometimes choose not to follow directions. Whether God-like or not, physicians are socially sanctioned authority figures who may sometimes come to believe Hippocrates' alleged saying "keep watch also on the faults of the patients, which often make them lie about the taking of things prescribed" (Wright, 1993). This frequently quoted statement does not appear in Thomas Coar's compilation of the Aphorisms of Hippocrates (Coar, 1822). What does occur are statements more consistent with a need for a negotiated alliance such as "A regimen too strict and unsubstantial is always dangerous ... when it does not agree with the patient."

The dialectic about an allegedly authoritarian physician and an ideally autonomous patient has waxed and waned with the sociopolitical zeitgeist (Steele, Blackwell, Gutmann, & Jackson, 1987). During the 18th and 19th centuries in the prescientific era of medicine, the public was exhorted to take care of its own health by such religious leaders as John Wesley. In his popular text "Primitive Physic" Wesley chastised the medical profession for mystifying its work in order to distance itself from people. The rise of scientific medicine in the early twentieth century reinforced medical authority and marked what Paul Starr (1982) called "the retreat of private judgment." Patient acquiescence was assumed and compliance was taken for granted. When problems were identified, they were often dealt with dismissively.

Following the Second World War, the pendulum began to swing back with a growing distrust of authoritarianism. The move towards individual autonomy was epitomized by the civil rights, women's rights, and patient's rights movements. Distrust of the purely biomedical approach was expressed, the biopsychosocial model was espoused, and both public and professional opinions began to advocate patient partnership in treatment. As these social changes took place, the physician's unique prerogative to prescribe was eroded. Other health professionals became more active in understanding and participating in treatment. These included pharmacists, nurses, psychologists, educators, sociologists, epidemiologists, and anthropologists.

Towards the late sixties and early seventies, social changes coalesced with scientific advances. The discovery of modern major pharmaceuticals including antibiotics, anti-inflammatory agents, steroids, synthetic analgesics and psychotropic drugs brought many diseases under control. As the acute treatable disorders were managed and the population aged, interest shifted to more chronic conditions and the emphasis was less on cure and more on risk reduction, disease prevention, and lifestyle change. This resulted in treatment regimens that were long-term, complex, and which created quality of life considerations for the consumer.

All of these social and scientific events resulted in a dramatic upsurge in interest in what had been an ancient but largely neglected topic (Blackwell, 1992). The word "compliance" entered the medical lexicon for the first time in 1975 when it replaced the older term "patient drop out" in the Index Medicus. The first two international conferences on compliance were held at the McMaster University in 1974 and 1977 (Haynes, Taylor & Sackett, 1979). These defined the parameters of the field and documented an exponential increase in the number of research studies and reviews. Several textbooks appeared, including one devoted to community care of people with persistent mental illness (Barofsky & Bulson, 1980). Despite this initial burst of energy, the level of interest dwindled and within less than ten years one of the principal architects of the early enthusiasm noted that "the wind seems to have gone out of the sails of the compliance research enterprise" (Haynes, Wang, & Da Mota Gomes,

1987). There has never been a third international conference. The reasons for this slackening of interest will become evident when we review the difficulties and shortcomings of attempts to study or modify the treatment alliance.

Perhaps the crudest index of interest in an area is to survey the number of articles published about the topic. When the McMaster group first undertook this type of census, they produced a graph which demonstrated the dramatic increase in articles on compliance from an average of less than 30 a year in the decade 1960 to 1970 to a total of between 100 and 200 in the three years 1975 through 1977 (Haynes, 1979).

Review of Medline data since that time reveals that these numbers continued to escalate until they reached about 700 articles a year in 1986. Since then, the rate of growth has slowed considerably and although it increased somewhat in 1989, it has remained almost unchanged for the last five years at between 800 and 900 articles annually. During this period of growth, the number of journals surveyed by Medline has doubled (from 1800 to 3600) adding emphasis in favor of a relative slowing of output.

WHAT'S IN A NAME?

Ambivalence about this topic is apparent from its semantics; some cultures (where authority is less often questioned) lack words to convey the concept of compliance. In more egalitarian societies advocates complain that the word is coercive, perhaps even politically incorrect. As long ago as 1979, Haynes noted the disfavor attached to the term "because it conjures up images of patient or client sin and serfdom" (Haynes, 1979).

The suggestions for alternative names have included adherence, congruence, or treatment alliance. Nevertheless, compliance has remained the preferred term in the scientific literature — less than a quarter of one percent of the most recent articles (11 out of 570) use the most preferred alternative word "adherence" in their title. Feinstein (1990) has made the tongue-in-cheek observation that "adherence seems too sticky, fidelity has too many connotations and maintenance suggests a repair crew."

One way to reconcile these disparate viewpoints is to make clear that compliance is best considered in a context of the treatment alliance thus ridding it of its coercive connotation. A recent essay in an ethics journal (Holm, 1993) concludes that "new terminology will not be sufficient, a change of the underlying attitudes is absolutely necessary." There is some evidence that such a change may be occurring, at least in some cultures. In America the National Council on Patient Information and Education (NCPIE), an organization of 280 health professionals, government, consumer and industry organizations, recently stated their belief that physicians now understand the complexity of the compliance problem and are willing to implement the organization's simple slogan "communicate before you medicate" (Bachman, 1993). A review of compliance with rehabilitation recommendations (Merrill, 1994) goes still further to suggest that successful therapists like "successful salespeople know their product, learn the patient's dominant buying motive, combine facts with benefits and present arguments that fit the person's belief system and norms."

DOES COMPLIANCE MATTER?

Beyond the semantic issues is a more fundamental question — does compliance matter? Both patients and providers underestimate the scope and significance of the issue. In an unpublished national survey of ophthalmologists who treat glaucoma, we found that only one out of two hundred estimated that their own patients were less compliant than the national norm. Similarly, patients consistently underestimate their forgetfulness when their own estimates are compared to more objective measures. In one study, 83% of parents claimed that their children were taking penicillin when 92% of urine samples had no antibiotic activity (Bergsman & Werner, 1963).

Some experts have espoused the opinion that noncompliance may be viewed as a protective device or a rational decision to shield the patient from the iatrogenic consequences of overprescribing (Donovan & Blake, 1992). Eraker, Kirscht, & Praker (1984) pointed out that the public is repeatedly subjected to medical controversies and contradictions. Charney (1975) made the tongue-in-cheek observation that compliance was balanced with "prescribance" when he argued that "some sort of rough and ready natural law seems to be at work. The physician will be expected to prescribe with only approximate accuracy, and the patient will be expected to comply with only modest fidelity." At least 20% of health care expenditures are on unnecessary procedures or services (HCFCA Statistics, 1992) and somewhere between a fifth and a third of patients admitted to hospitals have suffered an iatrogenic event (Leape, 1994).

These caveats serve as a reminder that doctors do not always know best. They must also be balanced against the equally obvious harm done by inadequate treatment. Computations of the extent of the damage are crude and culture specific. One American review estimated the annual cost of poor compliance was well in excess of one hundred billion dollars accounted for by unnecessary hospital or nursing home admissions, lost work productivity, premature deaths and outpatient treatment costs (Reston, 1992).

Whatever the overall social costs may be, the individual consequences will reflect that person's particular disease and the effectiveness of available treatment. As long as treatments were largely panaceas, neglect of compliance was hardly surprising or a matter of much interest. Now that so much therapy is effective, the personal and social costs compel our concern. An individual denied a scarce kidney or heart transplant because of suspected compliance problems receives a death sentence. A society that shuns preventative methods to check the spread of HIV infection embraces genocide.

Finally, attempts to improve compliance are not without potential adverse consequences. For example, intervention at the work site to improve compliance with antihypertensive treatments may increase absenteeism and decrease productivity, presumably as a result of enhancing the individual's sense of vulnerability and secondary sick role behavior (Alderman & Lamport, 1990). Another example, based on economic arguments, is that adopting an unrealistically high criterion for participation in screening programs may prove detrimental by diverting resources from additional at risk populations (Torgerson & Donaldson, 1994).

WHAT DOES "COMPLIANCE" MEAN?

Whatever word is used to describe this problem, there remains the need to precisely define its meaning. Probably the best and the most resilient definition of compliance is that adopted at the first international conference on compliance with therapeutic regimens in May 1974. This states that compliance is "the extent to which a person's behavior (in terms of taking medications, following diets, or executing lifestyle changes) coincides with medical or health advice" (Haynes, 1979). Although this definition is relatively free from fixing blame, it may not go far enough to meet Holm's recommendation that "It is not patients who should comply with their doctors' demands, but doctors who should comply with their patients' informed and considered desires" (Holm, 1993).

THE MULTIPLE MANIFESTATIONS OF NONCOMPLIANCE

This relatively succinct definition hints at the many manifestations of the compliance problem. First, it is necessary to define which behavior is involved beginning with the reluctance to initiate treatment, including rejection of screening procedures, not filling prescriptions or failure to attend an initial appointment ("no shows"). After engagement in therapy, compliance problems may include irregular attendance, premature termination (dropouts or "against medical advice") or failure to follow recommendations. The latter may involve diet, lifestyle, or prescriptions. Faulty compliance with medication may include errors of purpose, timing or dosage as well as total or partial omission or use of inadvertent combinations (Blackwell, Gutmann, & Jackson, 1981).

MEASUREMENT — PROBLEMS AND METHODS

A major problem is that compliance problems diminish under scrutiny. The fact that people modify their behavior in response to being observed or visiting a health care provider is known as the "toothbrush" or "white coat" effect. This reactivity makes it difficult to

Table 1.1 Methods of Measurement

---

1. CLINICIAN RATING
   Little better than chance accuracy

2. COLLATERAL OBSERVATION

3. INTERVIEW
   Subject to response bias, reduced by standardized, skilled, frequent interviews

4. PILL COUNTS
   Requires reliable dispensing, known amounts, complete return, truthfulness

5. BIOLOGICAL — Urine or Blood
   Metabolites or markers
   Best suited for 'yes-no' determinations

6. MEDICATION EVENT MONITORING (MEMS) — Microcircuitry
   Avoids reactance but creates ethical issues

7. SELF-MONITORING (diaries, dispensers, etc.)
   Helpful in problem-solving; provides feedback and self-correction

---

study compliance in ways that relate to real life. Added to this is the problem of minimization alluded to earlier; both patients and providers underestimate the scope of the problem.

It has been noted in the compliance field that simple measures are not accurate and accurate measures are not simple. The various methods used are listed in Table 1.1, together with brief comments on their advantages and drawbacks. Since no one method is without its drawbacks, some experts have recommended that more than one be used in any study of compliance. Of particular interest are the newer electronic methods in which time recording microcircuitry is installed in pill containers, eye droppers or oxygen equipment to record medication events (so-called medication event monitoring systems — MEMS) (Matsuyama, Mason, & Jue, 1993). This method permits accurate observation by subterfuge and therefore eliminates reactivity but it raises novel ethical issues concerning informed consent (Levine, 1994). These can be partly avoided by post-observation debriefing provided it is not deceptive or does not inflict unwanted insights on the patient.

HOW MUCH COMPLIANCE IS ENOUGH?

However accurately compliance is measured, it remains necessary to quantify how much is enough. This can be done in a number of ways and varies from one situation to another. The crudest method is categorical statements of good, fair, poor or nonadherent, each of which requires definition. Quantitative measures describe the percentage of the regimen adhered to in terms of medication, appointments, or risk reduction behaviors. The most sophisticated are index measures which take into account composite behaviors, for example, prescribing the appropriate drug and taking it in adequate amounts to a defined outcome.

Whatever method of quantification is selected, there remain a number of difficulties to be considered. In quantifying compliance, time is also a factor — whether or not deviation from a particular regimen is consistent, intermittent, or sporadic. It is not uncommon for individuals to subscribe to the idea of "giving their body a rest" from medication. Whether or not such "drug holidays" adversely affect outcome depends on the disorder and method of treatment.

How much compliance is enough also varies from one situation to another. Satisfactory blood pressure control is usually obtained with 80% compliance; the same level of adherence to a weight reduction regimen might result in significant weight gain. Even if a person is 100% compliant, blood pressure may remain poorly controlled if that person is overweight, under considerable stress, absorbs the drug poorly or metabolizes it rapidly. Finally, Urquhart (1993) has proposed the interesting concept of drug "forgiveness" as a factor in assessing the impact of noncompliance. Not all drugs are equal in this regard. The extent to which treatment outcome correlates with compliance depends on a drug's metabolism, mechanism of action, desired outcome and the immediacy with which withdrawal is manifested. This concept can be illustrated by contrasting two drugs: alprazolam used for the treatment of anxiety and fluoxetine used for the treatment of depression. Alprazolam is rapidly metabolized and induces its effect by immediate receptor binding. Its action is dramatic and the effects of cessation are virtually immediate. As a result, alprazolam is so unforgiving that it has been nicknamed "the American Express" pill — "don't leave home without it." Physiologic addiction ensures perfect compliance. By contrast, fluoxetine is very slowly metabolized and its mechanism of action is due to delayed receptor regulation. Its effects are therefore insidious and the results of cessation are delayed and prolonged. As a consequence, an occasional missed dose of fluoxetine is immaterial — the drug is very "forgiving".

RESEARCH ON COMPLIANCE

Research Standards — One of the contributions of the McMaster Group was to define optimal research standards in the compliance field (Haynes, Taylor, Snow, & Sackett, 1979). When these criteria were applied to the early studies, the results were not impressive. The best that could be said was that about half of the studies did at least define the term compliance but less than one in five had an

Table 1.2 Data Base Comparison — Conditions Studied

TOP FIVE TOPICS (%)

Pre 1977 (N = 853)		*1993–1994 (N = 579)*	
Pediatrics	(11)	Pediatrics	(8)
Psychiatry	(11)	Psychiatry	(8)
Hypertension	(8)	Screening	(8)
Smoking	(8)	Asthma/COPD	(7)
Screening	(7)	Diabetes	(6)

Relative decrease of interest in Hypertension and Smoking.

Relative increase of interest in Asthma/COPD and Diabetes.

APPEARED ONLY IN 1993–1994 (%):

HIV (2.4)
Organ Transplantation (1.2)

APPEARED ONLY PRE 1977 (%):

Seat Belt Use (2)

---

adequate design. Unfortunately, there is no way of knowing for certain how this compares to other fields of inquiry or even whether matters have improved significantly over the last 20 years.

Conditions Studied — Over 50 different diseases and conditions have been studied. Table 1.2 compares the major areas of interest pre-1977 with the most recent Medline data for October 1993 through September 1994.

Because interest in compliance is ubiquitous, no single subject accounts for more than 11% of the total output. In both time periods, separated by almost two decades, the two top areas are the same (pediatrics and psychiatry). There has been a relative decline of interest in hypertension, replaced by an increase in two other chronic medical conditions, asthma and diabetes. Various types of preventative screening have remained popular but interest in smoking has declined somewhat. One significant topic present pre-1979 that has disappeared is interest in seat belt use but HIV and organ transplantation have appeared as new areas of concern.

Outcome Factors — All aspects of the therapeutic alliance have been studied including disease factors, referrals and appointments, the therapeutic regimen, the patient-therapist interaction, and characteristics of the patient that contribute to outcome (Haynes, Taylor, & Sackett, 1979). With regard to what has been studied, two general statements could be made (Blackwell, Gutmann, & Jackson, 1981). The first is the obvious fact that what is easiest to study has been most studied. Disease factors and sociodemographic patient characteristics have often been included. Secondly, considerably more attention has been paid to patient characteristics and patient education than has to modifying or understanding physician behaviors.

WHAT HAS BEEN LEARNED?

Over 12,000 articles have been published on the topic of compliance in the past 25 years. About half of these are review articles and the remainder contain original data. Virtually every area of medicine has been studied and those of most interest have remained remarkably consistent. There is, however, a dearth of studies from developing countries about the problems particular to the Third World (Homedes & Ugalde, 1994).

Understanding Compliance — Five major models have been described in attempts to understand compliance problems (Leventhal & Cameron, 1987). The oldest and most basic is the biomedical approach, which focuses on the more technical or mechanistic problems and potential solutions. It emphasizes aspects of the treatment regimen and ignores more subtle interpersonal determinants of behavior. The second is the operant behavioral model. It emphasizes structuring the environment as well as teaching specific skills. This model lacks an individualized approach and fails to consider less conscious cognitions not linked to immediate rewards. A third model is the educational one, which aims to enhance communication between provider and patient. It stresses the significance of timing, construction and comprehension of information but tends to ignore powerful attitudinal, motivational and interpersonal factors that disrupt the transfer of knowledge into action. The fourth and particularly popular model is the health beliefs model, which views compliance as based on a rational appraisal of the balance between the perceived benefits of treatment and barriers to obtaining it. This model yields modest associations between its assumptions and compliance behavior in some situations but fails to do so when risk reduction behaviors are linked to more socially determined or unconscious motivations. A fifth model is the self-regulatory systems approach. This considers both the cognitive and the emotional response to a perceived threat of illness and examines the congruence between patient and practitioner with respect to illness representation, coping behavior and appraisal of action. This model is the most comprehensive but is difficult to apply because of its multivariate and transactional nature.

Limitations on interpretation of the data in this area of inquiry include problems of definition, measurement and reactivity. At least half the studies on compliance have failed to yield a positive relationship between the outcome factors being measured and compliance. Sociodemographic variables most easily studied have been least rewarding while psychosocial factors less amenable to manipulation have more often yielded positive outcomes. There is often a lack of generalizability; a factor found to exert a positive influence in one situation fails to do so in another (Blackwell, 1989). For example, factors that influence failure of clinic attendance differ considerably from those which determine adherence to medication regimens (Melnikow & Kiefe, 1994). Most research is cross-sectional but life is longitudinal. Within an individual compliance may alter radically across the life cycle. A juvenile diabetic who is passively compliant with parental wishes during latency may rebel by rejecting treatment during adolescence. In early adult life, the rewards of a healthy lifestyle may seem compelling but in old age the burdens of treatment may exceed the perceived benefits of longevity.

Knowledge of this literature leads to the conclusion that the determinants of compliance are ever changing and kaleidoscopic. There is no stereotypic noncompliant person or situation.

Despite these limitations in the data, there are areas of consensus. The degree of noncompliance tends to be similar across medical disorders with frequently cited estimates involving 25% of inpatients and 50% of outpatients. Although it is often assumed that patients with persistent psychiatric disorders have more problems, the evidence suggests that they do not differ from other populations afflicted with chronic medical conditions (Barofsky & Bulson, 1980).

Other areas of consensus include the fact that medication compliance is more readily achieved than modification in lifestyle, particularly when the latter requires long term readjustments. Some factors have generally (but *not* invariably) been found to have a positive or negative influence on compliance outcome (Blackwell, 1989). On the positive side, compliance is more likely if the patient's expectations are met, if they are satisfied or supervised, if there is continuity of care, and if they view the disease as a serious one to which they are susceptible. Family or friends often make a significant contribution as does an individual's previous compliance behavior. Poor compliance is fostered by lengthy treatment, particularly of asymptomatic disease, and is worsened by complicated regimens, side effects and social stress, isolation or alcoholism.

As with all areas of research, interest is sustained by new findings. Recent studies have yielded the provocative conclusion that individuals who comply with placebo have better outcomes than those who do not. This finding has been confirmed in a variety of conditions including treatment of myocardial infarction, alcoholism, schizophrenia, and antibiotic prophylaxis in patients with cancer (Horwitz & Horwitz, 1993). Even when taking a placebo adherent subjects may have improved health outcomes because they are better adapted to the stress of illness, more committed to treatment, or more engaged in behaviors that extend beyond the taking of medication.

Finally, there is an emerging consensus concerning the place of compliance in determining the outcome of research studies. In Phase II studies when it is important to confirm pharmacologic superiority of one agent over another, adherence run-ins are helpful in weeding out noncompliant subjects whose behavior may dilute a difference between treatments. By contrast, in Phase III studies, when the drug is known to be effective, "intention to treat" analysis allows noncompliance to play its real-world part in determining outcome. Although compliance is still only assessed by valid measures in a third of drug

Figure 1.1 Categorization of Interventions and Outcomes

Intervention		Intermediary Goals	Final Outcome(s)
EDUCATION	{ Didactic, Interactive }	KNOWLEDGE CONGRUENCE	COMPOSITE COMPLIANCE (TO CRITERION)
SUPERVISION	{ Professional, Social }	APPOINTMENT KEEPING	
CONVENIENCE	{ Regimen, Access to Care }	MEDICATION TAKING	AND
SKILLS TRAINING	{ Tailoring, Risk Reduction }	RISK REDUCTION	AUTONOMY (AN IDEAL)
PATIENT PARTICIPATION	{ Monitoring, Self-Management }	ACTIVE PATIENT	

trials, the number has doubled since 1974 (Bosley, Coucher, & Cochrane, 1993).

Influencing Compliance — Compliance interventions can be conceptualized in three stages. There is an initial phase of information exchange (education) followed by a negotiated alliance (supervised compliance) leading to the ideal of autonomous self-care (active patient participation). There is a subtle but profound difference between the open and parenthetical language which highlights a contemporary shift from passive compliance to an active alliance between patient and provider.

When it comes to a choice among interventions, two principles apply. We have learned that parsimony pays; some changes are relatively simple to make. For example, modifying the treatment regimen, reducing clinic waiting times and combining verbal with written information. Other factors may be more difficult to influence or change, such as memory impairment in the elderly or the patient's underlying attitudes and beliefs which modify their expectations toward treatment. As Mark Twain noted "You can't throw a habit out the window, you have to coax it down the stairs one step at a time."

Secondly, although single interventions contribute to outcome, sustained success requires the kind of multimodal approach shown in Figure 1.1 which characterizes interventions, intermediary goals and outcomes that are part of a truly comprehensive approach.

The primary intervention is educational and should be designed both to increase comprehension and facilitate recall (Ley, 1977). Unfortunately, research has shown that while education is necessary it is not sufficient. Even when patients have learned about their disease to a criterion, compliance often decreases to baseline when supervision is withdrawn (Wilber & Barrow, 1969; McKenney, Slining, Henderson, Devins, & Barr, 1973). Also problematic is the use of fear-provoking admonitions. Excessive fear encourages avoidance; it is necessary to deliver the proper dose of fear in order to facilitate the "work of worrying". For example, a patient with high blood pressure who is preoccupied by the risk of a stroke feels less anxious when they "forget" to take medication. If the same person is trained to measure their own blood pressure, they learn that treatment controls the symptoms and lessens the risk.

Some form of support or supervision is often essential to successful treatment. This may come from providers, family members, significant others or from peers in support groups (Levy, 1980). There remain many unanswered questions concerning the optimal amounts or components of support and its differential effects on individuals or outcome measures (for example, clinic attendance versus pill taking).

Often a significant source of support is the provider. For a successful alliance to develop, there needs to be congruence between the participants and their mutual expectations and understandings of treatment. Also helpful is a pleasant affective interaction and a negotiation concerning the patient's degree of active participation in treatment. Although autonomy is an ideal, not all people are eager or able to assume complete independence and not every physician is comfortable or willing to relinquish control.

Analysis of research studies in hypertension (Haynes, 1980) reveals that a large number of single interventions have been attempted to improve compliance but few produce sustained success compared to a control. Such single interventions include education, behavioral diaries, organizational strategies, counseling by health educators, home visits, self-monitoring, tangible rewards, group discussion and tailored regimens. In contrast, multiple or combined interventions demonstrate benefits in the range of 20 to 30% over controls. Successful interventions often include some degree of "active" patient involvement. Unfortunately, these multimodal studies require large sample sizes and complex statistical analysis. It often remains unclear to what extent the benefits are additive or due to synergism or segmentation ("different strokes for different folks").

THE BEST IS YET TO COME

Limited findings and difficulties of doing research have led to concerns about waning interest in compliance. But the volume of research remains substantial and there are new developments that will sustain the field into the next century. Ageing populations afflicted with chronic conditions are seeking longevity and improved quality of life. Our conceptualization has shifted from a narrowly defined interest in compliance and single solutions to a broader view of the treatment alliance and complex multimodal interventions. As with all areas of inquiry, this one will be stimulated by innovation. Microchip circuitry and computer technology are already providing the means for this to occur (Stehr-Green et al., 1993).

In a recent New England Journal of Medicine editorial, "The Next Transformation in the Delivery of Health Care," Kassirer (1995) talks of the computer Internet and its potential future use: "Ideally, responsibility for decisions could be shared by the patient and the physician. The patient could tap into authoritative medical data bases, including textbooks and newsletters formulated expressly for lay audiences ... if it was done right, the online computer system would function as a 'virtual physician' in a new kind of house call."

Both the patients who suffer from severe mental illness and the families who support them are likely to benefit from the advances yet to come.

REFERENCES

Alderman, M. H., & Lamport, B. (1990). Labelling of hypertensives: a review of the data. *Journal of Clinical Epidemiology, 43*, 195–200.

Bachman, R. M. (1993). Better compliance: physicians making it happen (editorial). *American Family Physician, 48*, 717–718.

Barofsky, I., & Bulson, R. D. (1980). In *The chronic psychiatric patient in the community: principles of treatment.* Jamaica, NY: Spectrum Publications.

Bergsman, A. B., & Werner, R. J. (1963). Failure of children to receive penicillin by mouth. *New England Journal of Medicine, 268,* 1334–1338.

Blackwell, B. (1989). Compliance — measurement and intervention. *Current Opinion in Psychiatry, 2,* 787–789.

Blackwell, B. (1992). Compliance. *Psychotherapy and Psychosomatics, 58,* 161–169.

Blackwell, B., Gutmann, M., & Jackson, T. (1981). An update and overview of compliance in hypertension. In A. C. Arntzenius, A. J. Dunning, & H. A. Snellen (Eds.), *Blood pressure measurement and systemic hypertension,* (pp. 295–309). IMS Breda Holland: Medical World Press.

Bosley, C. M., Coucher, J., & Cochrane, G. M. (1993). Letter to Editor. *The Lancet, 342,* 1427.

Charney, E. (1975). Compliance and prescribance. *American Journal of Diseases of Children, 129,* 1009–1010.

Coar, T. (1822). *The aphorisms of Hippocrates.* London: Longmen.

Donovan, J. L., & Blake, D. R. (1992). Patient non-compliance: deviance or reasoned decision-making? *Social Science and Medicine, 34,* 507–513.

Eraker, S. A., Kirscht, J. P., & Praker, M. H. (1984). Understanding and improving patient compliance. *Annals of Internal Medicine, 100,* 258–268.

Feinstein, A. R. (1990). On white-coat effects and the electronic monitoring of compliance (editorial). *Archives of Internal Medicine, 150,* 1377–1378.

Haynes, R. B. (1979). Introduction. In R. B. Haynes, D. W. Taylor & D. L. Sackett (Eds.), *Compliance in health care* (pp. 1–7). Baltimore: Johns Hopkins University Press.

Haynes, R. B. (1980). A review of tested interventions for improving compliance with antihypertensive treatment. In R. B. Haynes, M. E. Mattson, & T. O. Engebretson (Eds.), *Patient compliance to prescribed regimens: a report to the National Heart, Lung, and Blood Institute* (pp. 83–112). NIH Publication No. 81-2102.

Haynes, R. B., Taylor, D. W., & Sackett, D. L. (Eds.). (1979). *Compliance in health care.* Baltimore: Johns Hopkins University Press.

Haynes, R. B., Taylor, D. W., Snow, J. C., & Sackett, D. L. (1979). Appendix I: Annotated and indexed bibliography on compliance with therapeutic and preventive regimens. In R. B. Haynes, D. W. Taylor, & D. L. Sackett (Eds.), *Compliance in health care* (pp. 337–474). Baltimore: Johns Hopkins University Press.

Haynes, R. B., Wang, E., & Da Mota Gomes, M. (1987). A critical review of interventions to improve compliance with prescribed medications. *Patient Education & Counseling, 10,* 155–166.

Holm, S. (1993). What is wrong with compliance? *Journal of Medical Ethics, 19,* 108–110.

Homedes, N., & Ugalde, A. (1994). Research on patient compliance in developing countries. *Bulletin of the Pan American Health Organization, 28,* 17–33.

Horwitz, R. I., & Horwitz, S. M. (1993). Adherence to treatment and health outcomes. *Archives of Internal Medicine, 153,* 1863–1868.

Kassirer, J. P. (1995). The next transformation in the delivery of health care (editorial). *The New England Journal of Medicine, 332,* 52–54.

Leape, L. L. (1994). Error in medicine. *Journal of the American Medical Association, 272,* 1851–1857.

Leventhal, H., & Cameron, L. (1987). Behavioral theories and the problem of compliance. *Patient Education & Counseling, 10,* 117–138.

Levine, R. J. (1994). Monitoring for adherence: ethical considerations. *American Journal of Respiratory Critical Care Medicine, 149,* 287–288.

Levy, R. L. (1980). The role of social support in patient compliance: a selective review. In R. B. Haynes, M. E. Mattson, & T. O. Engebretson (Eds.), *Patient compliance to prescribed regimens: a report to the National Heart, Lung, and Blood Institute* (pp. 139–158). NIH Publication No. 81–2102.

Ley, P. (1977). Psychological studies of doctor-patient communication. In S. Rachman (Ed.), *Contributions to medical psychology.* Oxford: Pergamon Press.

Matsuyama, J. R., Mason, B. J., & Jue, S. G. (1993). Pharmacists interventions using an electronic medication-event monitoring devices adherence data versus pill counts. *The Annals of Pharmacotherapy, 27,* 851–855.

McKenney, J. M., Slining, J. G., Henderson, H. R., Devins, D., & Barr, M. (1973). The effect of clinical pharmacy services on patients with essential hypertension. *Circulation, 48,* 1104–1111.

Melnikow, J., & Kiefe, C. (1994). Patient compliance and medical research: issues in methodology. *Journal of General Internal Medicine, 9,* 96–105.

Merrill, B. A. (1994). A global look at compliance in health/safety and rehabilitation. *Journal of Orthopaedic & Sports Physical Therapy, 19,* 242–248.

Reston, V. A. (1992). Emerging issues in pharmaceutical cost containment. *National Pharmaceutical Council, 2,* 1–16.

Starr, P. (1982). *The social transformation of American medicine.* New York: Base Books.

Steele, D., Blackwell, B., Gutmann, M., & Jackson, T. (1987). Beyond advocacy: a review of the active patient concept. *Patient Education & Counseling, 10,* 3–23.

Stehr-Green, P. A., Dini, E. F., Lindegren, M. L., & Patriarca, P. A. (1993). Evaluation of telephoned computer-generated reminders to improve immunization coverage at inner-city clinics. *Public Health Reports, 108,* 426–430.

Torgerson, D. J., & Donaldson, C. (1994). An economic view of high compliance as a screening objective. *BMJ, 308,* 117–119.

Urquhart, J. (1993). Variable patient compliance in ambulatory trials — nuisance, threat, opportunity. *Journal of Antimicrobial Chemotherapy, 32,* 643–649.

U.S. Department of Health and Human Services. *1992 HCFA Statistics.* Health Care Financing Administration, Bureau of Data Management and Strategy. (HCFA Publication No. 03333).

Wilber, J. A., & Barrow, J. G. (1969). Reducing elevated blood pressure. *Minnesota Medicine, 52,* 1303–1305.

Wright, E. C. (1993). Non-compliance — or how many aunts has Matilda? *The Lancet, 34,* 909–913.

2

From Compliance to Social-Self-Regulation: Models of the Compliance Process[1]

HOWARD LEVENTHAL, JENNIFER FALCONER LAMBERT, MICHAEL DIEFENBACH and ELAINE A. LEVENTHAL

Interventions to improve compliance appear to be as varied as the diseases and regimens they are designed to effect. More serious, perhaps is that the outcomes are equally varied both across different interventions and for the same intervention over different sites and times. These variations should not be interpreted, however, as indications of capriciousness or lack of order in behavioral processes. Rather they reflect the fact that behavior is affected by a multiplicity of determinants which differ over sites and time. As a consequence, the very same determinant (e.g., public knowledge, social support, economic constraints), may have greater or lesser impact on adherence to a specific aspect of a treatment regimen at a specific site depending upon the population, the disease, and temporal context. Thus, adherence interventions are more likely to succeed and their outcomes to be understood if they are based upon a careful analysis of the determinants of the specific behavioral target for a given sample at a given place and time. These analyses are more likely to be informative if they are generated from the perspective of a comprehensive, theoretical framework.

[1] Authors can be contacted at the Institute for Health, Health Care Policy and Aging Research, 30 College Ave., PO Box 5062, New Brunswick, NJ 08903-5062. Preparation of this manuscript was supported in part by grant AG03501, H.L. and E.A.L. CoPI's.

OUR VIEW OF THE COMPLIANCE PROBLEM

We believe that sound behavioral theory is essential to minimize the dangers of non-compliance. Three themes are central to our approach. First, the theory should be comprehensive and should include both individual factors (biological and psychological) and contextual factors (cultural, institutional and social). Second, the theory should provide a logical way of representing the relationships among individual and contextual factors. This is essential if we are to anticipate how a newly discovered contextual factor might affect the compliance process. Finally, the model must depict both the patient's and the clinician's understanding of the disease and its treatment and it must identify the factors which affect mutual communication and the development of *shared and biologically valid perspectives* on treatment. In order to achieve maximum success, a treatment alliance must be formed between the patient and practitioner.

We conceive of the treatment alliance as a relationship in which the practioner serves as an expert adviser and consultant to the person (patient) who is in charge of the day by day execution of the treatment regimen. To be effective in any such relationship, the consultant must understand: 1) the patient's view of the problem; 2) the tactics the patient is using to solve it; and 3) the criteria and cues the patient is using to evaluate success. Given this understanding, the consultant can provide information respecting each of these three facets of the adherence process. The consultant's aim is to make use of both objective, medical data and the patient's subjective experience and behavior to generate a valid and shared representation of the illness, the goals and procedures for its treatment, and rules for appraising outcomes. A shared view will emerge when this is done with active collaboration and continued feedback from the treatment manager: the patient. The generation of a shared representation increases the likelihood that the treatment manager understands and adheres to the treatment plan and participates in its necessary adjustments.

As treatment for chronic physical and mental illness is extended in time and subject to modifications (e.g., medication dosage adjustments) an effective alliance requires mutual, long-term commitment. Changes in the symptomatology and physiology of a chronic illness require continual monitoring by both patient and practitioner as these changes may alter the match of the treatment regimen to the disease as well as the patient's perception of the disease-treatment match. Whether the change in the match of treatment to disease is "real" or merely "perceived", it can detract from continued adherence if these perceptions are not shared with the practitioner and evaluated in a mutually satisfactory manner. Thus, achieving an effective alliance will be enhanced by regular appointments with the same provider, following up on progress, minimizing and appropriately interpreting side effects, and simplifying and tailoring regimens to the patient's lifestyle. Thus, the treatment alliance is the focal point for conceptual elaboration, and it is a natural touchstone for evaluating the utility of existent compliance models. Models which fail to represent the content of the patient and practitioner's views of a disease and its treatment, and/or to examine the processes involved in the communication and sharing of these views, need to be revised and/or have their positive contributions incorporated into a more comprehensive framework. Finally, the alliance concept requires reconsideration of attributions of responsibility for treatment.

EXISTENT MODELS OF THE COMPLIANCE PROCESS

Our review of existent models of compliance is designed to summarize the main themes underlying these models (for a comprehensive review, see Leventhal, Zimmerman & Gutmann, 1984) and to identify those elements that should be incorporated into a more comprehensive theory of the adherence process. We then propose a perceptual-cognitive framework as a comprehensive model of the compliance process, and suggest ways in which this model can be elaborated and be of special value for understanding problems with treatment adherence for the patient with severe mental illness.

Bio-Medical Model

Early bio-medical models of compliance were couched in terms of institutionally defined roles of authority (doctor) and supplicant (patient): the doctor prescribes, the patient complies. This autocratic outlook viewed non-compliance as a failing of the patient; due to a deficit of knowledge, motivation and/or will. Vestiges of this orientation are visible in expressions such as, "The patient failed the treatment." These biases were unsupported by data (no specific patient characteristics consistently relate to non-adherence), and are inconsistent with the formation of a working alliance.

There are several facets of the model that must be preserved. First, the bio-medical perspective makes a critical contribution to compliance models by specifying multiple dependent measures for assessment of compliance outcomes. Among these is the prescribed treatment regimen as the criterion against which behavior is to be evaluated. It is essential that this be communicated to the patient. In addition, a measure of treatment outcome may be critical as variation in treatment outcome will reflect both compliance and the efficacy of the treatment regimen (Sackett, 1978). The medical approach also focussed on medication side effects as undesirable outcomes that affected adherence and the efficacy of treatment. Finally, medicine recognized the importance of situational barriers for compliance, such as problems of access and understanding (Finnerty, Mattie, & Finnerty, 1973).

Psychological Models for Compliance

Psychological models of the compliance process have their origin in two quite different traditions, learning-behavior theory and cognitive-social psychological theory. The two themes are fused in the more recent social-learning and cognitive-behavioral models which guide most intervention research in preventive health behavior.

Learning-behavioral theories. Learning-behavioral models emphasize the acquisition of behavior through repetition and reward such as operant conditioning of goal seeking behaviors or classical conditioning (Pavlovian) of emotional responses which may be critical for establishing and maintaining the desire to engage in and adhere to treatments (see Leventhal, 1970). The approaches focus on the cues that elicit behavior and on rewards that strengthen or extinguish behavior. Three features of the learning models are important for any comprehensive model: 1. The need to focus upon and measure the response that one wants to strengthen or reward; 2. Recognition that conditions for the acquisition of motivation and the conditions for the acquisition of response skills are likely to differ; 3. Realizing that the cues and rewards for eliciting and strengthening responses in the clinic may differ from those in the patient's environment.

Social psychological models. Social psychological models posit cognitive and emotional processes as mediators of learning and adherence. Mental processes were introduced in two ways. The first recognized that adherence reflects a decision based upon perceptions of vulnerability to a threat, a mental analysis of the costs and benefits of the possible actions for coping (Maiman & Becker, 1974; Rosenstock, 1974), and attitudes of other persons (Ajzen & Fishbein, 1980). These models introduced values and beliefs generating motivation for compliance.

The second way in which mental processes were introduced was in the specification of the steps required before information can affect behavior (McGuire, 1968). This includes the preparation and transmission of the message, its reception, comprehension and retention, its impact on attitudes, and finally, the impact of the message, if any, on behavior. The model pointed to the importance of evaluating outcomes at each communication step.

Cognitive-behavioral or social learning models. Cognitive behavioral (Meichenbaum, 1977) and social learning (Bandura, 1977) models combine cognitive and learning factors in their analysis of adherence behavior. While most of their concepts overlap with those in the social psychological models, they give greater emphasis to the concepts of self-competence (Leventhal, 1970) or self efficacy, that is the perceived ability to perform a response (Bandura, 1977). As the cognitive-behavioral models developed in a therapeutic framework, they presented numerous procedures to ensure the greatest likelihood of developing self efficacy to promote adherence to specific treatment regimens. These procedures are designed to encourage the patient's active participation, to increase their attention to outcome, and to provide continuous feedback to the clinician.

Positive and Negative Aspects of Existent Theory

The models reviewed raised at least 7 important themes that should be incorporated in a comprehensive approach to medication adherence for patients who have severe mental illness. They are:

1. Specification of multiple outcomes, including outcomes for compliance and for successful treatment.

2. Recognition of barriers to treatment and preventive services.

3. Generating motivation to comply.

4. Awareness that the cues and rewards for responding in the clinic and external reality may differ and conflict.

5. Recognizing the importance of evaluating adherence at every step of communication.

6. Developing a sense of efficacy to perform the target behavior.

7. Encouraging active exchange of information between patient and clinician that makes the patient an active participant in treatment.

These positive contributions are balanced, however, by the following 5 factors which are ignored or ill defined in all of the models.

1. None of the models specify the features of health threats or the values that are involved in health relevant motivation.

2. The models fail to specify the specific procedures that people use to enhance health or to avoid, control or remove disease threats.

3. None of the models provide a sufficient picture of the ongoing processes involved in the updating and/or changing of attitudes and actions, and none specify how the outcome of actions alter beliefs.

4. The models ignore how similarities and differences in the patients' and practitioners' views of the illness threat and treatment regimens, and the distribution of responsibility affect communication of information and adherence (i.e., they ignore the psychological aspects of the treatment alliance). The cognitive behavioral model is a partial exception.

5. The models do not clearly differentiate between the problems involved in teaching self regulation of conscious-deliberative versus unconscious-automatic thoughts and actions and emotional versus non-emotional thoughts and actions.

A SELF REGULATION MODEL

While models of self regulation have been in the literature for decades (e.g., Kanfer, 1977; Leventhal, 1970; Carver & Scheier, 1982), the earlier versions are content free and fail to correct many of the deficiencies which we have attributed to behavioral-cognitive models. The common-sense model of health threats which we will elaborate on in this section takes three, critical steps toward correcting these deficiencies: 1) It incorporates constructs respecting the representation of health threats and treatments; 2) It distinguishes different types and/or levels of control; and 3) It postulates that contextual factors affect adherence by their effects on self regulation. Four basic premises are critical for understanding how self regulation is conceptualized:

1. People (patients) are active problem solvers: they strive to make sense of their worlds and they search for convenient and effective ways of controlling and adapting to it (Kelly & Scott, 1990).

2. People's representations of health threats are generated by a multi-level processing system, one of which is perceptual and automatic (bottom-up processing) and the other deliberative or cognitive and reason(ing) based (top-down processing). The self-regulation model recognizes that symptom fluctuations are concrete givens and readily attributed to medication or other interventions; hence they are powerful, bottom-up reinforcers to encourage or discourage behavior (Leventhal, Meyer & Nerenz, 1980). On the other hand, abstract "top-down" factors such as the meaning assigned to symptoms also shape the positive or negative reward value of symptom experiences and the responses producing them (Leventhal, Diefenbach & Leventhal, 1992). For example, the noxious effects of lithium can be interpreted to mean that it is doing a poor job at controlling illness and making one well.

3. Emotional reactions and the cognitive representations of a disease and treatment are generated more or less simultaneously, (in parallel), and may yield different, and sometimes conflicting goals for action (Leventhal, 1970).

4. Contextual factors, including the cultural environment, formal and informal social relationships, and personality dispositions, influence the way in which individuals construe health threats and manage them.

These four premises led us to structure our self-regulation framework in the following way. First, we distinguish between the *problem domain* and its *context*. The former represents the individual's ongoing perceptions, thoughts, feelings, and actions to regulate the health threat. The problem domain is differentiated into three components; the *representation* of the health threat, the *procedures for threat management*, and the *rules for outcome appraisals*. The *context* includes the *environmental* and *personal* factors which feed information into the system and moderate the procedures for threat management. Finally, we identify several important rules of systems operation and the way in which the context can affect and conflict with internally generated programs.

The self-regulatory model is particularly relevant to patients who have severe mental illnesses. Their "illness" representations and the ruminations stimulated by them, are likely to be vastly different in content and structure than that of the practitioner, and to be less informed by clinical reality. Santiago et al. (1990) found that among a subgroup of patients with severe mental illness, the greater the difference between the patient's and therapist's perceptions of the illness, the greater the likelihood that the patient would drop out of treatment. Re-shaping the interpretations patients give to their concrete experiences and the procedures and criteria they use to test and validate their interpretations, will be critical for aligning the system with the realities of both the disease and the environment. Once this is achieved, compliance with treatment should improve. While we have tried throughout this section to focus on factors relevant to adherence to treatment for those with severe mental illness, many of the examples we use are from studies of adherence to treatment for physical illnesses. This choice reflects the limited number of compliance studies of mental illness from this framework. The choice does, however, allow us to contrast the problems in dealing with adherence issues in two very different areas.

The Problem Domain

Representation of the illness. The representation of the illness establishes targets (goals) for action and criteria for evaluating response efficacy: it is the framework which generates motivation for self-regulation. Investigators have identified five attributes of illness representations: 1. Identity, or the symptoms and the name or label applied to them; 2. Cause, or the individual's perceptions and beliefs about the factors causing the problem (infectious agent, constitutional weakness, chemical imbalance, witchcraft, etc.) 3. Time-line, or the time for the development of the disorder and its symptoms and its expected duration; 4. Consequences, or the experienced and anticipated physical, psychological, social and economic impact of the disease; and 5. Control, or beliefs about the susceptibility of the disease to various interventions by oneself, family and friends, and medical experts. These attributes are working hypotheses rather than fixed beliefs, and vary across persons and over time for the same person. There will also be differences in the degree to which these beliefs are changeable for different illnesses and persons.

Representations reflect the hierarchical nature of the processing system as they are anchored in both concrete perceptions and abstract labels or propositions. The concrete perceptual level is the basic groundwork that connects the individual to both the external and internal environment. Individuals' perceptions will be similar when environmental cues are rich. When cues are ambiguous, which is characteristic of most somatic experiences, the structure and content of the individual's experience will more strongly reflect abstract, personal interpretations (Leventhal, 1985). As the overall representation of illness is both concrete and abstract, each of these levels can generate goals for coping and self regulation can be directed towards *multiple and at times conflicting,* targets.

Adherence to anti-hypertension regimens illustrates how conceptual knowledge is over-ruled by concrete experience. Meyer, Leventhal and Gutmann (1985) found that over 80% of patients in hypertension treatment agreed with the statement that, "People can't tell when their blood pressure is elevated." Later on in the interview, 90% of these same participants responded that they could tell when their blood pressure was up. They reported symptoms such as warm face or heart beating, as valid indicators of elevated pressure. These ideas were not merely hypothetical: adherence to medication was

excellent and blood pressure control good to very good for those patients who believed that treatment had a positive effect on their symptoms while adherence was problematic and blood pressure control
fair to poor for the majority of these patients who reported that the
treatment did not have a beneficial effect on their symptoms. This
and other studies provide convincing evidence of a symmetrical relationship of labels and symptoms: when patients are symptomatic,
they seek to label their condition, and when diagnosed and labeled
they will notice and report symptoms even in conditions that professionals believe are asymptomatic (Baumann, et al., 1989).

While the difference between somatic sensations or symptoms and
disease labels provides the simplest illustration of this bi-level nature
of representation, it applies to every one of the representational attributes including time-line. For example, it has been shown that
patients are much more likely to drop out of treatment if they concep-
tualize their illness as an acute rather than a chronic condition; acute
conditions are cured once their symptoms disappear (Meyer, et al.,
1985). The practitioner must, therefore, address both the symptoms
the patient uses as indicators of the presence of the disease and the
time-frame for both symptoms and the underlying condition to insure adherence to treatment. Treatment with anti-depressants provides an even better example of the "concrete" nature of experienced
time. The conceptual rule is daily use of anti-depressants for a minimum of 1 to 2 weeks before experiencing any change in mood, with
other symptoms needing more or less time to be alleviated. The immediate, concrete experiences of dry mouth, sedation, and other possible effects such as urinary retention, hypotension, and disturbance
of cardiac rhythm, provide concrete evidence of the time of onset of
drug action. The absence of sought for changes in mood within the
time-frame of drug action defined by these medication "side-effects"
is evidence to the patient that the drug is ineffective in achieving its
targeted outcome. This picture might even be more complicated due
to variations in the amount of time needed for the alleviation of different types of symptoms (e.g., sleep disturbances or feelings of anxiety) with different drugs. It the patient is unaware of the effects and
time-lines for each of these medications, i.e., if he or she does not have
clear expectations of the sequence of effects, and a means of justifying
the delay in experiencing the sought after outcome, he or she is very
likely to misjudge the effectiveness of the drug regimen.

Causal time-lines is an area in which we expect changes in representations over experience with a mental illness. For example, a
person might attribute repeated episodes of depression to recent
stressful life-events, failing to acknowledge the ongoing biochemical
vulnerability to his/her disorder. By contrast, once a person enters
mental health treatment, or sees his/her depression as based on a
chemical imbalance, specific episodes of depression may be attributed to an underlying, ongoing disorder. If the latter is true, the time
frame of the illness will be defined by years since the first episode.
Shifting beliefs about time-lines are likely to be a critical source of
many of the compliance problems seen in patients with severe mental illness. For example, patients who have achieved control over

their depression with medications may come to believe that their ill-ness was acute and has been "cured". They may then relapse by ex-posing themselves to excessive stimulation (Brown & Harris, 1978) or discontinuing treatment despite recommendations by their clinician to continue with maintenance doses. After one or more relapse episodes they may come to revise their understanding of the disorder, and accept the idea that the underlying condition is recurrent. In short, time-lines and changing time lines associated with different causal attributions can have important influences on adherence and it is important for the practitioner both to inform the patient about likely sequences and time frames for symptom experiences and to inoculate against likely misinterpretations of these experiences.

Procedures and appraisals for threat management. A wide range of compliance producing procedures may be involved in a treatment regimen. Our hierarchical model of the processing system suggests that some procedures must address the patients' conscious concep-tual planning, while others must address automatic reactions. For example, conscious planning, such as list and appointment making, is necessary to obtain and fill prescriptions, while automatic, envi-ronmentally elicited responding is best for consistent pill taking (e.g., keeping medication with one's breakfast cereal). While adherence is relatively effortless under automatic control, it will become effortful when there is a need to shift to deliberate control (e.g., when the medication is exhausted). Developing procedures for shifting control, from automatic to deliberate and back again, will be a major chal-lenge for the design of effective, adherence interventions.

Every procedure implies a set of outcome expectations, with de-fined time-lines, and self-efficacy beliefs. Outcomes consistent with expectations confirm the representation and increase the individu-al's commitment. The effects of inconsistent outcomes will vary depending upon the individual's confidence in each system compo-nent. For example, a negative outcome is likely to generate a search for a new procedure if confidence in the identity of the representa-tion (diagnosis) is greater than that in the specific treatment proce-dure. On the other hand, if the level of confidence is reversed, or if the individual is motivated to reject a diagnosis of mental illness be-cause it stigmatizes the family or the self (Kleinman, 1980), treatment failure can lead to doctor shopping and a search for a new, more ac-ceptable definition of the problem.

In summary, the representation of a threat, the procedures for its management and the associated outcome expectancies, form a system that is generated and integrated by common-sense logic. Common-sense generates expectations that one will perceive "rea-sonable" connections between disease (its location, symptoms, cause, etc.), treatment procedures and outcomes. These expectations have the appearance of obvious truths at the very same time that they may be objectively false. For example, a participant in a clinical trial test-ing the effects of vitamin supplements on the vigor of immune re-sponse may conclude that she was in the placebo arm of the trial because she experienced no increase in vigor after a few days of "treatment". This conclusion makes sense if one's common-sense/

logic presumes that treatment should produce a change in how one feels if it has protective value. Of course, these beliefs may be false as supplement induced somatic changes may be imperceptible or delayed (as are the effects of antipsychotic and antidepressant medication), and the protective outcome probabilistic rather than certain. Again, the validity of these common-sense beliefs in an objectively defined biological framework is often completely irrelevant to their potency as guides to the patient's self-treatment decisions.

THE CONTEXT AND ITS MULTIPLE ROLES

The representation of an illness and the coping procedures and appraisal criteria used in its regulation are an ever evolving product of the ongoing interaction between stimulus inputs and the individual's memory systems. Biologically generated sensations and symptoms play a major role in initiating thoughts about illness and seeking health care (Cameron, Leventhal & Leventhal, 1993). However, the inherent ambiguity of many, if not most somatic sensations allows social communication, including observations of other persons, discussions with friends, family members and physicians, and exposure to media and cultural symbols (e.g., disease labels and treatment institutions), to shape and give meaning to these experiences. The reciprocal relationship between the fee-for-service structure of the traditional medical care system and the common-sense view of diseases as acute, infectious conditions, is frequently given as an example of cultural shaping. The disease model and the institutional structure are mutually reinforcing and encourage a behavioral pattern of seeking treatment when symptoms appear and disrupt daily activities rather than seeking ways to enhance health and prevent illness (Knowles, 1977).

One can also detect cultural and linguistic influences on models of mental illness. For example, the term "nervous breakdown" is used to describe a number of mental disorders. This term implies an acute episode caused by excessive stress and/or anxiety. Therefore, the common sense remedy, suggested by the illness label "nervous breakdown", may be short-term rest rather than a long-term medication regimen. On the other hand, in many cultures, psychiatric labels stigmatize both the patient and the patients' family, and it is not surprising that such labels are rejected in favor of somatic diagnoses (Kleinman, 1980). Fear of being incarcerated for life in a mental hospital may also motivate rejection of both the diagnosis and treatment for a severe mental illness such as schizophrenia.

THE ALLIANCE WITH PATIENTS WHO HAVE SEVERE MENTAL ILLNESS

The self-regulation model suggests two sets of problems will be critical in the structuring of an alliance to assure medication adherence by patients with severe mental illness. 1. Identifying the content of the patient's self regulation system (i.e., how does he/she represent the illness, what procedures does he/she use to test and validate the representation and what is the nature of her motivation to change and/ or to rid him/herself of it). 2. Developing new procedures which when used by the patient will reshape his or her belief system, i.e., alter the interpretation, time-line, perceived cause and perceived control over symptoms. These procedures, their expected outcomes and outcome time-lines must be developed in concert and their outcomes need to be shared. This process should lead to a revised view of the problem and should be developed into an overall treatment plan.

IDENTIFYING CONTENT AND PROCEDURES OF MENTAL ILLNESS

There are differences in the content of representations, procedures for management and rules for appraising outcomes for physical and severe mental illness. These differences can have profound effects on the tasks faced in forming a treatment alliance and have important consequences for adherence. As mentioned earlier, accidental exposure to environmental pathogens is typically seen as the cause of acute, infectious illnesses. Even chronic conditions such as diabetes, stroke, and cancers, are often attributed to environmental causes, though the genetic revolution may change the cultural view of these diseases. By contrast, people seem more likely to attribute emotional and mental health problems to shortcomings or traits of the self. Indeed, internality is one of the three (internal, stable, and global) cognitions hypothesized to be antecedents to hopelessness induced depression (Abramson, Seligman & Teasdale, 1978). The sense of guilt and worthlessness that may accompany such internal attributions may create a significant barrier to the mutual exchanges needed for the definition of goals for change and the construction of an action plan for self management.

Diseases also differ in the degree to which people perceive them as susceptible to control (Lau & Hartmann, 1983). Persons afflicted with severe mental illnesses are particularly likely to see them as uncontrollable as the experiential features of these disorders, (e.g., severe depression, delusions and hallucinations), are private and able to intrude upon consciousness, yet independent of the executive self. Indeed, recommending medication confirms that these experiences are external to volitional control and acceptance of its use may deepen the individual's sense of failure and inability to control his/ her mental operations.

The individual's relationship to these intrusive feelings and thoughts must also be explored. Do they arouse distress and avoidance or are they "Friendly, though at times threatening"? What does the patient do to avoid, or in other ways modulate their content, intensity and frequency? What has the patient observed respecting their variation and what contingencies, if any, convince him/her that his/her beliefs about their meaning are valid? Motivation for treatment will vary as a function of these perceptions. Sensitivity and deliberate exploration of perceptions of cause, control, consequences, time-lines and procedures for management may be essential to illuminate the content of the patient's illness representation.

More complex problems may arise in defining mutual goals when patients suffer severe thought disorders. These may range from inability to maintain a common focus between patient and practitioner on treatment goals, to paranoid fears of manipulation. In severe cases the formation of an alliance would necessarily await the control of disordered thought by prior use of medication during hospitalization. As normalization takes place, therapists can take the steps to form an alliance to insure adherence to treatment post-discharge. It may prove necessary in many cases to develop protocols for controlling adverse side-effects of medication and to help the patient to recognize that side-effects could be signs that the treatment is working.

Creating a Shared Definition of the Problem

Developing a shared representation of a severe mental illness is a key both to the formation of a successful treatment alliance and an outcome of its success. Sharing means that practitioner and patient must communicate the content of their respective views and establish clear expectations for outcomes and time-lines of specific intervention procedures. With some exceptions, (e.g., when hospitalized), it is the patient who performs specific treatment procedures and it is the patient who observes the changes in his or her mental and somatic condition contingent upon these actions. Thus, it is necessary that the patient be encouraged to share these experiences with the practitioner. Successful sharing requires that the practitioner be a willing listener. Thus, he/she must be open and non-judgmental in response to the patient's reports and be clear in communicating his/her own interpretations of the meanings of these experiential changes. More importantly, perhaps, the practitioner must anticipate and predict the possible range of the patient's experience. This not only legitimates him/her as a medical expert, but as understanding the patient's subjective life.

Two critical aspects of this social process are that it include both the concrete, perceptual aspects of experience and its abstract, interpretive facets. Sharing the concrete substance of the illness experience means identifying and making public both mental and somatic symptoms, their perceived determinants, time-lines and consequences. This could be seen as a process of rationalizing the irrational. Sharing the abstract interpretive facets, means making public both the patient's understanding of his/her experience and the practitioner's interpretations of it. More important, perhaps, the common-sense model suggests that sharing will be more complete when the practitioner is able to anticipate and articulate both the patient's likely interpretations as well as his/her own explanations of these concrete experiences. For example: "When you take your tricyclic antidepressant, you will begin to feel thirsty within 24 hours, and once you start to feel thirsty and fatigued, you will know the drug is working and I have a hunch that you will think that you should feel better. Although I'm telling you that it will take 1 to 2 weeks for your depression to begin to lift, I suspect that you will think you should feel better once you notice any sign of the medication working. Once you feel its negative signs and know it is at work, you naturally expect to feel its benefits. But it does not work that way. The medication will produce some symptoms very quickly; as soon as it gets in your system. But it takes much longer for it to normalize the connections between your nerve cells." Recognizing both the symptom and its likely meaning should facilitate discounting interpretations that may be barriers to compliance and substituting interpretations that are facilitative of it.

The absence of an objective, medical indicator that the practitioner can share with the patient makes it a hard task for the practioner both to validate his or her representation of the problem, as well as to predict the changes in the patients somatic and mental experience. An oncologist, for example, can image the patient's tumor, understand how it will affect experience and performance, and predict changes in both areas as a function of the location and anticipated rate of growth. These perceptions and expectations can be shared with the patient and they will provide objective, public, biological validation, of a substantial area of the patient's experience. The patient, therefore, "knows" there is an objective basis for the current and evolving experience and this knowledge allows him/her to adopt new procedures to form and more fully confirm a biologically grounded representation of cancer. Of course, not all physical disorders have objective features that are so readily shared.

Severe mental illness offers yet more complex challenges. What objective indicator can the practitioner point to and use to generate a shared model? If there is no such indicator, what else may be available? Are there procedures the patient can adopt, including medication use, that will provide an anchor for anticipating and sharing later, experienced changes? Moreover, how does the patient interpret the intervention? Does s/he see medication as dangerous, potentially addictive, or as the physician's tool for mind control? Adequate responses to these questions will represent major steps toward establishing a viable treatment alliance. One method commonly used in behavioral and cognitive therapies is self-monitoring. Patients are requested to keep records of the frequency, duration and/or intensity of their symptoms, behaviors, etc. From these records, a baseline is established and any progress can be charted over time and treatment adjusted accordingly. This method provides a means of quantifying and objectifying the patient's experiences and of providing data about treatment efficacy.

The alliance resides in the context of the social environment, including the family, work-place, and the larger culture. Patient and practitioner may find themselves bombarded with inputs from the surrounding context that agree or disagree with the perceptions of cause, interpretation of symptoms, time-lines, expectations for cure, and the management procedures they have negotiated. For example, family and friends may perceive the behavioral manifestations of mental illness as actions that are performed for no reason other than to irritate or annoy others, or as characterological flaws, rather than as consequences of a disturbance in biochemistry.

The socio-cultural view of the time-line for severe mental illness may also differ from reality. Once labeled as mentally ill, the individual may not be permitted normal work and social roles even when in remission. Resistance by employers and family members to the patient's return to "normal", every-day activities may be due to the stigma carried by labels such as schizophrenia and depression, or by resistance to yielding the activities and power acquired when performing roles vacated by the patient during the most recent episode. These conflicts can disrupt the alliance, interfere with medication adherence and exacerbate the patient's mental disorder.

The Common-Sense Framework as an Alternative to Prior Models

The self regulation model as we have conceived it, incorporates the central variables of prior models and fills in the gaps. More importantly, it places these variables within an organized structure which allows for more precise specification of their individual and joint relationship to adherence outcomes. For example, the medical model differentiates desired from undesired treatment outcomes ("side effects"), some of the latter benign and others warnings of danger. The self regulation model, adds the patient's perception of these outcomes. From this perspective symptoms might be viewed as benign when they are cues to danger, or vice versa. For instance, headaches in a patient taking a monamine oxidase inhibitor may be a benign, coincidental occurrence or may be due to a life threatening hypertensive crisis brought on by eating cheese. It is important that side effects be discussed and their etiology properly identified.

The concept of self-efficacy provides a second example. When this construct is embedded in the framework of the common-sense self-regulation model, it becomes apparent that beliefs in self-efficacy depend on more than the successful performance (adherence) of a preventive or treatment behavior. As the common-sense model suggests, the behavior must also produce its effect, and should not produce other, unanticipated side-effects whether or not these are medically desirable. Thus, our model suggests that a sense of efficacy in controlling threat emerges not only from the successful performance of a response, but from the confirmation of a broad set of expectations regarding response outcome. Evaluation against these latter criteria requires realistic temporal expectations, such as the fact that it may take 1 to 2 to weeks to experience symptomatic benefit from many psychotropic medications.

CONCLUDING COMMENT

This chapter reviews the main themes of existing models of the compliance/adherence process in order to select and integrate their contributions into a broad, social and self-regulation framework applicable for patients with severe mental illness. In this framework, compliance is a product of the meanings the individual assigns to his or her mental health problem and the perceived relevance and/or reasonableness of the recommended treatment procedures to the defined problem. This "problem domain" contains the key meanings defining the individual's phenomenological view of his/her illness and treatment. The problem domain is nested within a series of overlapping, social contexts such as that between patient and practitioner, that between the treatment dyad and the family, and of both to media and the larger culture. The forging of an effective treatment alliance, in which practitioner and patient share a common view of the mental health problem and the most effective procedures for its management, is no simple task when one member of the treatment dyad suffers from the cognitive and affective distortions of a mental disorder.

Given these complexities, it is unreasonable to expect any single factor or treatment regimen to produce substantial improvements in compliance for patients with severe mental illness. Complexity should not be equated, however, with chaos. Viewing seemingly contradictory studies within the context of a comprehensive framework should allow us to recognize order where inconsistency seems to reign. Thus, within the context of a comprehensive, self regulation model, differences across studies will be seen as variations reflecting the operation of moderator variables. When comparing the effects of a variable such as symptom severity upon compliance in a study of hypertensives to the effects of symptom severity on compliance in a study of patients with severe mental illness, inconsistencies may well appear. They should be resolvable as interactions, however, when we treat the disease labels as contextual or moderator variables which alter the meaning of symptoms, their implications for motivation for treatment, and the perceived and/or expected effect of symptom alleviation on treatment acceptance.

The common-sense model as we have elaborated it, puts the sharing of the illness representation at the center of the alliance. This focus does not imply that we ignore other social psychological factors that can impact adherence. For example, it is possible that an exceptionally strong and trusting relationship between doctor and patient could assure compliance in the absence of a shared view of disease and treatment. In days past it was not uncommon for the physician to be a valued and trusted member of the patient's family, and compliance with his recommendations was assured. While relationships of this type can achieve high levels of compliance in the absence of shared representations of a health problem, they are far less common, and indeed deemed inappropriate, in today's complex care systems. We have also paid little attention to the factor of social support, though it is clear that social contacts play an important role in seeking health care and have continuing effects upon compliance and the evaluation of treatment outcomes (Cameron, Leventhal, & Leventhal, 1993; Kelly & Scott, 1990). Similarly, a chaotic and unsafe environment can have major effects on compliance by blocking daily activities such as trips to the pharmacy, or by triggering severe episodes of mental dysfunction that make treatment seem ineffective. Ecological effects, which may be of great importance for compliance among patients with severe mental illness have received too little attention.

If there is a "major" lesson in our review, it is that theory must play a central role in compliance research. In a complex world of moderators and multiple causal pathways, an empirical approach dissociated from theory will yield a hodge-podge of conflicting outcomes and will result in diminishing patient care.

REFERENCES

Abramson, L. Y., Seligman, M. E. P., & Teasdale, J. (1978). Learned helplessness in humans: Critique and reformulation. *Journal of Abnormal Psychology, 87*, 49–74.

Ajzen, I., & Fishbein, M. (1980). *Understanding attitudes and predicting social behavior*. Englewood Cliffs, N.J.: Prentice Hall.

Bandura, A. (1977). Self-efficacy: toward a unifying theory of change. *Psychological Review, 84*, 191–215.

Baumann, L., Cameron, L. D., Zimmerman, R., & Leventhal, H. (1989). Illness representations and matching labels with symptoms. *Health Psychology, 8*, 449–469.

Blumhagen, D. (1980). Hyper-tension: A folk illness with a medical name. *Cultural and Medical Psychiatry, 4*, 197–227.

Brown, G., & Harris, T. (1978). *Social origins of depression: A study of psychiatric disorders in women*. New York: Free Press.

Cameron, L., Leventhal, E. A., & Leventhal, H. (1993). Symptom representations and affect as determinants of care seeking in a community dwelling adult sample population. *Health Psychology, 12*, 171–179.

Carver, C. S., & Scheier, M. F. (1982). Control theory: A useful conceptual framework for personality, social, clinical, and health psychology. *Psychological Bulletin, 92*, 111–135.

Dollard, J., & Miller, N. E. (1950). *Personality and Psychotherapy*. New York: McGraw Hill.

Finnerty, F. A., Mattie, E. C., & Finnerty, III, F. A. (1973). Hypertension in the inner city. *Circulation, 47*, 73–75.

Kanfer, F. H. (1977). The many faces of self-control, or behavior modification changes its focus. In R. B. Stuart (Ed.). *Behavioral self-management: Strategies, techniques and outcomes*. New York: Brunner/ Mazel.

Kelly, H. H. (1972). The processes of causal attribution. *American Psychologist, 28*, 107–128.

Kelly, G. R. & Scott, J. E. (1990). Medication compliance and health education among outpatients with chronic mental disorders. *Medical Care, 28*, 1181–1197.

Kleinman, A. (1980). *Healers and patients in the context of culture: The interface of anthropology, medicine, and psychiatry*. Berkeley: University of California Press.

Knowles, J. H. (Ed.) (1977). *Doing better and feeling worse: Health in the United States*. New York: Norton.

Lau, R. R., & Hartmann, K. (1983). Common sense representations of common illnesses. *Health Psychology, 2,* 167–185.

Leventhal, H. (1970). Findings and theory in the study of fear communications. *Advances in Experimental Social Psychology, 5,* 119–186.

Leventhal, H. (1985). Commentary: The role of theory in the study of adherence to treatment and doctor-patient interactions. *Medical Care, 23,* 556–563.

Leventhal, H., Meyer, D., & Nerenz, D. (1980). The common sense representation of illness danger. In S. Rachman (Ed.), *Contributions to medical psychology* (Vol. II, pp. 7–30). New York: Pergamon Press.

Leventhal, H., Zimmerman, R., & Gutmann, M. (1984). Compliance: A self-regulation perspective. In W. D. Gentry (Ed.), *Handbook of Behavioral Medicine* (pp. 369–436). New York: Guilford Press.

Leventhal, H., Diefenbach, M. A., & Leventhal, E. A. (1992). Illness cognition: Using commonsense to understand treatment adherence and affect cognition interactions. *Cognitive Therapy and Research, 16,* 143–163.

Levine, D. M., Green, L. W., Deeds, S. G. et al. (1979). Health education for hypertensive patients. *Journal of American Medical Association, 241,* 1700.

Maiman, L. A., & Becker, M. H. (1974). The health belief model: Origins and Correlates in Psychological Theory. In M. H. Becker (Ed.), *The health belief model and personal health behavior* (pp. 9–26). New Jersey: Slack, Inc.

McGuire, W. J. (1968). Personality and susceptibility to social influence. In E. Borgotta and W. Lambert (Eds.), *Handbook of Personality Theory and Research.* Chicago: Rand McNally.

Meichenbaum, D. (1977). *Cognitive-behavior modification: An integrative approach.* New York: Plenum Press.

Meyer, D., Leventhal, H., & Gutmann, M. (1985). Common-sense models of illness: The example of hypertension. *Health Psychology, 4,* 115–135.

Rosenstock, I. M. (1974). The health belief model and preventive health behavior. In M. H. Becker (Ed.), *The health belief model and personal the behavior* (pp. 27–59). New Jersey: Slack, Inc

Sackett, D. L. (1978). Patients and therapies: Getting the two together. *New England Journal of Medicine, 298,* 278–279.

Santiago, J. M., Berren, M. R., Beigel, A., Goldfinger, S. M. et al. (1990). The seriously mentally ill: Another perspective on treatment resistance. *Community Mental Health Journal, 26*(3), 237–244.

3

Medication Noncompliance in Schizophrenia: *Effects on Mental Health Service Policy*

PETER WEIDEN, MARK OLFSON and
SUSAN ESSOCK

SCOPE OF THE NONCOMPLIANCE PROBLEM

Introduction

The introduction of antipsychotic drugs in the 1960's brought hope that most institutionalized mentally ill patients could successfully return to the community. In hindsight, such optimism was naive. In retrospect, one of the reasons for overestimating the impact of better medications was the failure to anticipate the noncompliance problem. The lesson here is that it is essential to consider the impact of medication noncompliance on treatment services, and vice versa.

The goal of this chapter is to help you better understand the two-way interactions between noncompliance and mental health care services. Because of the complexity and scope of this topic, we will narrow our focus to compliance with **maintenance antipsychotic drugs** for outpatients with schizophrenia. Advantages of such a focus include the presence of an extensive outcome literature on maintenance antipsychotics for people with schizophrenia. The first part of this chapter will define noncompliance and estimate its public health impact. The second part will look at **clinical-barriers** to patient compliance. The third part will discuss **services-barriers** to compliance, and the final section will offer our recommendations. Because some readers may want to modify our definitions, criteria sets, or recommendations, we will present our working assumptions and rationales in considerable detail and in tabular formats.

Benefits and Limitations of Medication

Noncompliance is a problem only when treatment is effective. Therefore, the first step in understanding medication noncompliance is to understand medication efficacy. For the standard maintenance antipsychotic drugs (e.g. haloperidol or chlorpromazine, but not including risperidone, clozapine or newer antipsychotics), the efficacy picture is decidedly mixed. Because medication efficacy in schizophrenia is not unidimensional, the degree of benefit will depend greatly on which aspect of outcome is being considered. The most favorable aspect of maintenance antipsychotic medication is relapse prevention. Relapse rates are approximately 8% per month for the first 24 months after discharge without maintenance medication and approximately 3.5% per month on optimal doses of maintenance medication (Weiden and Olfson 1995). The magnitude of the difference in relapse rates between medicated and unmedicated patients is at least as good as the effectiveness of antibiotics for tuberculosis (Davis et al., 1993).

On the other hand, maintenance antipsychotics have major problems. Most patients continue to have symptoms of schizophrenia despite being on medication (Diamond 1985), and many others will relapse despite ongoing medication treatment (Schooler et al., 1980). Furthermore, antipsychotics have well-known, serious and distressing neurologic side effects such as drug-induced parkinsonism, akathisia, and tardive dyskinesia (Van Putten et al., 1976). While the newer "atypical" antipsychotics such as clozapine and risperidone are less likely to cause neurologic side effects, they are not devoid of them (Weiden 1995b). Therefore, even compliant, "medication-responsive" patients with schizophrenia are usually disappointed by the limitations of drug therapy.

Is it fair to call someone noncompliant when the benefits of treatment are so limited? Patient advocacy groups have justifiable concerns about the perjorative implications that come from calling people "noncompliant". One answer to these patient concerns that can also address policymakers' concerns is to emphasize medication's role in relapse prevention. Relapse prevention should be a shared goal of both patients and providers. Rehabilitation and recovery process cannot take place without symptom stabilization. For the vast majority of people with schizophrenia, long periods of stabilization are not possible without being on continuous antipsychotic medication (Hogarty et al., 1974; Schooler 1991).

CLINICAL BARRIERS TO COMPLIANCE

Operational Criteria for Medication Noncompliance

Most people do not take their medications as prescribed. At what point does irregular medication-taking behavior get called "noncompliance"? A sensible definition of noncompliance needs to be linked to the pharmacologic profile of the drug. Noncompliance needs to be extensive enough to cause plasma drug levels to fall below the minimally effective level. Dose/response data is essential in making this determination. Maintenance antipsychotics have a very wide dose/response curve, and for many people with schizophrenia, a small dose can be very effective. Many (but not all) patients can do quite well on lower doses than are commonly prescribed. On the other hand, the maintenance data also shows that complete cessation of antipsychotics leads to unacceptably high relapse rates (Johnson 1976) and that intermittent dosing strategies are not an acceptable substitute for continuous maintenance treatment (Herz et al., 1991). Accordingly, we suggest that the primary criterion for noncompliance to maintenance antipsychotics be **complete cessation** of medication. While it is hard to predict the consequences of stopping a portion of the neuroleptic regimen, complete cessation of medication almost always leads to relapse (Weiden et al., 1995a). In addition, we suggest that there be two consecutive weeks of medication cessation to establish that the noncompliant behavior is not transient and can be expected to continue until relapse.

The suggested **behavioral criteria** for noncompliance shown in Table 3.1 have the advantage of being relatively easy to detect and document. Table 3.1 also lists a more complicated but comprehensive criteria set for noncompliance that takes into account services-barriers to compliance.

Epidemiology of Medication Noncompliance

The epidemiology of noncompliance makes it possible to estimate the public health impact of the compliance problem. First, a cautionary note about an epidemiologic trap when evaluating noncompliance rates. Patient selection bias is a major confound among stable outpatient populations (e.g. a continuous day treatment program). Very often, clinic samples have already lost their most noncompliant patients before an evaluation of noncompliance rates is started. The remaining patients are more likely to continue to be compliant and bias the research into finding artificially high compliance rates (Sackett 1979). This epidemiologic trap has fooled many sincere but methodologically unsophisticated clinicians into believing that their own program is particularly adept at maintaining patient compliance. To circumvent this problem, noncompliance rates presented here are limited to prospective field studies with defined cohorts who are new to the outpatient treatment service being studied.

Table 3.1. Suggested Criteria for Defining Noncompliance

Criteria for *Noncompliant Behavior*

1. There has been complete cessation of all antipsychotic medication.
2. The medication has been stopped for at least two weeks.

Additional criteria that consider *Services Barriers to Compliance*

1. The diagnosis of schizophrenia or related psychotic disorder is correct. In particular, for first episode cases, there has been careful consideration of affective disorder or substance abuse disorder.
2. The patient and family has been given culturally and educationally appropriate diagnostic and accurate treatment information.
3. The medication treatment is effective based on:
   a. For patients with prior medication histories, from the past treatment history
   b. For patients without past medication histories, from pertinent clinical research studies.
4. The benefits of maintenance treatment based on Criteria 3a or 3b above outweigh the risks of treatment. Factors to be considered the risk/benefit determination include:
   a. Likelihood of relapse on and off maintenance antipsychotic drugs.
   b. Consequences from relapse including disruptiveness, risk of injury to self or others.
   c. Past history of neuroleptic malignant syndrome, presence of current side effects such as chronic parkinsonian symptoms and risk of future side effects (tardive dyskinesia).
5. The patient is not choosing an alternative *effective* treatment. Often, a reasonable alternate is a trial of an atypical antipsychotic (clozapine or risperidone) for those individuals who have intolerable neurologic side effects (Criteria 4c above.)
6. The noncompliance is extensive enough to adversely affect outcome. In general, patient-initiated dosage lowering, without complete cessation, should not be categorized as noncompliance.
7. There are no significant Systems Barriers to compliance, including:
   a. Problems with adequate quality of care
   b. Affordability of treatment
   c. Access to treatment services
8. The thresholds established for reasonable access and affordability (Criteria 7a and 7b above) take into account limitations imposed by symptoms of the illness.

Treatment no-show rates: Medication compliance depends on continued contact with the prescribing mental health care professional. Inpatients who fail their first outpatient appointment almost certainly are or will soon become noncompliant to their medication. Although little research has been conducted on no-show rates for the specific diagnosis of schizophrenia per se, high treatment no-show rates have been

Table 3.2. Monthly Noncompliance Rates after Discharge

Author	Year	N	Follow-Up (Months)	Noncompliance Rates (% Per Month)
Parkes et al.	1962	53	12	5.5%
Renton et al.	1963	124	12	5.0%
Raskin & Dyson	1968	45	6	17.7%
Serban & Thomas	1974	516 (Chronic)	24	6.5%
Serban & Thomas	1974	70 (Acute)	24	5.3%
Caton	1982	119	12	13.8%
Gaebel et al.	1985	64	12	5.4%
Frank & Gunderson	1990	72	18	5.4%
Weiden et al.	1991	72	24	5.4%
Thomas et al.	1992	384	6	8.5%
Zygmunt & Weiden	1993	115	12	6.3%
Summary		1,634	15.8 (± 6.7)	7.6%

(Caton 1982; Frank and Gunderson 1990; Gaebel and Pietzker 1985; Raskin and Dyson 1968; Renton et al. 1963; Serban and Thomas 1974; Thomas et al. 1992; Weiden et al. 1991)

reported from a range of mental health populations and treatment settings. No-show rates to the first clinic/aftercare appointment range from 20–60% (Gould et al., 1970; Kluger and Karras 1983).

Medication noncompliance rates: Table 3.2 above shows the post-discharge medication noncompliance rates found in community samples with follow-up lengths between 6 months and two years (Weiden and Olfson 1995). These studies represent "standard care" programs, which typically would include medication management and some supportive therapy but not intensive outpatient services (e.g. ACT/PACT models of care). Noncompliance rates averaged 7.6% per month, which translates to approximately 50% for the first post-discharge year and 75% after two years post-discharge. These studies show that medication noncompliance after discharge is a predictable feature of the illness. A key epidemiologic risk factor for these high noncompliance rates is discharge from the hospital. Noncompliance rates eventually decrease for patients who have remained out of the hospital for several years (Curson 1985).

The implication for mental health services is the need to anticipate that, within a year of discharge, at least 50% of neuroleptic-responsive patients with schizophrenia will stop their medication and another 50% will stop during the second year. Therefore, the 50% per year medication noncompliance figure might be a suitable yardstick by which to compare the compliance effectiveness of outpatient programs treating discharged patients with schizophrenia. In contrast, a considerably lower noncompliance rate should be expected from programs treating patients who have not recently been hospitalized.

Consequences of Medication Noncompliance

Medication noncompliance has a range of detrimental consequences.

Effects on "real world" relapse rates: When discharged patients stop their medication, relapse rates go up from about 3.4% a month to about 12% per month (Weiden and Olfson 1995). By modeling known noncompliance rates and relapse rates on and off medication, we estimate that noncompliance accounts for at least 40% of all episodes of "revolving-door" relapse and rehospitalizations.

Economic cost: The 40% relapse rate estimate can be used to estimate cost of hospital treatment due to medication noncompliance. There were approximately 257,000 short-term (<90 days) hospitalizations per year for multiple-episode patients with schizophrenia diagnoses during 1986 (the last year this data is available). The aggregate direct hospital cost (in 1991 dollars) was 1.9 billion, making the direct inpatient hospital cost of noncompliance to be over 750 million dollars per year.

Effects on long-term outcome: There is some evidence the intermittent pattern of medication treatment from noncompliance may actually increase the risk of tardive dyskinesia. Prolonged, untreated psychosis may diminish the effectiveness of medication treatment (Wyatt 1991). Noncompliant relapse is associated with longer hospitalizations (Bartko et al., 1987), as well as suicidal behavior (Virkkunen 1974).

Social costs: Relapse that is caused by medication noncompliance may be more dangerous than relapse occurring in the context of compliance (Johnson et al., 1983). Compared to the relapse that occurs when patients with schizophrenia are taking medication, relapse among noncompliant patients is often more severe and disruptive. Medication noncompliance, especially in combination with substance abuse, has also been associated with assaultive and dangerous behavior (Torrey 1994).

To summarize, there is compelling evidence that medication compliance achieves two major goals. For the person with schizophrenia, medication compliance usually assists in his or her personal goals staying out of the hospital and getting on with life. From a public health viewpoint, improving compliance rates will decrease recidivism, and help reduce the economic and social cost of this disorder.

Type of Antipsychotic Prescribed

Over the last few years, there have been major changes in maintenance drug treatment that have increased treatment options. There is a reemergence of interest in the depot route of medication delivery, and clozapine and risperidone are recently introduced "atypical" antipsychotics. Both of these treatment approaches — atypical antipsychotics (Addington et al., 1993; Hale 1993) and long-acting depot drugs (Glazer and Kane 1992; Weiden et al., 1995b) have the potential to improve compliance rates compared with the standard neuroleptic drugs. As new antipsychotics are introduced, one of the challenges will be patient selection to match the best medication treatment to the compliance issues of the individual patient (Weiden 1995a; Weiden 1995b).

Depot route and compliance: One critical issue is whether the long-acting (depot) route of medication delivery, compared with oral medication, is associated with better compliance. Depot neuroleptic agents are not used as commonly in the United States as they are elsewhere. Current practice in the US today is based, in large part, on the results of several influential double-blind studies which showed no statistical differences in relapse rates between depot and oral drug, although a meta-analysis of these studies showed superiority of the depot route on relapse rates occurring in the second year (Glazer and Kane 1992). Other studies used a 'mirror-image' methodology and compared a patient's clinical course for a matched time period before and after starting the depot neuroleptic route. This kind of study showed strikingly positive effects on relapse rates after switching patients from using the oral to the depot route. A recent study by Weiden and colleagues (Weiden et al., 1995b) showed time-limited compliance benefits from depot conversion. Inpatients converted to a depot neuroleptic had significantly better compliance one-month postdischarge compared to matched patients on oral medication; however, the compliance benefit in this study did not persist. The depot route seemed to facilitate medication compliance during the transition to aftercare, but other interventions are needed to maintain compliance over time.

New antipsychotics and compliance: The second question is how the newer "atypical" antipsychotic medications (e.g. clozapine or risperidone) will affect long-term compliance. Some studies have found reductions in relapse rates when patients are maintained on the atypical antipsychotic drugs compared with standard neuroleptics (Addington et al., 1993; Essock et al. (1996)). It is unclear whether the superiority in relapse is due to patient selection biases, superior efficacy, or better compliance. Preliminary data and clinical experience suggest that noncompliance will remain a problem for the newer atypical drugs even despite better efficacy and/or better side effect profiles. At this point, there is an urgent need to study compliance with new antipsychotic medications.

Policy implications: There will be intense financial pressure to place arbitrary limits on pharmacy budgets, or try to ration use of expensive antipsychotic agents. In our opinion, such an approach is misguided. Because relapse is so expensive and loss of efficacy and noncompliance are the major causes of relapse, there will be little conflict between the goals of good patient care and cost-containment. Medication selection should be based solely on 1) efficacy (not only relapse but broader quality of life outcomes) and 2) likelihood of promoting compliance. Mental health policies need to encourage long-term treatment planning where medications are selected systematically to address target goals of persistent symptoms and/or noncompliance. For the patient with compliance problems, the first step is to assess the underlying reasons for compliance and noncompliance. Once known, it is possible to choose the type of drug that can best address the reason for noncompliance. For example, a disorganized patient with little supervision might be a candidate for the depot (long-acting) medication route, whereas an atypical drug might be better for someone who stops medication because of neurologic side effects. The opportunity here is to develop long-term policy strategies that integrate the noncompliance assessment into treatment selection options. Mental health planners should not expect to solve compliance problems by medications alone, but consider medication selection to be an essential part of a treatment program designed to facilitate patient compliance.

Risk Factors for Patient-Initiated Noncompliance

"Patient-initiated noncompliance" is a shorthand term meant to describe those risk factors for medication noncompliance arising from either the individuals' attitude, psychiatric symptoms, or response to treatment. Table 3.3 below lists of some of the more prominent noncompliance risk factors that are related to symptoms of schizophrenia and/or limitations of antipsychotic treatment. The mental health policy implications of how these psychiatric symptoms and limitations of medication interact with compliance will be discussed in later parts of this chapter.

Table 3.3. Symptom and Medication Risk Factors for Noncompliance

Psychiatric Symptom	Mechanism Impairing Compliance
Denial of illness	1. Leads to unawareness of benefits of medication. 2. Side effects are less tolerated when there is no perceived need for medication.
Paranoia	1. Limits trust in treatment or medication recommendations. 2. Limits ability to use public transportation.
Grandiosity	1. Decreases "signal" that there is a psychiatric problem. 2. Medication response means loss of grandiose "high".
Cognitive disorganization	1. Impaired ability to follow complex medication regimes.
Cognitive impairments	1. Diminished ability to learn from experience (e.g. understanding the connection between stopping medication and relapse).

Table 3.3. Continued

Psychiatric Symptom	Mechanism Impairing Compliance
Motivational deficits	1. Leads to problems with appointment attendance. 2. Indifference to benefits of medication.

Limitations of Medication Treatments

Relapse despite compliance	1. Decreases faith in the effectiveness of medication. 2. Diminishes credibility of clinicians who overpromise medication benefits.
Side effects	1. Direct cause of distress and discomfrot. 2. Visibile neurologic side-effects increase stigma. 3. Decreases family support of continuous medication therapy.
Persistent positive symptoms	1. Directly causes lack of insight. 2. Leads to "vicious-cycle" of noncompliance worsening psychotic symptoms which aggravate loss of insight.
Persistent negative symptoms	1. Decreases motivation to stay on medication. 2. Life goals are not accomplished despite medication. 3. Diminishes family support of medication.

(Amador et al., 1994; Babiker 1986; Bachrach 1981; Baekeland and Lundwall 1975; Barofsky 1978; Barofsky and Connelly 1980; Blaska 1990; Buchanan 1992; Diamond 1985; Diamond 1983; Fink and Heckerman 1981; Heinrichs et al., 1985; Hogan and Awad 1992; Kelly and Scott 1990; Keown 1985; Parkes et al., 1962; Van Putten and May 1978; Weiden et al., 1995a; Weiden et al., 1994)

SERVICES BARRIERS TO COMPLIANCE

Conceptual Issues

Taking a broad view, compliance represents a successful linkage between the patient, features of his or her illness and treatment, and a
treatment service (Blackwell 1992; Goldfinger et al., 1984). To better
understand interactions between the patient and the mental health
service, we will contrast patient-initiated noncompliance with services barriers that make medication compliance more difficult to
achieve. Medication compliance can be thought of as a successful link
between patient and treatment service (Talbott et al., 1986). This linkage is illustrated as the overlapping area on the Venn diagram shown
in Figure 3.1. Overlapping areas represent a successful match between the patient and treatment service and nonoverlapping areas
represent unsuccessful matches. This diagram makes the important
point that, on a macro level, there are at least two conceptual approaches to improve medication compliance. Where the traditional
medical model approach would view medication noncompliance as
a result of patient-initiated behavior, a services model would tend to
view the same behavior as failure to achieve a fit between the patient
and the patient's treatment service. The net effect of this shift from a
medical model to a services model is to pay more attention to the
patient-treatment interaction than to the patient's particular attitude
or behavior.

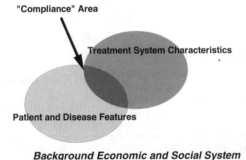

Figure 3.1. *Schematic diagram of overlap of Patient & Disease Features with Treatment System Characteristics necessary for patient "compliance".*

Patient/Services Interactions

The boundaries between patient-initiated noncompliance and services barriers to compliance may be quite hazy. There are a myriad
of interactions between the patient and his or her treatment service
that can exacerbate compliance problems. The exact sequencing of

events can be difficult to disentangle. The following case example illustrates how patient attitudes, psychiatric symptoms, and limitations in the delivery of care interact as an episode of medication noncompliance unfolds.

Mr. A is a 28 year man suffering from schizophrenia with a history of three prior hospitalizations. Over the last year, Mr. A. has accepted the need for medication, and, until recently, has been taking it regularly. He is now hospitalized after stopping his medication. Compliance problems began three months ago, when Mr. A. decided to seek vitamin therapy to supplement his medication with the eventual goal of stopping antipsychotic medication. Several weeks after starting the vitamins, Mr. A got confused over the prescribed antipsychotic regimen. He called his psychiatric clinic and got an extra appointment for later that month. In his confusion, however, Mr. A decided to stop all of his medications while waiting for his appointment. Shortly before his appointment, Mr. A. became increasingly paranoid. He was unable to travel to the clinic because of fears that the passengers on the bus were plotting to kill him. Mr. A. rescheduled his appointment which, not surprisingly, he failed again. Eventually, Mr. A. threatened his neighbors and was brought to the hospital by the police.

Mr. A's noncompliance started off as **patient-initiated** (seeking vitamins as an alternate therapy) and then increased due to **symptom exacerbation** (disorganization and confusion). His clinic couldn't schedule him right away (**services barrier**), and he soon was unable to travel (**symptom exacerbation**). Even though it was apparent that Mr. A. was relapsing, the clinic was unable to provide outreach to his home (**services barrier**). It is worth attempting to disentangle these factors to develop a practical set of criteria that can be used to evaluate and modify services barriers to compliance.

Operationalizing Services Barriers to Compliance

Table 3.4 below lists some common barriers to compliance that frequently arise in mental health treatment settings. In many ways, these services barriers to compliance are the mirror image to patient-initiated noncompliance. The operational definition of a services barrier to compliance is the presence of a problem in the treatment service that may be the cause of the patient's medication cessation. In other words, a patient with a severe mental illness should not be categorized as "medication noncompliant" if the person's mental health care service has prominent deficits making it much more difficult to achieve medication compliance.

Barriers to Treatment Access and Availability

Health care delivery services in the United States are structured so that individuals typically either receive their care in the private

Table 3.4. Suggested Criteria for Services
Barriers to Patient Compliance

Medication noncompliance is more likely to occur when the following services components are missing or deficient.

1. Presence of mental health professionals with clinical skills for treating schizophrenia.
   a. Accuracy of diagnosis.
   b. Medication and side effect management skills.
   c. Ability to give patient and family psychoeducation.
   d. Relationship skills to develop alliance with people with major mental illness.

2. Ability to provide reasonable continuity of care.
   a. Minimizing changes of outpatient clinician or clinical team. When staff changes occur, adequate continuity of clinical history and case supervison.
   b. Adequate communication between inpatient and outpatient clinicians.
   c. Availability of medical records with readable and coherent summaries.
   d. Reasonable stability of treatment location.

3. The capacity to prescribe and monitor all major classes of psychotropic medications without major practical or bureaucratic hurdles.
   a. Depot antipsychotic medications (fluphenazine and haloperidol decanoate).
   b. Atypical antipsychotics (clozapine and risperidone).
   c. Full range of side effect medications (e.g. propranolol for akathisia).
   d. Concurrent medicines for chronic medical conditions (e.g. insulin for diabetes).

4. Availability of a full range of essential psychiatric services.
   a. Emergency and crisis services.
   b. Inpatient beds or crisis services during relapse.
   c. Prompt scheduling (no more than a week interval) of first outpatient appointment after discharge or upon reentering treatment service.
   d. Services for co-existing substance abuse problems.
   e. Providing lines of communication with involved family.

5. Adapting treatment delivery to symptoms of schizophrenia, including:
   a. Travel constraints that arise from symptoms of schizophrenia.
   b. Symptom-based difficulties obtaining benefits.
   c. Symptom-based difficulties in obtaining or regularly taking medication.
   d. Affordability of medication, especially in co-pay situations.
   e. Available medical services that are sensitive to needs of severely mentally ill.

6. Matching patient goals and treatment options.
   a. Having the flexibility to provide, or omit, psychosocial therapies with medication treatment.
   b. Provision of other basic supportive therapies that will enhance compliance through maintaining a therapeutic alliance.

---

sector with payment via third parties, such as private insurers or Champus, or in the public sector, with payment by the State with some State payments augmented by Federal Medicaid payments. Because the traditional private and public sectors are so different, they will be discussed separately. For this discussion, agencies such as group homes and private managed care programs that contract for patients financed by public sector funds are considered as being within a public sector treatment (Essock and Goldman 1995).

Treatment in a traditional private sector system: Individuals with diagnoses of schizophrenia are underrepresented in traditional private fee-for-service or pre-paid HMO services. For example, Johnson & McFarland (1994) found treatment rates for schizophrenia within a large HMO to be .16% of the covered population, less than one-half of the ECA estimate of an overall treatment rate of .4% in the community. Not only are fewer patients treated in the traditional private sector, those who are treated typically have third-rate insurance benefits for their mental illness. HMO patients may receive only the most basic medication services from general psychiatric clinicians who do not routinely treat schizophrenia. Traditional fee for service plans usually do not provide comparable benefits for private psychiatric care relative to medical care, even if the psychiatric condition is as serious as schizophrenia. Even when medication coverage is provided, there often is a shocking lack of knowledge on private insurers' part about treatment basics. One striking example of a private patient with schizophrenia being treated by one of the authors was a repeated rejection of a claim for weekly white blood count monitoring for a clozapine patient as being excessive!

There are several reasons for the relatively high barriers to treatment for severe mentally illness within the traditional private sector. First, the private sector's coverage of severe mental illness is sparse even while individuals are still eligible for those services. Second, schizophrenia is a chronic and disabling illness, and most people with schizophrenia rapidly become poor enough to qualify for public-sector care, which often is more comprehensive than the services offered by the private insurer. Third, private sector mental health care has evolved to provide services to the most common mental health problems (e.g., depression) where the individual requiring treatment usually recognizes the need for treatment, can come in for treatment, and can afford medication and treatment co-payments. In short, there are many converging reasons why individuals with schizophrenia who begin treatment in the private sector usually end up receiving care in the public sector.

Treatment in a public sector system: States play a central role in providing mental health care for the severely mentally ill, far exceeding their role in the delivery of general health care services (Essock and Goldman 1995). Therefore, beginning in the 1960s, with Medicaid and Medicare, states began to deliver public mental health services using a mix of state dollars and federal third-party payments. When considering public sector treatment, we are really considering programs that are at least partly determined within each state; thus, there will be considerable variability in the program specifics from state to state. Looked at from a national perspective, Narrow and colleagues (1993) estimated a 69.5% one-year outpatient utilization rate for patient with schizophrenia for 'mostly' publically-funded ambulatory specialty mental health services. This group averaged 16.0 outpatient visits per year, suggesting that, on average, during 1983 patients with schizophrenia have access to biweekly or monthly clinic-based maintenance treatment services. A corollary is that intensive or daily treatment services were not the norm. The overall conclusion from the ECA data is that basic public sector services are available but that intensive, community-based rehabilitation programs are not. Consistent with the ECA data, a study of multiple episode patients in an urban setting (Caton et al., 1984) found that basic medication clinic services tended to be available after discharge, whereas other, more intensive aftercare services such as supportive housing were not.

ACT/PACT Services: While many patients can remain compliant and do well with low-intensity, medication-oriented clinic settings, there is a large subgroup of patients who are unable to comply with traditional clinic settings. Many of these can be successfully engaged by a more comprehensive and assertive program. The state of the art can be found in comprehensive programs where severely disabled clients are treated by an assertive community treatment (ACT) team (Stein 1993). An example of the kind of intervention an ACT team makes is to travel to the client's home and deliver medications when the person is too symptomatic to travel. While the ACT treatment model is more widely implemented than when the ECA study was conducted, the majority of outpatient services remain clinic-based and do not have the resources to make outreach interventions. Unfortunately, even when public mental health systems contain state of the art components such as ACT teams and supported housing programs, spaces in such programs are usually fewer than the number of people who would benefit from such care. While most states fund some ACT programs, at this time (1995) more than one-half of the programs are concentrated in just two states (Michigan and Wisconsin), and the vast majority of severely mentally ill in need of such services do not have it available at this time. As states move away from inpatient services towards ACT/PACT models, there is real danger of fallout during the transition period. If state hospital beds are closed before the ACT/PACT teams are up and running, it will be much harder for the severely ill to get reasonable care. "Service planning and capital investment need to precede, not follow, changes in organization and practice of care" (Kavanagh et al., 1995).

Disincentives to Caring for Noncompliant Patients

Private sector disincentives: Historically, private sector mental health delivery systems have had few fiscal incentives to develop integrated treatment services like the ACT model. From the private payer's point of view, individuals suffering from schizophrenia are likely to "cost out" either because benefit maximums had been reached, or because the individual was no longer eligible for coverage (e.g., no longer employed, no longer an eligible dependent). From the payers' perspective, the sooner a person with schizophrenia 'costs out', the better. The case of 'Sylvia Frumpkin' is a well-known example of how expensive schizophrenia is for private payors. Her illness started when she was covered on her parents' policy. Her hospitalizations cost private 3rd party payors over 600,000 (1983) dollars until her care eventually was transferred to the public state mental health system (Moran et al., 1984).

It is not surprising that the private sector has used noncompliance with treatment (independent of the type of treatment offered) to deny further coverage. Noncompliance with medication has been suggested as a criterion for benefit termination by managed mental health care vendors (Gerson 1994). Such a policy could easily become a self-fulfilling prophesy and makes about as much clinical sense as denying further treatment to a person with diabetes who has not been able to maintain a stable blood sugar level. Yet, medication noncompliance can be a perfect way for private payors to gracefully extricate themselves from the financial responsibility of paying the huge treatment costs associated with schizophrenia (Petrila 1995). Therefore, medication and treatment noncompliance helps the private payors hand the treatment of schizophrenia back to the public sector. Until the private sector is held responsible for noncompliance (e.g. capitation with continued clinical responsibility for **noncompliant** patients), private payors will continue to hold the door wide open as the patient walks away from private treatment.

Public sector disincentives: There are also many disincentives for public systems to accept noncompliant patients with schizophrenia. Noncompliant individuals will often require more treatment resources than compliant individuals. However, because they are noncompliant, they may be more erratic in their attendance, or be more likely to disappear from treatment. Therefore, a public program treating the severely mentally ill on a fee-for-service schedule would get less steady income from noncompliant individuals compared to "easier" compliant referrals. Even when payments are structured so that a program does not have a fiscal disincentive to serve more difficult clients, other referral barriers may exist. For example, a group home's contract with the State mental health authority may contain a "no reject" clause stating that the program cannot refuse any referral, but some clients may not accept the group home placement because of features of their illness (e.g., their discomfort living in such a communal situation may exacerbate their symptoms) or because of a mismatch between the service and person being referred (e.g., because the ethnic mix in the group home or in the group home's neighborhood is uncomfortably foreign to the client).

Another disincentive in the treatment of noncompliant patients in the public sector is concern over the legal responsibility for dangerous behavior during relapse. Relapse from noncompliance is more frequent, less manageable, and often more dangerous than relapse among compliant patients. Mental health providers assume

greater malpractice risks from accepting such patients, or from trying to work with the person or family after he or she stops medication. Termination of treatment ("closing the chart") because of
medication noncompliance is often a tacit way of discharging medical responsibility. While understandable, it exacerbates continuity
of care problems and increases the likelihood of disaster from the
next relapse. From a policy perspective, there is an urgent need to
remove such disincentives to caring for noncompliant patients.

Quality of Care Barriers

We will highlight three areas where major problems exist that are
amenable to mental health policy interventions.

   Clinical skills: Any service needs a team of clinicians trained in
psychiatric diagnosis, medication management, psychoeducation, and
forming and maintaining relationships with patients/consumers and
their families. While the use of antipsychotic medication is now almost
universally accepted, significant problems remain in their optimal
use. Essock and colleagues (in press) found that in a state hospital
system in 1991, 45% of "treatment-unresponsive" patients never
had received two separate antipsychotic trials (the two trial criterion
is widely regarded as a minimum before defining a person as
"treatment-unresponsive") (Kane et al., 1988). Also, there are major
skills problems with outpatient medication management. Many
clinicians prematurely stop the antipsychotic medications for maintenance therapy of outpatients with schizophrenia, especially for first-
episode schizophrenia (Kissling 1991), or may underestimate the
devastating impact of relapse on the person's life (Johnson et al., 1983).
Clinicians may fail to recognize or properly treat the distressing
extrapyramidal side effects of antipsychotic drugs (Weiden et al.,
1987), which in turn can undermine any working relationship between
patients and their doctors. Clinicians underestimate and under-
diagnose concurrent medical conditions (Roca et al., 1987). In part this
is because people with schizophrenia tend to underreport medical
symptoms (Dworkin 1994), and in part because of lack of accessible
medical services for the severely mentally ill (Roca et al., 1987). Finally,
many of the service settings are far away from teaching centers, and
'front-line' clinical staff rarely have opportunities for ongoing medical
education and updating of clinical skills.

   Continuity of care: Continuity of care is an essential part of quality
treatment (Bachrach 1981). Communication and coordination between the referring and receiving services have been shown to improve referral completion and subsequent patient functioning (Caton
et al., 1984). It seems that transitions in care of a person with schizophrenia (e.g. going from inpatient to outpatient care, or changing outpatient clinics) will be associated with a high "no-show" rate. The
obvious quality of care implication for mental health policy is to foster linkages between inpatient and outpatient services, and to convey
the message that continuity of care and good communication between
services is a valued outcome.

Communication with family members: A continuing quality of care problem is the frequency with which mental health personnel fail to involve family members in treatment planning and psychoeducation. Most disconcerting is the unwillingness of many treatment services to respond to the family member's observation that the client is relapsing. The rationale on the clinicians part is concern about confidentiality; however, such notions are inappropriate during emergencies and usually reflect outdated psychoanalytic notions about treatment privacy. While it is hard to get quantitative data on this, there was so much concern over lack of communication between treatment teams and families in New Hampshire that this state recently passed legislation mandating clinicians to respond to family calls in a timely fashion.

Medication Cost and Co-Payment Barriers

Medication cost is an obvious barrier to compliance, especially for the mentally ill who are often disabled and poor. The few studies looking at how medication costs affect compliance in severe mental illness have had paradoxical findings, especially with out-of-pocket medication expenses. While inconclusive, earlier studies indicated that patients who were able to get full medication reimbursement through Medicaid did better than groups who had even small out-of-pocket medication co-payments (Cody and Robinson 1977; Davis et al., 1977). Both authors felt that the real issue involved the fact that the Medicaid patients had the wherewithal or social support to seek and obtain Medicaid, while those who paid out of pocket were too psychiatrically disabled or lacked support. In a more recent study of severe mentally ill in rural Mississippi, Sullivan (Sullivan et al. (1995)) found that even low co-payment costs created significant compliance barriers. The most striking effect of changing medication costs was shown by Soumerai and colleagues (1994) who documented a 21% decrease in antipsychotic drug use for outpatients treated for schizophrenia in New Hampshire CMHCs after legislation that capped Medicaid drug reimbursement to three prescriptions per month. During the period when the capping was in effect, there was a corresponding 50% increase in CMHC visits. Similar to the tone in the other articles, the Soumerai article hinted that one reason for this large an effect was that patients with schizophrenia were not particularly adept at circumventing the capping restrictions.

In summary, seemingly minor changes in co-payment or access to medication can create major services barriers to treatment. This sensitivity to price or access changes seem to be from symptoms of schizophrenia that lead to disorganization and poverty. These results suggest that patients with schizophrenia are not as adept as chronic medical patients in coping with medication co-payments or circumventing medication restrictions. There is convincing evidence that any co-payment plan (or other medication restriction) targeted for the person with schizophrenia will boomerang and result in unacceptable increases in relapse rates.

RECOMMENDATIONS

The remainder of this chapter will attempt to integrate the patient and service issues already mentioned; in particular, how to set up a service that takes the schizophrenic illness into account such that non-compliance is not induced by the services barriers. Obviously, the suggestions here are based from the earlier assumptions; changes in the assumptions will lead to modifications in recommendations.

In Theory, Closed Systems of Care are Preferable to Open Systems

A key patient problem in evaluating the role of treatment service is the frequency that patients with schizophrenia lose insight about symptoms or deny their illness. Denial of illness is a complex issue that is by no means limited to mental illness, nor is it always pathologic (for further details, see Chapter 4 on Insight and Compliance). Nonetheless, there is substantial evidence that the denial of illness seen in people suffering from schizophrenia is more persistent than in other diagnoses. Denial of illness creates a major problem in how to evaluate the treatment service provided. For example, denial of a problem will lead to drop out and save a third-party payor considerable money. It is unlikely that patients who are told they suffer from cancer would drop their insurance coverage at the time of the evaluation and diagnosis. Yet, exactly such a scenario is common for patients diagnosed with psychotic disorders. The question then is, to what extent is a mental health treatment service obliged to locate, or reach out to, its drop-outs? Should a treatment service be allowed to terminate its responsibility to treat when a patient no longer accepts or acknowledges the need for continued treatment despite overwhelming evidence to the contrary? Currently, there are incentives for service systems to retain compliant and less demanding patients and be relieved when an uncooperative patient finally leaves. If costs can be shifted to another player — such as a State hospital — the incentive for a single entity to minimize total mental health expenditures disappears. A capitated approach theoretically should help counteract the denial of illness problem, and there have been reports of how these payment arrangements have improved the quality of services (Harris and Bergman 1988). A cautionary note is in order. The above analysis is theoretical and omits a crucial problem with capitation. It naively leaves out the harmful effect of capitation when used as a vehicle to reduce overall services to maximize profits (See Shadish (1989) for an excellent discussion of the problem of profit vs. good care).

Develop Provider Incentives to Improve Compliance Rates

Even if a closed system is not feasible in the short run, an alternate approach is to use compliance outcome in contract negotiations and reimbursement. Clinicians should be paid more to treat noncompliant patients than compliant ones. To the extent that one can expect to get what one pays for, contracts for broad services for people with schizophrenia should create incentives for the service provider to maximize patients' medication compliance by including performance measures geared to services believed to enhance compliance. If psychoeducation about medication, transportation, free medication, continuity of prescribing physician, reminder phone calls, and other interventions are thought to enhance compliance and avoid costly hospitalizations and their sequelae, then contracts can include clauses to encourage these services (e.g., "at least X% of patients receiving medication management sessions see the same psychiatrist at least once every Y weeks for at least Z months).

Promote Flexibility of Treatment Services

The best of today's public mental health services match available services to clients' needs and preferences, rather than the other way around. Medication clinics equipped with the best and brightest array of physicians and pharmaceuticals are of no use to someone with schizophrenia who does not have the bus fare or cognitive capacity to get to the clinic. Greer Sullivan's work in rural Mississippi demonstrated that even minimal co-payments for medication created a significant barrier to having a prescription filled, as did transportation hurdles (Sullivan et. al (1995); Nageotte et. al. (in press)). As payers come to recognize that delivering free medication to people with schizophrenia can avoid expensive, life-disrupting hospitalizations, we can expect to see payment mechanisms evolve for such services so long as the same payor is responsible for the community and hospital services. Most States now fund at least some assertive case management services such as ACT teams, and, as more States contract with managed mental health care firms to provide services to people with serious mental illnesses, we can also expect to see more flexible services evolving in the private sector than has previously been the case. Such flexibility can be expected to occur only when the contract between the payer and the service provider (or the service provider's agent, as in the case of a managed mental health care vendor) creates fiscal incentives to provide flexible services. If payment is limited to inpatient and outpatient treatment, as is the case in many private sector benefit plans, then there will be no incentive for a provider to develop novel services such as a system of reminder phone calls to encourage medication compliance. On the other hand, if a contract calls for such features, or if the contract creates incentives for providers to "flex" benefits and provide individualized services to promote care in the least restrictive settings, then payment mechanisms exist for such services to evolve.

Checklist of Specific Recommendations

Table 3.5 below is a checklist of specific aspects of treatment that, in our opinion, should be a goal for mental health service providers.

Table 3.5. Checklist to Minimize Services-Barriers to Compliance

---

1. Illness/Service Interactions.

   a. Having a medication orientation consistent with modern psychiatric nosology and psychopharmacology.
   b. Maintaining adequate medication management skills, including ability to prescribe newer psychotropic medications such as risperidone or clozapine.
   c. Not excluding patients who have substance abuse comorbidity from basic medication services.
   d. Availability of clinical and laboratory services for depot medications, atypical neuroleptic medications, and mood stabilizers.
   e. Access to medical services that are familiar with and sensitive to the medical needs of the severely mentally ill patient population.
   f. Maintaining flexibility of interventions; in particular, not forcing patients/clients into programs above and beyond their basic medication needs.

2. Psychoeducation and family services.

   a. Providing basic psychoeducation regarding severe mental illness and/or referral to peer or advocacy groups such as local consumer (patient) groups and the local affiliates of the National Alliance for the Mentally Ill.
   b. Maintaining communication with actively involved family members to alert staff to changes in clinical condition.
   c. Providing patients and families ways to obtain consultation and having a regular mechanism for consumer groups to provide feedback.

3. Emergency services.

   a. Availability of 24-hour backup for emergencies and crises.
   b. Maintaining ongoing communication with the inpatient (or crisis) service to coordinate long-term treatment planning.

4. Management of treatment drop-outs.

   a. Assessment of reason for drop-out.
   b. Attempt to reengage patient in treatment
   c. Notification of involved family members.
   d. Availability of rapid reaccess to treatment after a drop-out and relapse cycle.
   e. Availability of acute services during relapse.
   f. Allowing reentry back to former treatment system after relapse.

5. Logistical interventions.

   a. Adequate transportation taking into account travel limitations imposed by psychiatric symptoms.
   b. Flexible hours for "drop-in" patients receiving long-acting "depot" medications but who are irregular with appointments.

SUMMARY

To avoid repeating the mistakes of deinstitutionalization, medication compliance should be a primary concern in mental health policy decisions. Mental health policymakers need to consider the impact on compliance with each change or new policy being considered. Regarding the potential of mental health policy or systems interventions to improve upon the currently abysmal rates of medication noncompliance, it seems that we are currently in a "good news/bad news" situation.

The good news is that the medication and psychosocial treatments are better, and can improve compliance rates. On the medication front, the newer atypical antipsychotics, compared to those previously available, are very promising. They may reduce the noncompliance toll caused by side effects and, if more effective for psychiatric symptoms, may reduce the "catch-22" of persistent symptoms driving medication noncompliance. Also, in the United States, there is a reemergence in the use of depot medications. Compared to oral standard neuroleptic medication, the depot route improves compliance rates, and helps track when patients become medication noncompliance. From a services delivery vantage, there are many practical, relatively low cost services interventions that are known to improve compliance rates. These interventions include clinician training in medication management skills, patient and family psychoeducation, improving communications between inpatient and outpatient services, or ensuring that antipsychotic medications are very easy to obtain at no cost. In addition, there are intensive community treatment approaches such as the ACT/PACT model that, while expensive to implement, would be able to reach many of the most persistently noncompliant patients. The bad news is that there are major gaps between what is theoretically possible and conditions of actual clinical practice. Moreover, current mental health financing, along with a fragmented system, contains far too many disincentives for treating the noncompliant patient. It seems likely that the current pressure to decrease treatment costs will exacerbate the disincentive problem unless there is a counterbalancing incentive for mental health programs to treat their most noncompliant patients.

Mental health systems are changing more rapidly than any time since the deinstitutionalization period of the 1960's, and many existing systems are under intense scrutiny with an eye towards better care and/or cost reduction. We hope that this chapter has provided you with a better understanding of the risk factors for medication noncompliance, the existing services barriers to compliance, and how essential it is to have mental health policies that better meet the needs of those patients who have difficulty obtaining or accepting proper treatment.

REFERENCES

Addington, D. E., Jones, B., Bloom, D., Chouinard, G., Remington, G., & Albright, P. (1993). Reduction in hospital days in chronic schizophrenic patients treated with risperidone: A retrospective study. *Clinical Therapeutics, 15,* 917–925.

Amador, X. F., Flaum, M., Andreasen, N. C., Strauss, D., Yale, S. A., Clark, S. C., & Gorman, J. M. (1994). Awareness of illness in schizophrenia and schizoaffective and mood disorders. *Archives of General Psychiatry, 51,* 826–836.

Babiker, I. E. (1986). Noncompliance in schizophrenia. *Psychiatric Developments, 4,* 329–337.

Bachrach, L. L. (1981). Continuity of care for chronic mental patients: A conceptual analysis. *American Journal of Psychiatry, 138,* 1449–1456.

Baekeland, F., & Lundwall, L. (1975). Dropping out of treatment: A critical review. *Psychological Bulletin, 82,* 738–783.

Barofsky, I. (1978). Compliance, adherence, and the therapeutic alliance: Steps in the development of self-care. *Social Science and Medicine, 12,* 369–376.

Barofsky, I., & Connelly, C. E. (1980). Problems in providing effective care for the chronic psychiatric patient. In I. Barofsky & R. D. Budson (Eds.), *The Chronic Psychiatric Patient in the Community: Principles of Treatment* (pp. 83–129). New York: SP Medical and Psychiatric Books.

Bartko, G., Maylath, E., & Herczeg, I. (1987). Comparative study of schizophrenic patients relapsed on and off medication. *Psychiatry Research, 22,* 221–227.

Blackwell, B. (1992). Compliance. *Psychotherapy and Psychosomatics, 58,* 161–169.

Blaska, B. (1990). The myriad medication mistakes in psychiatry: A consumer's view. *Hospital and Community Psychiatry, 41,* 993–998.

Buchanan, A. (1992). A two-year prospective study of treatment compliance in patients with schizophrenia. *Psychological Medicine, 22,* 787–797.

Caton, C., Goldstein, J. M., Serrano, O., & Bender, R. (1984). The impact of discharge planning on chronic schizophrenic patients. *Hospital and Community Psychiatry, 35,* 255–262.

Caton, C. L. M. (1982). Effect of length of inpatient treatment for chronic schizophrenia. *American Journal of Psychiatry, 139,* 856–861.

Cody, J., & Robinson, A. M. (1977). The effect of low-cost maintenance medication on the rehospitalization of schizophrenic outpatients. *American Journal of Psychiatry, 134,* 73–76.

Curson, D. A. (1985). Long-term depot maintenance of chronic schizophrenic outpatients: The 7 year follow-up of the Medical Research Council fluphenazine placebo trial. II. Incidence of compliance problems, side effects, neurotic symptoms, and depression. *British Journal of Psychiatry, 146,* 469–474.

Davis, J. M., Kane, J. M., Marder, S. R., Brauzer, B., Gierl, B., Schooler, N., Casey, D. E., & Hassan, M. (1993). Dose response of prophylactic antipsychotics. *Journal of Clinical Psychiatry, 54 Suppl,* 24–30.

Davis, K. L., Estess, F. M., Simonton, S. C., & Gonda, T. A. (1977). Effects of payment mode on clinic attendance and rehospitalization. *American Journal of Psychiatry, 134,* 576–578.

Diamond, R. (1985). Quality of life: The patient's point of view. *J of Clinical Psychiatry, 46,* 29–35.

Diamond, R. J. (1983). Enhancing medication use in schizophrenic patients. *Journal of Clinical Psychiatry, 44,* 7–14.

Dworkin, R. (1994). Pain insensitivity in schizophrenia: A neglected phenomenon and some implications. *Schizophrenia Bulletin, 20,* 235–255.

Essock, S., & Goldman, H. (1995). States' embrace of managed mental health care. *Health Affairs, 14(3),* 34–44.

Essock, S., Hargreaves, W. A., Dohm, F. A., Goethe, J., Carver, L., & Hipshman, L. (1996). Clozapine eligibility among state hospital patients. *Schizophrenia Bulletin, 22,* 15–25.

Fink, E. B., & Heckerman, C. L. (1981). Treatment adherence after brief hospitalization. *Comprehensive Psychiatry, 22,* 379–386.

Frank, A. F., & Gunderson, J. G. (1990). The role of the therapeutic alliance in the treatment of schizophrenia. *Archives of General Psychiatry, 47,* 228–235.

Gaebel, W., & Pietzker, A. (1985). Multidimensional study of the outcome of schizophrenic patients 1 year after discharge: Predictors and influence of neuroleptic treatment. *European Archives of Psychiatry and Neurological Sciences, 235,* 45–52.

Gerson, S. N. (1994). When should managed care firms terminate private benefits for chronically mentally ill patients? *Behavioral Healthcare Tomorrow,* 31–35.

Glazer, W., & Kane, J. (1992). Depot neuroleptic therapy: An underutilized treatment option. *Journal Clinical Psychiatry, 53,* 426–433.

Goldfinger, S. M., Hopkin, J. T., & Surber, R. W. (1984). Treatment resisters or system resisters?: Toward a better service system for acute care recidivists. *New Directions in Mental Health Services, 21,* 17–27.

Gould, R. L., Paulson, I., & Daniels-Epps, L. (1970). Patients who flirt with treatment: The silent patients. *American Journal of Psychiatry, 127,* 524–529.

Hale, A. (1993). Will the new anti-psychotics improve the treatment of schizophrenia? *British Medical Journal, 307,* 749–750.

Harris, M., & Bergman, H. (1988). Capitation financing for the chronic mentally ill: A case management approach. *Hospital and Community Psychiatry, 39,* 68–72.

Heinrichs, D. W., Cohen, B. P., & Carpenter, W. T. (1985). Early Insight and the Management of Schizophrenic Decompensation. *Journal of Nervous and Mental Disease, 173,* 133–138.

Herz, M. I., Glazer, W. M., Mostert, M. A., Sheard, M. A., Szymanski, H., Hafez, H., Mirza, M., & Vana, J. (1991). Intermittent vs maintenance medication in schizophrenia. *Archives of General Psychiatry, 48,* 333–339.

Hogan, T. P., & Awad, A. G. (1992). Subjective response to neuroleptics and outcome in schizophrenia: A re-examination comparing two measures. *Psychological Medicine, 22,* 347–352.

Hogarty, G. E., Goldberg, S., Schooler, N., & al., e. (1974). Drug and sociotherapy in the aftercare of schizophrenic patients.II. Two-year relapse rates. *Archives of General Psychiatry, 31,* 603–608.

Johnson, D. A. W. (1976). The duration of maintenance therapy in chronic schizophrenia. *Acta Psychiatrica Scandinavia, 53,* 298–301.

Johnson, D. A. W., Pasterski, G., Ludlow, J. M., Street, K., & Taylow, R. D. W. (1983). The discontinuance of maintenance neuroleptic therapy in chronic schizophrenic patients: Drug and social consequences. *Acta Psychiatrica Scandinavia, 67,* 339–352.

Johnson, R. E., & McFarland, R. E. (1994). Treated prevalence rates of severe mental illness among HMO members. *Hospital and Community Psychiatry, 45*, 919–924.

Kane, J., Honigfeld, G., Singer, J., & al., e. (1988). Clozapine for the treatment-resistant schizophrenic: A double-blind comparison with chlorpromazine. *Archives of General Psychiatry,* 789–796.

Kavanagh, S., Opit, L., Knapp, M., & Beecham, J. (1995). Schizophrenia: Shifting the balance of care. *Social Psychiatry and Psychiatric Epidemiology, 30*, 206–212.

Kelly, G. R., & Scott, J. E. (1990). Medication compliance and health education among outpatients with chronic mental disorders. *Medical Care, 28*, 1181–1197.

Keown, C. F. (1985). Contextual effects on people's ratings of seriousness for side effects of prescription drugs. *Perceptual and Motor Skills, 61*, 435–441.

Kissling, W. (1991). The current unsatisfactory state of relapse prevention in schizophrenic psychoses — suggestions for improvement. *Clinical Neuropharmacology, 14*, 33–44.

Kluger, M. P., & Karras, A. (1983). Strategies for reducing missed initial appointments in a community mental health center. *Community Mental Health Journal, 19*, 137–143.

Moran, A. E., Freedman, R. I., & Sharfstein, S. S. (1984). The journey of Sylvia Frumpkin: A case study for policy makers. *Hospital and Community Psychiatry, 35*, 887–893.

Nageotte, C., Sullivan, G., Duan, N., & Camp, P. (in press). Medication compliance among the seriously mentally ill in a public mental health system. *Social Psychiatry and Psychiatric Epidemiology.*

Narrow, W. E., Regier, D. A., Rae, D. S., Manderscheid, R. W., & Locke, B. Z. (1993). Use of services by persons with mental and addictive disorders service system: findings from the National Institute of Mental Health Epidemiologic Catchment Area program. *Archives of General Psychiatry, 50*, 95–107.

Parkes, C. M., Brown, G. W., & Monck, E. M. (1962). The general practitioner and the schizophrenic patient. *British Medical Journal, 1*, 972–976.

Petrila, J. (1995). Who will pay for involuntary civil commitment under capitated managed care? An emerging dilemma. *Psychiatric Services, 46*(10), 1045–1048.

Raskin, M., & Dyson, W. L. (1968). Treatment problems leading to readmission of schizophrenic patients. *Archives of General Psychiatry, 19*, 356–360.

Renton, C. A., Affleck, J. W., Carstairs, G. M., & Forrest, A. D. (1963). A follow-up of schizophrenic patients in Edinburgh. *Acta Psychiatrica Scandinavia, 39*, 548–581.

Roca, R., Breakey, W., & Fisher, P. (1987). Medical care of chronic psychiatric outpatients. *Hospital and Community Psychiatry, 38*, 741–44.

Sackett, D. L. (1979). Bias in analytic research. *Journal of Chronic Disease, 32*, 51–63.

Schooler, N. R. (1991). Maintenance medication for schizophrenia Strategies for dose reduction. *Schizophrenia Bulletin, 17*, 311–324.

Schooler, N. R., Levine, J., Severe, J. B., Brauzer, B., DiMascio, A., Klerman, G., & Tuason, V. B. (1980). Prevention of Relapse in Schizophrenia: An evaluation of fluphenazine decanoate. *Archives of General Psychiatry, 37*, 16–24.

Serban, G., & Thomas, A. (1974). Attitudes and behaviors of acute and chronic schizophrenic patients regarding ambulatory treatment. *American Journal of Psychiatry, 136,* 991–995.

Shadish, W. (1989). Private sector care for chronically mentally ill individuals. *American Psychologist, 44,* 1142–1147.

Soumerai, S., McLaughlin, T. J., Ross-Degnan, D., Casteris, C. S., & Bollini, P. (1994). Effects of limiting Medicaid drug-reimbursement benefits on the use of psychotropic agents and acute mental health services by patients with schizophrenia. *New England Journal of Medicine, 331,* 650–655.

Stein, L. I. (1993). A systems approach to reducing relapse in schizophrenia. *Journal of Clinical Psychiatry, 54 (Supp),* 7–12.

Sullivan, G., Wells, K. B., Morgenstern, H., & Leake, B. (1995). Identifying modifiable risk factors for rehospitalization in a seriously mentally ill population: A case-control study in Mississippi. *American Journal of Psychiatry, 152,* 1749–1756.

Talbott, J., Bachrach, L., & Ross, L. (1986). Noncompliance and mental health systems. *Psychiatric Annals, 16,* 596–599.

Thomas, B. H., Ernst, C., & Ernst, K. (1992). Wie erricht man compliance? Zur nachbehandlung psychischkranker nach dem klinikaustritt. *Nervenarzt, 63,* 442–443.

Torrey, E. F. (1994). Violent behavior by individuals with serious mental illness. *Hospital and Community Psychiatry, 45,* 653–662.

Van Putten, T., Crumpton, E., & Yale, C. (1976). Drug refusal in schizophrenia and the wish to be crazy. *Archives of General Psychiatry, 333,* 1443–1446.

Van Putten, T., & May, P. R. A. (1978). Subjective response as a predictor of outcome in pharmacotherapy (The consumer has a point). *Archives of General Psychiatry, 35,* 477–480.

Virkkunen, M. (1974). Observations on violence in schizophrenia. *Acta Psychiatrica Scandinavia, 50,* 145–151.

Weiden, P. (1995a). Understanding depot therapy in schizophrenia. *Journal of Practical Psychiatry and Behavioral Health, 1,* 182–184.

Weiden, P. (1995b). Using atypical antipsychotics. *Journal of Practical Psychiatry and Behavioral Health, 1,* 115–119.

Weiden, P., Dixon, L., Frances, A., Appelbaum, P., Haas, G., & Rapkin, B. (1991). Neuroleptic Noncompliance in Schizophrenia. In C. Tamminga & C. Schulz (Eds.), *Advances in Neuropsychiatry and Psychopharmacology, Volume 1: Schizophrenia Research* (pp. 285–296). New York: Raven Press.

Weiden, P., Mott, T., & Curcio, N. (1995a). Recognition and management of neuroleptic noncompliance. In C. Shriqui & H. Nasrallah (Eds.), *Contemporary Issues in the Treatment of Schizophrenia* (pp. 463–485). Washington, D.C.: American Psychiatric Press.

Weiden, P., Rapkin, B., Zygmunt, A., Mott, T., Goldman, D., & Frances, A. (1995). Postdischarge medication compliance of inpatients converted from an oral to a depot neuroleptic regimen. *Psychiatric Services, 46,* 1049–1054.

Weiden, P. J., Mann, J. J., Haas, G., Mattson, M., & Frances, A. (1987). Clinical nonrecognition of neuroleptic-induced movement disorders: A cautionary study. *American Journal of Psychiatry, 144,* 1148–1153.

Weiden, P. J., & Olfson, M. (1995). Cost of relapse in schizophrenia. *Schizophrenia Bulletin, 21,* 419–429.

Weiden, P. J., Rapkin, B., Mott, T., Zygmunt, A., Goldman, D., & Frances, A. (1994). Rating of medication influences (ROMI) scale in schizophrenia. *Schizophrenia Bulletin, 20,* 297–310.

Wyatt, R. J. (1991). Neuroleptics and the natural course of schizophrenia. *Schizophrenia Bulletin, 17,* 325–351.

4

Insight and Compliance

ROISIN KEMP and ANTHONY DAVID

INTRODUCTION

What is Insight?

Insight into illness can be considered as one of the most important targets for therapeutic intervention. Aubrey Lewis characterised insight as a "correct attitude to morbid change in oneself" (Lewis, 1934). More recently it is conceptualised as a multi-dimensional phenomenon (David, 1990; Amador et al., 1991) with several overlapping aspects. The individual with poor insight disregards his illness, fails to recognise his dysfunction for what it is, and fails to seek or accept treatment. It was traditionally considered that severe mental illness or psychosis precluded insight, but Strauss (1969) considers psychosis to be on a continuum, so that intermediate phases may exist, especially during onset and recovery where insight into psychosis may be possible; so-called "double awareness" (Sacks, 1974). Insight in severe mental illness is often partial and may, confusingly, be present at one level, but absent on another. Awareness of morbid change does not automatically lead to acceptance of treatment. Conversely, it is evident that patients may have no insight, yet still accept and derive benefit from treatment.

MEASUREMENT OF INSIGHT

Can this elusive concept be measured? Most studies have focused on schizophrenia, but have used different diagnostic criteria, making comparison difficult. Amador (1991) has reviewed five methods of assessment:

1. clinical descriptions of free responses

2. clinical descriptions of free responses to a controlled stimulus

61

3. systematized scoring of free responses

4. systematized scoring of responses to a standard stimulus

5. multiple choice.

The oldest studies used descriptions of patient's beliefs. Others have used chart review for the clinician's assessment, often relegated to curt statements such as, "patient has poor insight". More quantitative and qualitative data have been obtained from patients' responses to a semi-structured interview (Greenfeld et al., 1989; McGlashan et al., 1976), sometimes made more systematic by rating scales (see Wciorka, 1988).

Two commonly used psychopathology rating scales contain items addressing insight, the Hamilton Depression scale (Hamilton, 1960) and the Positive and Negative Syndrome Scale for schizophrenia (PANSS: Kay et al., 1987). The latter offers criteria for the measure (on a scale of 1 to 7), defined as: "impaired awareness of one's own psychiatric condition and life situation ... evidenced by failure to recognise past or present psychiatric illness or symptoms, denial of need for psychiatric hospitalization or treatment, decisions characterised by poor anticipation of consequences, and unrealistic short-term and long-range planning."

At least four groups have devised standardised instruments for assessment (methods 4 or 5 according to Amador). McEvoy proposed the Insight and Treatment Attitudes Questionnaire (ITAQ: McEvoy et al., 1989a), an 11 item questionnaire administered as an interview. It assesses congruence between the patient's and clinician's view of symptoms and treatment. Verbatim responses are rated for good/partial/no insight. McEvoy and colleagues reported a high inter-rater reliability ($r = 0.82$; $p < 0.001$), and high construct validity ($r = 0.85$; $p < 0.001$), obtained by correlation with interview and medication compliance (vide infra).

David (1990) developed the Schedule of Assessment of Insight (SAI) with probe questions to assess three separate dimensions: recognition of illness, relabelling of psychosis, and compliance with treatment, and investigated this in 91 patients (David et al., 1992). All three subcomponents correlated significantly with each other. A "hypothetical contradiction" (Brett-Jones et al., 1987) item was added which ascertains the patient's capacity to encompass another person's view of their illness experience such as the other's inability to hear 'the voices'. Inter-rater reliability was satisfactory. Concurrent validity was established by significant, moderate to strong correlations with the Present State Examination insight item (PSE; Wing et al., 1974) and all subcomponents of the SAI. The PSE insight item 104, measures insight on a 4-point ordinal scale: 0 = full insight; 1 = as much insight as education and intelligence will allow; 2 = agrees to a mental illness but the examiner is not convinced; 3 = denies illness entirely. This scale has also been extended to include items on awareness of change, difficulties resulting from mental condition, and key symptoms (Appendix).

Markova and Berrios (1992) devised a structured interview consisting of 32 statements addressing, "hospitalization, mental illness in general, changes in the self, perception of the environment, control over the situation, and wanting to understand one's situation". This is one of the few scales used to investigate insight in non-psychotic disorders. The authors compared patients with depression and schizophrenia, and found, surprisingly, higher scores (better insight) in patients with schizophrenia; reliability was satisfactory.

Amador et al. (1993) devised the Scale to Assess Unawareness of Mental Disorder (SUMD), which consists of 3 global ratings (awareness of illness, benefits of treatment, and social consequences of illness), as well as two scales to measure awareness and attribution, for each prominent symptom, for both past and current illness. Inter-rater reliability varied for the items on the subscales, between r = 0.11 to r = 0.98. Concurrent validity was established with moderate to strong correlations of the first three global items with the mental status examination insight rating and the insight item on the Hamilton Depression scale. The SUMD provides more information on a variety of different aspects than the ITAQ, but is more complicated, and reliability between raters more difficult to obtain. An abridged version of the scale has recently been used in a large study (Amador et al., 1994), resulting in improved reliability.

Finally, Birchwood et al. (1994) constructed a self-report scale, based on the 3 dimensions of insight proposed by David, containing 8 statements which the patient marks as true, untrue or unsure, e.g., "some of my symptoms were made by my mind". This has the advantage of being quick and easy and avoids observer bias. Again, concurrent validity was established with PSE item 104 and internal consistency was good (Cronbach's alpha was 0.75). Factor analysis revealed one factor accounting for 60% of the variance giving support to the insight construct. This group has used the scale to track recovery from acute psychosis in 30 patients, and suggest a use for the measure to monitor progress of cognitive-behaviour therapy.

Most studies have focused on insight in schizophrenia (Ghaemi and Pope, 1994), but recently there have been a couple of studies looking at insight in affective disorders. Michalakeas et al. (1994), found no difference between initial insight scores in patients with mania or schizophrenia (both poor), but insight showed a negative correlation with psychopathology in patients with schizophrenia only at final assessment, whereas a consistent relationship over the four assessments was evident in mania. Patients with depression on the other hand showed good insight scores. The authors suggested that insight was more consistently related to psychopathology in mania, but that other factors might be as important in schizophrenia. Insight deficits were found to differ according to diagnosis in the study by Amador et al. (1994). They found that overall, the group of patients with schizophrenia had poorer average insight scores and a higher incidence of severe insight deficits than did the other groups examined: patients with schizoaffective disorder, bipolar disorder and depression with and without psychotic features.

Table 4.1. Factors affecting compliance

The Person
Culture, family, values and prejudices
Experience and beliefs
Support network and milieu
Personality
Intelligence
Insight

The Illness	*The Treatment*
Psychosis	Doctor-Patient Relationship
Grandiosity	Treatment Setting
Depression	Effectiveness
Cognitive Impairment	Complexity
	Side-effects
	Stigma

FACTORS MEDIATING INSIGHT AND COMPLIANCE

When discussing putative links between insight and compliance, several interacting factors need to be considered, including loss of reality testing due to psychosis, cognitive deficits, and the subjective experience of treatment (see Table 4.1).

THE ILLNESS

Psychopathology

Refusal of treatment has been strongly linked to higher rates of psychopathology, including paranoia, hostility, perplexity and delusional beliefs about medication (Appelbaum & Gutheil, 1980; Marder et al., 1983; Hoge et al., 1990). David et al.'s 1992 study found that the PSE total score, an indication of global severity of illness, correlated moderately with the compliance component of the total insight score ($r = -0.35; p < 0.01$). Compliance may be problematic if a patient is very disturbed with a distorted view of reality. Additionally, it makes intuitive sense that negative symptoms such as impaired motivation will hinder compliance. Nevertheless, the relationship between severity of illness and insight is a complex one. Of the recent studies using standardised measures, four found a modest inverse correlation between degree of insight and severity of psychopathology (David et al., 1992; Amador et al., 1993; Markova & Berrios, 1992; Kemp & Lambert, 1995), two found no relationship (McEvoy et al., 1989a; David et al., 1995) or an indirect one (Michalakeas et al., 1994). Additionally two groups have recently posited a particular link with negative or deficit symptoms (Kemp & Lambert, 1995; Amador et al., 1994).

Likewise insight may not improve as symptoms are treated (McEvoy et al., 1989a). Not unexpectedly, insight has been found to be lower in patients confined involuntarily in at least two studies (David et al., 1992; McEvoy et al., 1989b).

Cognitive Impairment

The capacity to recognise the need for treatment may have some relationship to intelligence. David et al. (1992) found that there was a small but significant correlation between IQ scores and the compliance component of the total insight score ($r = 0.26$, $p < 0.05$). A subsequent larger survey of 150 recent onset patients with psychosis showed a strong association between higher verbal IQ and perfect insight on PSE item 104 but no corresponding association between poor insight and low IQ (David et al., 1995).

Low IQ may predispose an individual, when ill, to lack insight. Alternatively, cognitive impairment as a consequence of severe psychosis is liable to adversely affect understanding of the need for treatment. Two studies which surveyed large groups of patients with chronic illness in institutions revealed that the vast majority were unable to tell what medication they were on or its purpose, and that length of stay and evidence of cognitive impairment contributed independently to whether they could provide this information (MacPherson et al., 1993; Geller, 1982). The limited ability of patients who are psychotic to integrate and abstract information may also have a bearing on the extent to which they can consider the rationale for treatment. A study by Young et al. (1993), on 31 patients with chronic schizophrenia found that impaired performance on the Wisconsin Card Sorting Test (WCST), suggesting impaired frontal lobe function and poor mental flexibility, was associated with lack of awareness of symptoms. Lysaker and co-workers (1994) found that insight was related to lower IQ scores, more impaired performance on the WCST, and more bizarre/idiosyncratic thought on the Gorham's Proverb Test. A study by Cuesta and Peralta (1994) showed a relationship between poor insight and reduced scores on tests of memory but not frontal lobe tests.

Knowledge deficits may affect patients with severe psychiatric disorders more than those with chronic medical conditions. Soskis (1978) compared a group of 25 inpatients with schizophrenia with a matched group of 15 inpatients with medical disorders on knowledge about their treatment and condition using a structured interview. Only one patient with schizophrenia mentioned their diagnosis, and only 32% mentioned any problem areas requiring treatment, compared to 87% of medical inpatients. Medical patients were better informed about positive aspects of medication, such as name, dose, and relationship of drug treatment to a specific diagnosis whereas patients with schizophrenia were more aware of potential side-effects. Ninety-three percent of medical patients but only 56% of patients with schizophrenia said they would continue taking the medication if they had the choice.

THE TREATMENT

Positive and Negative Effects of Medication

Despite the overwhelming effectiveness of neuroleptic drugs in the treatment of psychosis, a substantial minority of patients — up to 40% in some series (Johnstone et al., 1991) — fail to respond, and approximately the same percentage of recovered patients will relapse within two years despite active maintenance treatment (Johnstone & Geddes, 1994). Furthermore, such agents can cause aversive symptoms such as dysphoria and sexual dysfunction. Relating compliance to objective measures of favourable and unfavourable responses to medication is a curiously neglected area of research. Van Putten (1974) has commented on the contribution of disabling extra-pyramidal side-effects, particularly akathisia, to the reluctance to take medications. However, he later reported that even when these were controlled for, and after treatment had been imposed, the initial medication refusers were rated as being more ill and less cooperative than the medication compliant patients (Van Putten et al., 1976). On reviewing evidence of this kind, Sellwood and Tarrier (1994) concluded that the importance of side-effects as a major determinant of non-compliance is minimal. Some studies have highlighted the positive association of compliance with perceived, indirect benefits from medication, such as, "it keeps me out of hospital", "it allows me to make friends", as well as benefits secondary to symptom relief (Adams & Howe, 1993). In Irwin et al.'s study (1985) of 33 consecutive patients admitted with a diagnosis of schizophrenia, acknowledgement of benefits from prior antipsychotic treatment was the most powerful predictor of consent to treatment.

Doctor-Patient Relationship

Greenfeld (1985) encourages us to consider the fears and ambivalent feelings of the person who is psychotic as normal reactions. He describes the patient's struggle to convince himself that the "breakdown" was an isolated incident, and the patient's need to think of him- or herself as "normal". Treatment may be regarded as humiliating or a stigmatizing, and the clinician viewed as an adversary. We are urged to anticipate difficulties in the therapeutic alliance especially in the earlier stages of treatment, and consider defensiveness and resistance as predictable issues.

THE PERSON

Marder's group (Marder et al., 1983) commented that people who refuse medication were more mistrustful of both the staff and their physician than patients who consent. Richard's study of reasons for refusal (1964), used semantic differentials to highlight the tendency of patients who refuse to resent authority and coercion. It seems likely that when patients are admitted to hospital involuntarily, they are both more disturbed and antagonistic to treatment.

Self and Social Psychology

Identifying oneself as having a psychiatric condition might be assumed to be a first basic step to accepting treatment. However, regardless of other factors impinging on insight, the 'narcissistic injury' that this may involve, leads to denial of illness. In a study by Thompson (1988) on a group of 65 young adult psychiatric patients, two-thirds characterised themselves as much more like a typical member of the community than like a mental patient. Although reporting less psychological distress, this group showed poorer compliance and more frequent hospitalisations.

Illness Attribution

Kane (1983) mentions the difficulty in appreciating the concept of prophylaxis and the trouble some patients have in accepting the risk of relapse. If patients attribute the acute illness to certain life stresses or emotional concerns, they may reject the need for continued treatment. Angermeyer and Matschinger (1994) highlighted the prominence of psychosocial over biological explanations for schizophrenia among the lay public in Germany, and a corresponding preference for psychological over pharmacological interventions. Acknowledgement of a biological factor in etiology may be very threatening as it may seem to remove the element of control. Additionally, the delay seen between discontinuation of treatment and relapse may blur the cause and effect relationship in the eyes of patients. Further, Kane (1983) draws attention to psychodynamic factors that may come into play, for example, the expression of anger or interpersonal or family conflicts which become manifest through noncompliance. Falloon (1984) has also commented on forgetfulness, particularly when treatment regimes are complex, and negative attitudes towards drugs from personal, family, and cultural prejudices.

A study by McEvoy et al. (1981) of 45 hospitalized patients with persistent schizophrenia showed that only 48% reported any need for medication and only 44% stated that they would need it in the future. A small but significant correlation existed between acceptance of illness and reported need for medication. One might predict that if a biological explanation for mental illness became more widely accepted, assuaging any sense of personal guilt at the expense of control, then compliance with biological treatment should become more acceptable. Beliefs about the cause of the problem have also been shown to affect compliance with psychotherapy. Sixty patients treated in the outpatient clinic of a large teaching hospital were given an inventory on causes of illness (Foulks et al.,

1986). Patients' beliefs were found to be related to two measures of compliance: number of visits and manner of termination of therapy. Subjects endorsing more medical beliefs were more compliant than those who endorsed more nonmedical beliefs about the cause of their illness, and demographic characteristics apart from age did not influence the result.

Perceived Benefits of Medication

Serban and Thomas (1974) have commented on the discrepancy between positive attitudes towards medication, aftercare and the need for employment and their noncompliance with these procedures. For example, although 68% of patients with chronic illness expressed the belief that medication would be beneficial, only 29% stated that they took medication between hospitalizations, and checks with informants revealed the true figure to be only 20%. The reasons expressed for discontinuation were: 1) if they felt they "no longer needed it"; 2) if taking medication interfered with their activities; 3) if taking medication made them feel different from others; 4) if they felt no difference in their condition after forgetting to take medication. However, up to 20% disclosed that increased supervision of medication would lead to them complying. These data suggest deficits in knowledge about the prophylactic value of medication, and possible scope for improved compliance through psychoeducational approaches combined with more effective supervision.

In summary there is a considerable body of literature which emphasises the different barriers to treatment of the severely mentally ill, and particularly patients who are psychotic. It is our experience that in the acute phase the most important factors involve illness-related variables and insight itself but that when the disturbance recedes, more enduring personal and cultural influences take hold. The following are a number of examples from a study in progress in which we have assessed compliance-related issues in over 60 patients.

Case 1. A young Afro-Caribbean woman with mania could not appreciate her expansiveness and elation as constituting a problem and therefore did not see the need for treatment. However, in part because of the increased people-seeking and hyper-sociability, she was able to engage in discussion and benefitted from educational input, especially on some of her more idiosyncratic views about medication. She was able to respond to feedback on the behavioural disturbance evident to others, and was more able to distinguish symptoms from side-effects. She eventually accepted treatment with lithium, and showed an improved ability to monitor her mood state.

Case 2. An intelligent young man had delusions of reference and grandiose delusions of being Christ. His level of insight fluctuated; delusional thinking responded to challenge by exposing illogicality, but when he experienced renewed auditory and visual hallucinations his conviction returned. The failure of medication to alleviate his symptoms and akinesia led to ambivalence about treatment. This was also affected by his experience of dysphoric mood, leading to demoralisation including negativity towards treatment, which may have been exacerbated by neuroleptic drugs.

Case 3. A middle aged man had been experiencing psychotic symptoms for 10 years but had avoided treatment. The index admission was involuntary and resulted from an episode of unprovoked violence. On admission he was guarded and generally suspicious. After several sessions, he revealed a difficulty he had in viewing himself as having a mental illness, mainly due to fear of not being helped and also his view that hospitals and doctors represented authority and could not be trusted. He was aware that at least some of his experiences were abnormal. Gradually the effectiveness of medication in reducing his feelings of unease and decreasing the auditory hallucinations, made him happier to discuss his symptoms and treatment.

In these cases, we see how different factors interact to affect insight and compliance. The final disposition to treatment may depend on a combination of the individual's preconceptions, psychopathology, effectiveness of medication in treating troubling symptoms, side-effects, a capacity to see their predicament objectively, as well as ability to engage with the clinician. The initial view of the problem may not be so important as willingness to discuss and consider other points of view.

INSIGHT AND THE THERAPEUTIC ALLIANCE

Reviewing data from over 60 cases in an ongoing study of insight and compliance led us to the following impressions. If the psychotic symptoms are frightening, there is a greater chance that the patient will seek help. If on the other hand, the delusions are self-enhancing, especially if low self-esteem, or depressive material appears to underlie them, there will be greater resistance. Patients who have thought disorder have great difficulty conceptualizing their psychological difficulties and the need for treatment.

Mania typically involves global denial of problems. However, if there is mood lability and dysphoria, patients may see the benefits of treatment. Also, if the mania leads to increased affability and sociability, there is more chance of engaging in treatment. Grandiose patients tend to be less accessible. Paranoid symptoms often lead to suspiciousness of medication and the clinician. Perception of side-effects is often affected and requires clarification. Establishing trust and being consistent are crucial. Paranoia itself can be a focus for treatment, if the patient can be convinced of how misinterpreting others is painful or difficult, and that medication can help.

The effectiveness of medication in alleviating symptoms, especially those acknowledged as troublesome by the patient, is vital. Establishing a *consensus* of what constitutes the target symptoms for treatment is a useful objective, and strengthens the therapeutic alliance. Personal attributes of patients can exert an influence. Intelligence, affective warmth, acceptance of expert help and attitudes to authority figures, and capacity for objectivity, all impact on readiness for dialogue.

The physician's attitudes and behaviours have a role in facilitating such dialogue. Irwin et al. (1971) found the strength of the physician's belief in medication to correlate with compliance. Weiden et al. (1986) caution on some counter-transference issues which can worsen non-compliance — doctor's experiencing patients with schizophrenia as being hopeless or incurable, and consequently, developing an indifferent attitude to the patient or to the morbidity arising form neuroleptic side-effects; or being unable to empathise with the reasons why patients might be reluctant to take medication. They specifically warn against the oppositional stance which can develop between doctor and patient, precluding future compromises. Meichenbaum and Turk, (1987) in their recommendations to facilitate treatment adherence, offer a set of guidelines to follow. Their "first step" is to elicit and nurture the patient's confidence in treatment. They advise a "warm empathic manner, conveying competence, confidence, and knowledge concerning the treatment regimen, and a sense of hope and optimism."

INSIGHT AND TREATMENT ADHERENCE

Next we examine studies which directly tested the relationship between insight and compliance. Many authors have assumed that one of the components of insight is a recognition of the benefit of hospitalisation and need for treatment, and hence that insight should be a predictor of compliance. Measuring this becomes rather tautological if compliance is used to assess insight. David et al. (1992) in their study of 91 patients with psychotic disorders, found that compliance correlated with the ability to recognise an illness in oneself ($r = 0.50$; $p < 0.001$), but did not correlate with, "the ability to recognise delusions and hallucinations and relabel them as abnormal". Similarly Amador et al. (1993), in their study of 43 patients with schizophrenia and schizoaffective disorder found moderate correlations between compliance ratings (on McEvoy's 4-point rating scale) and several components of the SUMD insight scale (current and past awareness of mental disorder, and the benefits of medication).

Lin et al. (1979) examined 100 patients with schizophrenia and assessed insight on the basis of whether they responded positively to questions on need for hospitalization, or to see a psychiatrist. Perceived benefit from medication combined with good insight was the best predictor of compliance (as determined by self-report and information from the psychiatrist). Only 12 of 69 (17%) patients with poor insight were compliant, whereas 14 of 30 (45%) patients with good insight were compliant ($p < 0.01$). Half the patients reported perceiving benefit of medication, and of these, 18 (36%) were compliant, whereas of those who perceived no benefit, only 8 (15%) were compliant ($p = 0.04$).

A one-year follow-up study of 72 patients, mostly with schizophrenia, was conducted by Weiden et al. (1991). Subjective experience, insight and attitudinal factors were assessed. During the year following index hospitalization, 48% became noncompliant for at least one week. Among the factors significantly associated with noncompliance were denial of illness, and perceived stigma or coercion. Compliance could be predicted by positive experience of the relationship with the clinician, benefit from medication, and fear of relapse.

Bartko et al. (1988) rated insight and psychopathology at discharge from hospital in a group of 26 compliant and a group of 32 non-compliant patients with schizophrenia. Their 4-point insight scale assessed denial of illness, failure to acknowledge pathological behaviour and emotions, and denial of necessity for treatment. Compliance was rated a year later based on defaulting on appointments and missing depot neuroleptics. The noncompliant group had lower mean ratings of insight (p < 0.01), nonsignificantly higher ratings on the Brief Psychiatric Rating Scale (BPRS), and moderately lower on ratings of global functioning (49.1 vs. 62.2, p < 0.05). Interestingly the compliant group rated as significantly more depressed, and the noncompliant group scored more highly on the BPRS grandiosity item.

This link with affect was also borne out in the study by Van Putten and colleagues (1976). From a population of patients with persistent schizophrenia, 29 were characterised as habitual drug-refusers, and 30 as compliers, on the basis of information from the patient's main therapist. Only 7 of the 29 medication noncompliers compared to 18 of the 30 compliers showed insight according to an operational definition, and rated as present or absent (p < 0.01). However, the authors felt that grandiose delusions were a better predictor, since they were present in a significantly larger proportion of the noncompliers. McEvoy et al. (1989c) examined the relationship between insight and compliance over the course of an exacerbation in 52 patients with schizophrenia admitted to hospital following noncompliance. Insight ratings were made using the ITAQ and compliance ratings using a 4-point rating scale from (1) active compliance to (4) overt refusal. A moderate inverse correlation was found at initial assessment (r = –0.35; p = 0.06), and at day 14 (r = –0.36; p = 0.05), but was not found at discharge. They felt this may have been due to a reduced range of scores and high overall compliance rate by discharge. Good compliance was observed in a proportion of patients who lacked insight, probably due to socialization to expected behaviours. The conclusion was that insight did largely predict compliance, but that ultimately compliance in hospitalized patients may reflect other factors.

Forty-six patients were followed up by McEvoy's group around 3 years after discharge from the index hospitalisation. Compliance ratings were based on information from their treating clinicians on attendance at appointments and adherence to prescribed medications. Data on readmissions were collected as well as global estimates of "aftercare environment", that is the degree to which there was a supportive living arrangement, and facilitative treatment program. At 30-day follow-up, 75% of patients were compliant but this fell to 53% over the duration of the follow-up, and 61% of patients were re-hospitalized at least once. Those with supportive aftercare were significantly more likely to be compliant at 30-day and longer-term follow-up. There was a trend for patients with more insight to be compliant with treatment at 30-day follow-up; patients with more insight were significantly less likely to be re-admitted. The effects of insight and aftercare environment on outcome appeared to operate independently.

The link between insight and reduced rates of rehospitalization has been reported by Heinrichs et al. (1985). They found that "early insight", the recognition by the patient in the early stages that he is becoming unwell, facilitated the seeking of treatment and successful outpatient resolution of the episode.

A 2-year follow-up study of 61 patients with schizophrenia was conducted by Buchanan (1992). Prior to discharge, insight was investigated by analysing responses to 6 questions, including, "Did you think that you had been unwell during this admission?" and "Will you take treatment after your discharge?". Compliance was rated as "good", "average", or "poor" on the basis of attendance and medication received, as well as urine analysis. Fifty-nine per cent were compliant after one year, and 51% after two years. Those who stated that medication had helped were significantly more likely to remain compliant, as were those willing to take medication after discharge. A previous history of compliance with treatment, absence of drug-induced akinesia, and voluntary status during admission were also predictors while socio-demographic factors, illness variables, and treatment setting were not. There was a trend for those discharged to their families to be more compliant.

There is a paucity of work on the relationship between insight and adherence to rehabilitation programs. One such study, by Lysaker et al. (1994), investigated this issue in a group of 85 subjects with DSM-IIIR schizophrenia or schizoaffective disorder who were given job placements in a psycho-social rehabilitation program. Insight was rated with the PANSS insight item. Poorer insight at intake predicted poorer adherence, even when these patients expressed a desire to work. There was no association with impaired skills or motivation. Poor insight was related to a range of cognitive difficulties, stereotyped thought, and also with poor rapport with the interviewer. It predicted behavioural deficits in social skills and personal presentation 5 weeks later. The authors speculated whether the poorer compliance with the program reflected cognitive deficits leading to poor organization, or whether it was related to an interpersonal style which accompanies poor insight. They concluded that both factors could be relevant.

The majority of studies indicate that there is a positive relationship between insight and compliance. We conclude that aspects of compliance such as adherence to medication, or voluntary admissions reflect various dimensions of insight, such as treatment attitudes, and awareness of the disorder. However the relationship is far from straightforward, and in addition to the factors such as psychological attributes and culture, prior experience of treatment, relationship with treating professionals, supervision and community support assume importance.

CHANGE STRATEGIES FOR IMPROVING COMPLIANCE

Selective Review of the Literature

Interest in psychoeducational measures in medicine generally has increased significantly over recent years with a growing emphasis on viewing the patient as an informed consumer (McIntyre et al., 1989). It seems natural that clinicians would seek to improve compliance with techniques that aim to persuade patients of the rationale for treatment and help them to view adherence as a priority. For example, a statement of this belief by Matthews (1975) was that, "if the patient believes his illness is serious, that the drug is doing something, that he may experience future attacks, and that medical treatment will be effective, his compliance will improve." Support for the effectiveness of education in various medical disorders has come from a number of sources. Similar success with psychiatric patients is to be anticipated, though clearly problems with insight and co-operativeness make such efforts more challenging. Indeed Haynes (1976) has cast doubt on whether, in fact, there is any relationship discernible from the general medical literature on those patients' knowledge of disease or its therapy and compliance, and added that patients' intelligence or educational achievement may also have little bearing on compliance. Nonetheless, despite this scepticism, Goldstein (1992) has argued that an important first step for patients with severe psychiatric illnesses would be education about the disorder, while anticipating certain fears such as those of dependence and loss of control. He has quoted approvingly from several authorities supporting this view (Anderson et al., 1980; Falloon et al., 1982).

Many strategies to improve compliance have been suggested (Diamond, 1983; Falloon, 1984), but few have been systematically evaluated. Approaches have consisted of either behavioural interventions or psychoeducational measures to improve knowledge about illness and medication but the results have been mixed.

Boczkowski et al. (1985) compared the effects of a behavioural-tailoring (BT) and a psychoeducational (PE) intervention on 36 chronic schizophrenic outpatients (BT n = 12; PE n = 12; controls n = 12). Follow-up after 3 months showed that the BT group were significantly more compliant, as measured by pill-counts. The BT intervention included practical guidelines such as stimulus cues to facilitate remembering, and self-monitoring calendars. The PE intervention consisted of didactic information on the illness and reasons for taking medication. The individual sessions lasted a maximum of 50 minutes in total, too brief to draw any solid conclusions.

Seltzer et al. (1980) found improved compliance as measured by pill counts and urine tests in their group of 32 mixed psychotic patients compared with 35 controls, 5 months after a course of lectures and written information given to patients while in hospital. The intervention was considerably more intensive than that of Boczkowski and colleagues, consisting of 9 lectures given in small groups. The content included teaching about the nature of the disorder, patient experiences, side-effects, and the relationship between relapse and premature cessation of drugs. The compliant patients were less fearful of side-effects and addiction at follow-up. However the intervention was not randomized, the groups were not well matched, and only half the sample's compliance data were measured at follow-up.

Streicker et al. (1986) studied the effects of 6 sessions of didactic education providing mainly medication information, and 4 peer counselling sessions with recovered patients, in enhancing compliance in a mixed population (mostly patients with schizophrenia). There were 40 subjects and 35 matched controls, who attended a rehabilitation unit. This was an intensive educative program spread over 10 weeks. Knowledge about medication was improved and retained at 6-month follow-up. Attitudes to medication improved initially but worsened at follow-up. Unfortunately, actual compliance was not improved in the 10-month study period or beyond.

More recently, Eckman et al. (1990) investigated the potential of a behaviourally oriented programme in improving compliance and medication management skills in outpatients with schizophrenia. This was part of a comprehensive series of modules for training in social and independent living skills. This program aims to empower patients to take a greater role in their own treatment. In a multi-centre field trial, patients were administered a structured module by trained therapists, using behavioural techniques, in groups for about 3 hours a week over 4 months. The multimedia module uses videotaped demonstrations, focused instruction, role plays, social and video feedback, and practice in the "real world". The four skill areas targeted are (1) information on benefits of antipsychotic medication, (2) correct self-administration and evaluation of medication, (3) identifying side-effects, and (4) negotiating medication issues with health-care providers. The study showed that these skills could be learned and increasingly utilized over 3-month follow-up, as assessed on video role-play tests. Compliance as independently assessed, improved significantly, from about 60% to 80%. Therefore, this was a group with relatively good baseline compliance. The module has also been investigated in a randomised controlled trial with a smaller group (n = 41) (Eckman et al., 1992). A significantly greater improvement was seen in medication management knowledge and skills in subjects compared with controls, who received supportive group psychotherapy. The skills were retained over 1 year, without significant erosion. Compliance data were not reported here. Evidently this intervention is very promising but involves considerable input, which may not be easily adapted to the typical busy clinical setting.

In examining the rather mixed results from education programs, a few points need to be considered. First of all, gaining knowledge, especially when abstract, does not necessarily lead to changes in attitude. In Streicker's study (1986), there was an initial improvement in attitudes which decayed over time. This suggests a need for boosters or maintenance sessions to consolidate any gains made. Diamond (1983) has commented on the importance of tailoring medical recommendations with a patient's own perceptions. Talking in very general terms is likely to make less impact than specifically addressing an individual's idiosyncratic needs. Hence, there are grounds for investigating whether more individualised interventions are more effective. Also, Hogan et al. (1983) have commented on the problem in providing positive information about medication when patients' interoceptive cues from the effects of drugs are decidedly unfavourable. The need for greater collaboration in attempts to tackle compliance have been highlighted by Corrigan et al. (1990) with a discussion of the barriers that prevent partnership in treatment.

The Study

We have recently attempted to test a cognitive-type intervention in an inpatient setting (Hayward et al., 1995). The intervention used some of the principles of motivational interviewing (MI), a technique first developed to treat substance abuse (Miller and Rollnick, 1991). This has recently been used in a number of medical settings to help patients stop smoking, drink less and improve diet. It aims to help people work through ambivalence about behaviour change, and avoids the confrontation and stalemate of many conventional doctor-patient interactions. The therapist takes into account the patient's unique circumstances and experience which influence his/her conceptualisation of the need for treatment and advantages of treatment.

There were several adaptations to make this technique viable in working with psychotic patients: a more flexible session length, a more active therapeutic stance, an increased educational component, and cognitive approaches to tackle delusions, especially those regarding medication. Our package, called Compliance Therapy (Kemp et al., 1995) utilises key principles of MI:

Reflective listening
Avoidance of blaming
Exploration of the pluses and minuses of alternative courses of action.

The Sample and Methods

The study population was drawn from consecutive acute admissions to a ward of the Maudsley Hospital serving an inner London catchment area. Informed consent was sought and there was a 30% non-participation rate, due to refusal, rapid discharge, or communication difficulties (e.g., deafness, non-English speaking, etc). Patients with below normal intelligence were excluded. The remaining subjects were a mixed group of 47 patients with psychosis. Patients were randomly assigned to the intervention group, who received 4–6 sessions of the package described above, and a control group, who received an equal number of sessions of supportive counselling. Compliance was rated blindly by the patients' primary nurses according to a 7-point rating scale, from 1 — complete refusal to 7 — active participation / readily accepts / shows some responsibility for regimen.

Prior to treatment, the intervention group had significantly higher BPRS scores (more ill) than the control group 64.1 compared to 55.4, (t = 2.09, p < 0.04) and nonsignificantly higher doses of neuroleptics. The two groups were reasonably well-matched in terms of age, diagnosis and illness histories, and had similar scores on insight, attitudes to medication scales, and compliance ratings — these were 3.4 for cases vs 4.1 for controls (t = 1.35, p = 0.18), indicating rather poor initial compliance.

Both groups had substantially improved BPRS scores over the two assessments, 38.4 (SD 10) compared to 34.6 (SD 7) with no significant difference between them. There were improvements of about 40% on measures of insight and attitudes to medication in the intervention group, compared to only 10% in controls. Compliance was significantly better after treatment (t = 3.28, p < .001), and examination of the change scores revealed minimal change in the controls but a 57% improvement (t = 7.28, p < .001) in the intervention group. Thus these effects can be judged to result not merely from improvements in symptoms, which were the same in both groups.

We concluded that the improvement in insight and attitudes was reflected in improved compliance. The follow-up data are as yet incomplete, but 6-month follow-up results show little erosion. Thus it appears that deficits in insight and unfavourable attitudes are not immutable, and efforts to produce change in these are important levers to bring about improved compliance.

Problems Encountered with Strategies to Improve Compliance

There are practical difficulties involved in conducting such intervention trials. Recruiting sufficient numbers of subjects to demonstrate the potential treatment effect may prove difficult. Non-compliant, severely ill patients are by definition, difficult to engage. Involuntarily admitted patients who are paranoid are often very reluctant to participate in research. Patients may resent being involved in assessments and interviews. Those with least insight may not accept the study rationale or see the intervention as having any relevance for them. The very nature of the problem may preclude recruitment of the most affected group. In our study there was a preponderance of Afro-Caribbean patients declining to participate. This group have particular problems in accepting psychiatric treatment. For example, Perkins and Moodley (1993), in their study of 60 acute admissions to wards serving an inner city area of London, found that Afro-Caribbeans were more likely to deny they had any problems and be compulsorily admitted than whites. Similarly, Sellwood and Tarrier (1994), found extreme non-compliance to be more common in Afro-Caribbeans, particularly males.

High rates of non-participation in studies of maintenance treatment in schizophrenia have also been quoted (Kane and Borenstein, 1985). Apart from non-entry, another problem is patient drop-out over the course of the study, particularly when longer-term follow-up is attempted. In fact, drop-out rates of up to 40% in studies of psychosocial interventions have been noted (Corrigan et al., 1990). These factors limit the generaliziblity of research findings.

In assessing the outcome of these interventions, several points need to be considered. As Blackwell (1992) points out, compliance problems tend to disappear under scrutiny. Thus treatment effects may be harder to discern. Difficulties in measuring compliance have been covered in chapter one, with the relative merits and limitations of direct observation, pill counts and blood and urine assays. Ward observations of compliance behaviour may be misleading due to subjects conforming with the imposed regime, and bear little relationship to behaviour when the patient is discharged from hospital. Relying on patient report is obviously problematic, and information must be sought from a variety of sources.

INSIGHT AND COMPLIANCE: CONCLUSIONS

Improved insight and attitudes to medication augur well for improved compliance. If higher levels of insight are associated with depression, then the intervention needs to enhance self-efficacy, rather than aiming solely for greater acknowledgement of illness. We believe that the Compliance Therapy package addresses this. Improved medication management skills can be tested, as illustrated by the innovative work by Eckman and colleagues (Eckman et al., 1992). Such outcomes are obviously desirable in themselves whether or not compliance can be shown to improve simultaneously. We found that the psychoeducational input was welcomed by many patients; service utilisation may be another measurable outcome. Improved compliance leads to decreased relapse and readmission rates. More ambitiously, we hope that improved compliance may have a positive impact on global functioning and quality of life in patients with severe and recurrent psychiatric illnesses.

REFERENCES

Amador, X. F., & David, A. S. (in press). *Insight and Psychosis*. New York: Oxford University Press.

Adams, S. G., & Howe, J. T. (1993). Predicting medication compliance in a psychotic population. *Journal of Nervous and Mental Disease, 181*, 558–560.

Amador, X. F., Strauss, D. H., Yale, S. A., & Gorman, J. M. (1991). Awareness of illness in schizophrenia. *Schizophrenia Bulletin, 17*, 113–32.

Amador, X. F., Strauss, D. H., Yale, S. A., Flaum, M. M., Endicott, J., & Gorman, J. M. (1993). Assessment of insight in psychosis. *American Journal of Psychiatry, 150*, 873–879.

Amador, X. F., Flaum, M., Andreasen, N. C., Strauss, D. H., Yale, S. A., Clark, S. C., & Gorman, J. M. (1994). Awareness of illness in schizophrenia and schizoaffective and mood disorders. *Archives of General Psychiatry, 51*, 826–836.

American Psychiatric Association. (1987). *DSM111-R: Diagnostic and Statistical Manual of Mental Disorders*, 3rd Ed., revised. Washington D.C.

Anderson, C. M., Hogarty, G., & Reiss, D. J. (1980). Family treatment of adult schizophrenic patients: a psycho-educational approach. *Schizophrenia Bulletin*, 6, 490–505.

Appelbaum, P. S., & Gutheil, T. G. (1980). Drug Refusal: A study of psychiatric inpatients. *American Journal of Psychiatry*, 137, 340–346.

Angermeyer, M. C., & Matschinger, H. (1994). Lay beliefs about schizophrenic disorder: The result of a population survey in Germany. *Acta Psychiatrica Scandinavica*, 89 (suppl 382), 39–45.

Bartko, G., Herceg, I., & Zador, G. (1988). Clinical Symptomatology and drug compliance in schizophrenic patients. *Acta Psychiatrica Scandinavica*, 77, 74–76.

Birchwood, M., Smith, J., Drury, V., Healy, J., Macmillan, F., & Slade, M. (1994). A self-report insight scale for psychosis: reliability, validity, and sensitivity to change. *Acta Psychiatrica Scandinavica*, 89, 62–67.

Boczkowski, J. A., Zeichner, A., & DeSanto, N. (1985). Neuroleptic compliance among chronic schizophrenic outpatients: an intervention outcome report. *Journal of Consulting and Clinical Psychology*, 53, 666–671.

Brett-Jones, J., Garety, P., & Hemsley, D. (1987). Measuring delusional experiences: a method and its application. *British Journal of clinical Psychology*, 26, 256–257.

Buchanan, A. (1992). A two-year prospective study of treatment compliance in patients with schizophrenia. *Psychological Medicine*, 22, 787–797.

Blackwell, B. (1992). Compliance. *Psychotherapy and Psychosomatics*, 58, 161–169.

Corrigan, P. W., Liberman, R. P., & Engel, J. D. (1990). From noncompliance to collaboration in the treatment of schizophrenia. *Hospital and Community Psychiatry*, 41, 1203–1211.

Cuesta, M. J., & Peralta, V. (1994). Lack of insight in schizophrenia. *Schizophrenia Bulletin*, 20, 359–366.

David, A. S. (1990). Insight and psychosis. *British Journal of Psychiatry*, 156, 798–808.

David, A., Buchanan, A., Reed, A., & Almeida, O. (1992). The assessment of insight in psychosis. *British Journal of Psychiatry*, 161, 599–602.

David, A., Van Os, J., Jones, P., Fahy, T., & Harvey, I. (1995). Insight and course of psychotic illness: cross-sectional and longitudinal associations. *British Journal of Psychiatry*, 167, 621–628.

Diamond, R. J. (1983). Enhancing medication use in schizophrenic patients. *The Journal of Clinical Psychiatry*, 44, 7–14.

Eckman, T. A., Liberman, R. P., Phipps, C. C., & Blair, K. E. (1990). Teaching Medication Management skills to schizophrenic patients. *Journal of Clinical Pharmacology*, 10, 33–38.

Eckman, T. A., Wirshing, W. C., Marder, S. R., Liberman, R. P., Johnston-Cronk, K., Zimmerman, K., & Mintz, J. (1992). Technique for training patients in illness self-management: a controlled trial. *American Journal of Psychiatry*, 149, 1549–1555.

Falloon, I. R. H., Boyd, J. L., McGill, C. W., Razani, J., Moss, H. B., & Gilderman, A. M. (1982). Family Management in the prevention of exacerbations of schizophrenia: a controlled study. *New England Journal of Medicine, 306,* 1437–1440.

Falloon, I. R. H. (1984). Developing and maintaining adherence to long-term drug-taking regimens. *Schizophrenia Bulletin, 10,* 412–417.

Foulks, E. F., Persons, J. B., & Merkel, L. (1986). The effect of patients beliefs about their illness on compliance with psychotherapy. *American Journal of Psychiatry, 143,* 340–344.

Ghaemi, S. N., & Pope, H. G. (1994). Lack of insight in psychotic and affective disorders: a review of empirical studies. *Harvard Review of Psychaitry, 2,* 22–33.

Geller, J. L. (1982). State hospital patients and their medication; do they know what they take? *American Journal of psychiatry, 139,* 611–615.

Goldstein, M. J. (1992). Psychoocial strategies for maximising the effects of psychotropic medications for schizophrenia and mood disorder. *Psychopharmacology Bulletin, 28,* 237–240.

Greenfeld, D. (1985). *The psychotic patient: medication and psychotherapy.* New York: Free Press.

Greenfeld, D., Strauss, J. S., Bowers, M. B., & Mandelkern, M. (1989). Insight and interpretation of illness in recovery from psychosis. *Schizophrenia Bulletin, 15,* 245–252.

Hamilton, M. (1960). A rating scale for depression. *Journal of Neurology, Neurosurgery and Psychiatry, 23,* 56–62.

Haynes, R. B. (1976). A critical review of the "determinants" of patient compliance with therapeutic regimens. In Haynes, R. B., Sackett, D. L. (Eds.) *Compliance in health care,* (pp. 27–39) Baltimore: Johns Hopkins University Press.

Hayward, P., Chan, N., Kemp, R., Youle, S., & David, A. (1995). Illness self-management in psychotic patients. *J Mental Health, 4,* 513–519.

Heinrichs, D. W., Cohen, B. P., & Carpenter, W. T. (1985). Early insight and the management of schizophrenic decompensation. *Journal of Nervous and Mental Disease, 17,* 133–138.

Hogan, T. P., Awad, A. G., & Eastwood, R. (1983). A self-report scale predictive of drug compliance in schizophrenics: reliability and discriminative validity. *Psychological Medicine, 13,* 177–183.

Hoge, S. K., Appelbaum, P. S., Lawlor, T., Beck, J. C., Litman, R., Greer A., Gutheil, T. G., & Kaplan, E. (1990). A prospective, multi-center study of patients' refusal of antipsychotic medication. *Archives of General Psychiatry, 47,* 949–956.

Irwin, D. S., Weitzel, W. D., & Morgan, D. W. (1971). Phenothiazine intake and staff attitudes. *American Journal of Psychiatry, 127,* 1631–1635.

Irwin, M., Lovitz, A., Marder, S. R., Mintz, J., Winslade, W. J., Van Putten, T., & Mills, M. J. (1985). Psychotic patients' understanding of informed consent. *American Journal of Psychiatry, 142,* 1351–1354

Johnstone, E. C., Crow, T. J, Owens, D. J. C., & Frith, C. D. (1991). The Northwick Park "functional" psychosis study. Phase 2: maintenance treatment. *Journal of Psychopharmacology, 5,* 388–395.

Johnstone, E. C., & Geddes, J. (1994). How high is the relapse rate in schizophrenia? *Acta Psychiatrica Scandinavica, 89* (suppl 382) 6–10.

Kane, J. M. (1983). Problems of compliance in the outpatient treatment of schizophrenia. *Journal of Clinical Psychiatry, 44,* 3–6.

Kane, J. M., & Borenstein, M. (1985). Compliance in the long-term treatment of schizophrenia. *Psychopharmacology Bulletin, 21,* 23–27.

Kay, S. R., Fiszbein, A., & Opler, L. A. (1987). The positive and negative syndrome scale (PANSS) for schizophrenia. *Schizophrenia Bulletin, 13,* 261–276.

Kemp, R., Hayward, P., Applewhaite, G., Everitt, B., & David, A. (1996). Compliance Therapy in psychotic patients: a randomised controlled trial. *British Medical Journal, 312,* 345–349.

Kemp, R. A., & Lambert, T. J. C. (1995). Insight in schizophrenia and its relationship to psychopathology. *Schizophrenia Research, 18,* 21–28.

Lewis, A. (1934). The psychopathology of insight. *British Journal of Medical Psychology, 14,* 332–348.

Lin, I. F., Spiga, R., & Fortsch, W. (1979). Insight and adherence to medication in chronic schizophrenia. *Journal of Clinical Psychiatry, 40,* 430–432.

Lukoff, D., Nuechterlein, K. H., & Ventura, J. (1986). Manual for Expanded BPRS. *Schizophrenia Bulletin, 12,* 594–602.

Lysaker, P., Bell, M., Milstein, R., Bryson, G., & Beam-Goulet, J. (1994). Insight and psychosocial treatment compliance in schizophrenia. *Psychiatry, 57,* 307–315.

McEvoy, J. P., Aland, J., Wilson, W. H., Guy, W., & Hawkins, L. (1981). Measuring chronic schizophrenic patients' attitudes towards their illness and treatment. *Hospital and Community Psychiatry, 32,* 586–588.

McEvoy, J. P., Apperson, L. J., Appelbaum, P. S., Ortlip, P., Brecosky, J., Hammill, K., Geller, J. L., & Roth, L. (1989a). Insight in schizophrenia; its relationship to acute psychopathology. *The Journal of Nervous and Mental Disease, 177,* 43–47.

McEvoy, J. P., Appelbaum, P. S., Apperson, L. J., Geller, J. L., & Freter, S. (1989b). Wy must some schizophrenic patients be involuntarily committed? The role of insight. *Comprehensive Psychiatry, 30,* 13–17.

McEvoy, J. P., Freter, S., Everett, G., Geller, G. L., Appelbaum, P., Apperson, L. J., & Roth, L. (1989c). Insight and the clinical outcome of schizophrenic patients. *Journal of Nervous and Mental Disease, 177,* 48–51.

McGlashan, T. H., Docherty, J. P., & Siris, P. (1976). Integrative and sealing-over recoveries from schizophrenia. *Psychiatry, 39,* 325–328.

McIntyre, K., Farrell, M., & David, A. S. (1989). In-patient psychiatric care: the patient's view. *British Journal of Medical Psychology, 62,* 249–255.

MacPherson, R., Double, D. B., Rowlands, R. P., & Harrison, D. M. (1993). Long-term psychiatric patients' understanding of neuroleptic medication. *Hospital and Community Psychiatry, 44,* 71–73.

Marder, S. R., Mebane, A., Chien, C. P., Winslade, W. J., Swann, E., & Van Putten, T. (1983). A comparison of patients who refuse and consent to neuroleptic treatment. *American Journal of Psychiatry, 140,* 470–472.

Markova, I. S., & Berrios, G. E. (1992). The assessment of insight in clinical psychiatry: a new scale. *Acta Psychiatrica Scandinavica, 86,* 159–164.

Matthews, D. (1975). The noncompliant patient. *Primary Care, 2,* 2.

Meichenbaum, D., & Turk, D. C. (1987). *Facilitating treatment adherence: A practitioner's handbook.* New York: Plenum Press.

Michalakeas, A., Skoutas, C., Charalambous, A., Peristeris, A., Marinos, V., Keramari, E., & Theolgou, A. (1994). Insight in schizophrenia and mood disorders and its relationship to psychopathology. *Acta psychiatrica Scandinavica, 90,* 46–49.

Miller, W. R., & Rollnick, S. (1991). *Motivational Interviewing: Preparing People to Change.* New York: Guilford Press.

Perkins, R. E., & Moodley, P. (1993). Perception of problems in psychiatric inpatients : denial, race, and service usage. *Social Psychiatry and Psychiatric Epidemiology, 28,* 189–193.

Richards, A. D. (1964). Attitude and drug acceptance. *British Journal of Psychiatry, 110,* 46–52.

Sacks, M. H., Carpenter, W. T., & Strauss, J. S. (1974). Recovery from delusions: Three phases documented by patient's interpretation of research procedures. *Archives of General Psychiatry, 43,* 117–120.

Seltzer, A., Roncari, I., & Garfinkel, P. (1980). Effect of patient education on medication compliance. *American Journal of Psychiatry, 25,* 638–645.

Sellwood, W., & Tarrier, N. (1994). Demographic factors asociate with extreme non-compliance in schizophrenia. *Social Psychiatry and Psychiatric Epidemiology, 29,* 172–177.

Serban, G., & Thomas, A. (1974). Attitudes and behaviours of acute and chronic schizophrenic patients regarding ambulatory treatment. *American Journal of Psychiatry, 131,* 991–995.

Soskis, D. A. (1978). Schizophrenic and medical inpatients as informed drug consumers. *Archives of General Psychiatry, 35,* 645–647.

Strauss, J. S. (1969). Hallucinations and delusions as points on continual function. *Archives of General Psychiatry, 21,* 581–586.

Strauss, J. S., & Carpenter, W. T. (1972). Prediction of outcome in schizophrenia. *Archives of General Psychiatry, 27,* 739–746.

Streicker, S. K., Amdur, M., & Dincin, J. (1986). Educating patients about psychiatric medications: failure to enhance compliance. *Psychosocial Rehabilitation Journal, 4,* 15–28.

Thompson, E. H. (1988). Variation in the self-concept of young adult chronic patients. *Hospital and Community Psychiatry, 39,* 771–775.

Van Putten, T. (1974). Why do schizophrenic patients refuse to take their drugs? *Archives of General Psychiatry, 31,* 67–72.

Van Putten, T., Crumpton, E., & Yale, C. (1976). Drug refusal in schizophrenia and the wish to be crazy. *Archives of general Psychiatry, 33,* 1443–1446.

Wciorka, J. (1988). A clinical typology of schizophrenic patients attitudes towards their illness. *Psychopathology, 21,* 259–266.

Weiden, P. J., Dixon, L., Frances, A., Appelbaum, P., Haas, G., & Rapkin, B. (1991). Neuroleptic noncompliance in schizophrenia. In Schulz, S. C. (Eds.), *Advances in Neuropsychology and Pharmacology* (pp. 285–296). New York; Raven Press.

Weiden, P. J., Shaw, E., & Mann, J. (1986). Causes of neuroleptic noncompliance. *Psychiatric Annals, 16,* 571–575.

Wing, J. K., Cooper, J. E., & Sartorius, N. (1974). *Measurement and classification of psychiatric symptoms.* Cambridge: Cambridge University Press.

Young, D. A., Davila, R., & Scher, H. (1993). Unawareness of illness and neuropsychological performance in chronic schizophrenia. *Schizophrenia Research, 10,* 117–124.

APPENDIX

Schedule for the Assessment of Insight (SAI-E) — Expanded version

1. *"Do you think you have been experiencing any emotional or psychological changes or difficulties?"*

   often   = 2 (thought present most of the day, most days)
   sometimes = 1 (thought present occasionally)
   never   = 0 (ask why doctors / others think so)

2. *"Do you think this means there is something wrong with you?"* *(eg. a nervous condition)*

   often   = 2 (thought present most of the day, most days)
   sometimes = 1 (thought present occasionally)
   never   = 0 (ask why doctors / others think so)

3. *"Do you think your condition amounts to a mental illness or mental disorder?"*

   often   = 2 (thought present most of the day, most days)
   sometimes = 1 (thought present occasionally)
   never   = 0 (ask why doctors / others think so)

   If positive score on previous two questions, proceed to 4.

4. *"How do you explain your condition /disorder /illness?"*

   Reasonable account given based on plausible mechanisms
   (appropriate given social, cultural and educational
   background, eg. excess stress, chemical imbalance,
   family history)   = 2
   Confused account, or overheard explanation without
   adequate understanding or "don't know"   = 1
   Delusional or bizarre explanation   = 0

   If positive score on 1,2,3, proceed to 5.

5. *"Has your nervous/emotional /psychological /mental /psychiatric condition (use patient's term) led to adverse consequences or problems in your life?"*

   (eg. conflict with others, neglect, financial or accommodation difficulties, irrational, impulsive or dangerous behaviour)
   Yes (with example)   = 2
   Unsure (cannot give example or contradicts self)   = 1
   No   = 0

6. *"Do you think your .... condition (use patient's term) or the problem resulting from it warrants treatment?"*

Yes (with plausible reason)	= 2
Unsure (cannot give reason or contradicts self)	= 1
No	= 0

Use primary nurse to rate following two items

7. *How readily does patient accept treatment (includes passive acceptance)?*

often = 2 (may rarely question need for treatment)
sometimes = 1 (may occasionally question need for treatment)
never = 0 (ask why)

Treatment includes medication and/or hospitalisation and/or other physical and psychological therapies.

8. *Does patient ask for treatment unprompted?*

often = 2 (exclude inappropriate requests for medication etc.)
sometimes = 1 (rate if forgetfulness/disorganisation leads to occasional requests only)
never = 0 (ask why doctors/others think so)

9. *Pick the most prominent symptoms up to a maximum of 4 (eg. highest scoring on BPRS). Then rate awareness of symptom out of 4 as below.*

Examples:
"Do you think that the belief .... is not really true/happening (could you be imagining things)?"

"Do you think the 'voices' you hear are actually real people talking, or is it something arising from your own mind?"

"Have you been able to think clearly, or do your thoughts seem mixed up /confused? Is your speech jumbled?"

"Would you say you have been more agitated/overactive/speeded up /withdrawn than usual?"

"Are you aware of any problem with attention/concentration/memory?"

"Have you a problem with doing what you intend/getting going/finishing tasks/motivation?"

Definitely (full awareness)	= 4
Probably (moderate awareness)	= 3
Unsure (sometimes yes, sometimes no)	= 2
Possibly (slight awareness)	= 1
Absolutely not (no awareness)	= 0

Mean ....

10. *For each symptom rated above (up to a maximum of 4), ask patient ...*

"How do you explain .... (false beliefs, hearing voices, thoughts muddled, lack of drive etc.)

Part of my illness	= 4
Due to nervous condition	= 3
Reaction to stress / fatigue	= 2
Unsure, maybe one of above	= 1
Can't say, or delusional/bizarre explanation	= 0

Mean ....

Hypothetical contradiction (supplementary question):
"How do you feel when people do not believe you?" (when you talk about .... delusions or hallucinations).

They're lying	= 0
I'm still sure despite what others say	= 1
I'm confused and don't know what to think	= 2
I wonder whether there's something wrong with me	= 3
That's when I know I'm sick	= 4

TOTAL SCORE = 24 + 4 = 28

Roisin Kemp & Anthony David, July 1995

5

Compliance and Decision Making Capacity

ANSAR HAROUN and GRANT H. MORRIS

WHAT IS DECISION MAKING CAPACITY (DMC)?

Decision making capacity (DMC) is a relatively new term that is not defined in many major psychiatric textbooks. Although the 1995 edition of the Comprehensive Textbook of Psychiatry specifically refers to DMC, earlier editions did not (Ross & Halpern, 1995). Until recently, when clinicians considered a patient's capacity to make a decision or to perform a task, they would discuss the patient's "competence." Although "competence" has a specific legal definition, its definition in medicine is far more ambiguous.

At a time when paternalism ruled, doctors were often the final authorities on whether the patient could or could not refuse treatment. In essence, the doctor decided the patient's "competence." The doctor's pro-treatment bias influenced the assessment of the patient's competence. Typically the clinician would focus on the "reasonableness" of the patient's decision and would find the patient competent only if the patient made the "reasonable" or "responsible" decision to accept treatment. In essence, doctors equated the patient's legal competence with clinical competence.

Some clinicians, especially those with forensic training, now focus on the "rationality" of the patient's decision. Instead of using the clinician's subjective pro-treatment bias, a focus on "rationality" uses objective criteria, such as whether the patient's decision conforms to the rules of deductive logic.

Unreasonable decisions are not necessarily irrational. For example, a doctor may assert that a dying patient is making an "unreasonable"

85

decision to refuse a lifesaving blood transfusion. However, if the patient does so because of a religious belief, the decision is not irrational. As long as the patient understands the risk, i.e., that he or she will die, and has decided that life preserved by a blood transfusion is not worth living, the law demands that the patient's decision be accepted.

A poor decision, which we may characterize as a "wrong" or "bad" decision, is not necessarily an irrational one. Over forty million Americans continue to smoke cigarettes. Millions are overweight and continue to eat cholesterol-laden food. Society does not interfere with these decisions even though, objectively, they are not in the person's best interest.

Over the years, society has increasingly valued individual autonomy. Supreme Court decisions have expanded the right to privacy to include family planning decisions and abortions (*Griswold v. Connecticut*, 1965; *Roe v. Wade*, 1973). Courts have upheld the right of physically ill patients to give or withhold informed consent to medically appropriate treatments (*Cobbs v. Grant*, 1972).

In recent years, courts have ruled that when a patient's competence to make a treatment refusal is in question, the determination of competence is a legal decision to be made by a judge or hearing officer. Often, a medical expert is called upon to express his or her opinion regarding the mental state of the patient and how it affects the patient's decision making. The judge considers this opinion, and any other evidence presented, in reaching judgment. Although psychiatry recognizes that a patient's decision making ability may range on a gradient from very bad to very good, the legal decision maker decides the case on an all or nothing basis. The patient is determined to be either competent or incompetent to make the treatment refusal decision.

Historically, competence was assessed in global terms. A patient with severe mental disorder who was found "incompetent" would be deprived of various rights. Today, both law and medicine focus more narrowly on the specific deficit in decision making capacity so that a finding of incompetence deprives the individual only of rights that relate directly to that deficit. For example, a patient who lacks the competence to make every day decisions necessary to provide food, clothing, and shelter, may be subject to involuntary civil commitment. However, the patient may retain the competence to refuse psychiatric treatment that will improve his or her mental condition. Some civilly committed patients may be found incompetent to refuse psychotropic medication but competent to refuse other medical treatment.

CAN DMC BE MEASURED?

Although writers have suggested various tests of competency (Roth, Meisel, & Lidz, 1977), no instrument is available to score or quantify DMC in clinical practice. Rather, DMC is assessed in the same manner as is mental state. However, specific cognitive components that contribute to DMC may be individually quantified. For example, memory can be assessed through the Wechsler Memory Scale and attention can be scored through a Computerized Performance Test. Some researchers have developed forensic assessment instruments to assist clinicians in measuring specific legal competency questions. For example, Roth et al. (1982) developed a two-part consent form for use as a research tool to assess patients' competence to consent to ECT. This form has not been published although it is available from the authors. Weithorn (1980) developed an instrument to measure competency to render informed treatment decisions. The instrument was designed as a research tool and has not been published for clinical use.

DOES A LINK EXIST BETWEEN SERIOUS MENTAL ILLNESS AND IMPAIRED DMC?

Because DMC has not been quantified in a standard way, and because the boundaries of "serious mental illness" are imprecise, a scientific link between impaired DMC and serious mental illness has not been established. Nevertheless, impaired DMC is present in some, but not all, mental disorders regardless of severity. For example, disorders of attention, which prevent the patient from listening to and considering information, disorders of perception, which distort information, and thought disorders, which interfere with logic, are likely to cause impairments in DMC. In contrast, paraphilias are not likely to cause impairments in DMC. Anxiety disorders may or may not negatively impact DMC. Although anxiety may disrupt information processing, decision making may actually be enhanced by an increased alertness and attention to the situation. For example, in a combat-related situation, a person experiencing enormous anxiety from a possible imminent death, may, nevertheless, retain the capacity to think clearly and to make rational decisions necessary to preserve his or her life.

DOES A LINK EXIST BETWEEN DMC AND BEHAVIOR?

Psychiatrists believe that a person's behavior results from both conscious and unconscious, planned and unplanned, rationally considered and impulsive thoughts. Some behavior is clearly the result of planned decision making and some behavior appears to be senseless. Psychoanalysts emphasize the role of unconscious factors that contribute to decision making. The law, however, assumes that decisions are the result of a conscious process. That conscious process is presumed to involve rational thinking, unless the decision maker is shown to be incapable of rational thought.

A person may have the mental capacity to make rational decisions, but his or her actual decision making on a specific issue may not be rational. And even if the individual makes a rational decision, the decision may not produce rational behavior.

In the context of moral decision making and resultant moral behavior, Rest (1994) proposed a four-component, sequential model that explains why a person may engage in inappropriate behavior. This model can be adapted to explain a patient's medication noncompliance.

Component 1: Interpreting the situation.

A patient's willingness to comply with a medication regimen depends upon a correct understanding of the medical situation. Before a patient can be expected to consent to proposed treatment, the doctor must fully inform the patient of the medical problem; the risks, benefits, and alternatives to the proposed treatment; and the prognosis with and without the treatment. If the doctor has not informed the patient, if the patient did not understand the information, or if the patient lacks insight, noncompliance is likely.

Component 2: Judging between clinically right and wrong actions.

Assuming the patient understands the clinical situation, he or she decides whether to accept the intervention. From the doctor's perspective, the patient should reason: "I understand I suffer from a mental disorder. I understand that treatment choices include medication therapy, group therapy, milieu therapy, or no therapy. My doctor recommends psychotropic medication because he or she believes it will have the greatest potential benefit. Although the doctor has explained the medication's potential side effects, the doctor has convinced me that the benefits from this medication outweigh the risks. I believe my clinical interest is best served by my taking it." Ideally, doctors want patients to be guided by their recommendations. However, if a patient is legally competent to make the decision, the patient's decision governs even if the patient is only marginally competent. The doctor is expected merely to inform and educate the patient; the patient then exercises his or her autonomous judgment.

Component 3: Prioritizing Values.

Even if a patient has insight and is able to weigh the risks, benefits, and alternatives, he or she may disagree with the doctor's clinical judgment on the value of the proposed therapy. For example, a patient who has experienced neurological side effects from previous administration of psychotropic medication may be reluctant to experience a repetition despite his or her doctor's belief that this risk is outweighed by the benefit. Some patients have religious or other life style beliefs against taking medication. As citizens of a free country, people are at liberty to choose a value system that differs from a physician's conventional values.

Component 4: Having persistence.

Even if a patient has insight (Component 1), has the mental capacity to choose the clinically correct treatment (Component 2), and prioritizes a restoration to health above other values (Component 3), he or she may not actually comply with treatment. Impediments to compliance include the inconvenience of keeping scheduled appointments, time commitments and cost, discomfort or pain from treatment (e.g., from injection needles or from side effects). Not all patients are motivated, or have the organizational skills, to persist with treatment, and thus, may be noncompliant (Component 4). As illustrated by this model, compliance may be affected by impairment in DMC at any component stage.

WHAT IS THE RELATIONSHIP BETWEEN
DMC AND COMPLIANCE?

One might posit that a causal relationship exists between DMC and compliance: "Unimpaired DMC causes compliance; impaired DMC causes noncompliance." In testing that hypothesis, one could note that persons with severe mental illness who are likely to have impaired DMC, are overrepresented in the population of noncompliant persons. However, individuals whose DMC is not impaired may be either compliant or noncompliant. Thus, impaired DMC is neither a necessary nor a sufficient condition for noncompliance. Rather, it is one of many factors that may contribute to noncompliance.

The medical profession has no objective definition of unimpaired DMC. Often, doctors equate the quality of DMC with the willingness of the patient to agree with the doctor's decision. Such an approach is logically inconsistent. It is circular reasoning to assert that impaired DMC causes noncompliance if noncompliance is itself incorporated within the very definition of impaired DMC.

To more appropriately assess the relationship between DMC and compliance, one should consider four situations: (1) unimpaired DMC resulting in compliance, (2) impaired DMC resulting in compliance, (3) unimpaired DMC resulting in noncompliance, and (4) impaired DMC resulting in noncompliance.

From the doctor's perspective, the first situation is optimal. The patient understands the information provided by the doctor, and exercises his or her autonomous judgment to accept the doctor's recommendation. No conflict exists between doctor and patient, and the decision to comply results in a good outcome.

In the second situation, the patient complies with the doctor's treatment but does so for the wrong reason — the patient accepts medication without making a rational assessment of the risks and benefits. This situation is rarely addressed in the literature. Doctors are so delighted with the prospect of good compliance and a successful outcome, that they are unlikely to critically examine the quality of the patient's DMC. In fact, for patients who are likely to be compliant, some doctors actively discourage the patient's analytical thinking by failing to provide information that is essential for the patient's consideration. Often, doctors either do not fully disclose the risks and alternatives to therapy or they "sugar-coat" the information so that side effects and other risks are unfairly minimized.

Consider this example: A doctor treated a patient who had committed an assault in response to paranoid beliefs. The doctor wanted to prescribe Mellaril® to reduce the patient's paranoid thinking and decrease the risk of violence. The patient believed that he did not suffer from psychosis and did not need any antipsychotic medication. Knowing that the patient would reject a recommendation of antipsychotic medication, the doctor asked the patient whether he would consider taking Mellaril® to reduce stress or anxiety. The doctor knew that sedation is an effect of Mellaril® but did not inform the patient of the medication's antipsychotic effects. The patient noted that a friend of his told him that Mellaril® "makes him mellow." Because the patient wished to be mellow, he accepted the doctor's recommendation.

In this example, the patient's impaired DMC was produced both by the patient's mental disorder and by the doctor's failure to inform the patient of the antipsychotic effects of the medication. The doctor's ethical obligation was to minimize harm both to the patient and to potential victims. His legal obligation was to inform the patient of the antipsychotic effects of the medication so that the patient's decision would be informed. By withholding information, the doctor chose to fulfill his ethical obligation at the expense of his legal one.

In the third situation, the patient's decision making is unimpaired, but he or she rationally chooses noncompliance. In a free society, a person with unimpaired DMC has the right to make a foolish or clinically bad decision. Competent individuals may assess risks and benefits differently than do doctors. The law does not empower doctors to impose their clinical judgment by coercing treatment.

As previously stated, mental disorder does not necessarily equate with impaired DMC. Patients who are capable of rationally balancing the benefits of medication with its risks and alternatives are permitted to make their own judgment. The decision to accept or reject treatment is not determinative of unimpaired or impaired DMC. Rather, the quality of a patient's DMC is determined by the quality of the patient's reasoning. Thus, even patients who are psychotic may be capable of making unimpaired judgments if they base their decision making on a rational consideration of the risks and benefits of therapy.

In the fourth situation, when a patient has impaired DMC and is not compliant, the results may be detrimental to the patient and/or to others. Through involuntary civil commitment, and through hearings that establish the patient's incompetence to make treatment decisions, the law may empower the doctor to impose clinically correct decisions, even over the patient's objection.

DEALING WITH PATIENTS WHO DO NOT COMPLY

Doctors want their patients to comply with prescribed treatment. They do so, not out of any malevolent motive, but out of beneficence. They want to help their patients, and they need their patients' compliance for treatment to succeed. Doctors are trained to diagnose and treat disease. They believe that patients lack training to question their clinical judgments.

Until recently, paternalism was the dominant paradigm of medical school training. Doctors were assumed to know best, and patients, especially patients with psychiatric disorders, were considered incapable of questioning their doctors' judgment. As such, patients could be treated by doctors as children who are governed by their parents' decisions.

From a medical perspective, the doctor's obligation is to do what is clinically best for the patient, with or without the patient's consent. Just as parents are permitted to trick or bribe their sick children into getting medically needed injections, doctors are tempted to trick or bribe their patients into taking clinically needed medication. If full disclosure of the risks and alternatives to the proposed treatment would result in increased noncompliance, doctors are tempted to avoid disclosure.

In contrast to the doctor's paternalism stands the lawyer's concern for individual rights and autonomy. Restoration to health is only one value, and the individual may prioritize other values more highly. Lawyers do not want individuals to be deprived of their right to decide what medicines, if any, will be introduced into their bodies.

Whose viewpoint should prevail — the doctors' or the lawyers'? In any civilized society, varying viewpoints are ultimately resolved through court decisions and legislation that reflects the wishes of those who live in that society. Although many doctors consider laws to be an unnecessary and unwarranted intrusion on their medical judgment, they need to understand how and why these laws have evolved.

IS IMPAIRED DMC ESTABLISHED BY CIVIL COMMITMENT?

Historically, society's approach to the involuntary civil commitment of mentally disordered persons has fluctuated between a paternalistic or medical model and a libertarian or legal model. Before 1970, in most states a person could be hospitalized if a physician certified that he or she was mentally ill and needed treatment. Civilly committed patients were required to comply with their doctors' treatment orders.

The civil rights movement of the 1960s expanded opportunities for women, members of racial and ethnic minority groups, and criminal defendants. It also heralded reforms in the civil commitment process. In some states, a mentally disordered person could not be detained unless he or she was dangerous to self or others. The process for achieving commitment was made more difficult. Even the psychiatrist's authority to impose treatment on civilly committed patients was questioned.

The constriction of civil commitment by a rights-based model produced some deleterious consequences. Mental patients were no longer warehoused in large state hospitals, but they were abandoned in the streets of our cities (Stone, 1975). Seriously disturbed persons were not treated in well-financed community treatment centers. If they were treated at all, they were treated in jail. Recently, proposals have emerged that would reestablish a more paternalistic approach to civil commitment. The American Psychiatric Association has endorsed a proposal that would authorize detention of a person suffering from a severe, but treatable, mental disorder who is likely to harm himself or herself or to suffer substantial mental or physical deterioration. Under that proposal, civil commitment would also be conditioned on a finding of incapacity to make informed treatment decisions (Stromberg and Stone, 1983). Only a few states have adopted this proposal. Other proposals include: (1) outpatient commitment laws that condition the patient's freedom on compliance with treatment, and (2) mental health guardianships. Under the latter arrangement, a guardian is appointed who may substitute his or her judgment for that of the patient and consent to treatment. Typically, the patient must be found to lack DMC before outpatient commitment or a mental health guardianship can be imposed.

DEVELOPMENT OF THE LEGAL RIGHT
TO REFUSE TREATMENT

As long ago as 1914, the eminent jurist Benjamin Cardozo declared that an individual has a right to determine what shall be done with his or her own body, and therefore, that a doctor who performs an operation on a patient without that patient's consent commits an assault (*Schloendorff v. Society of New York Hosp.*, 1914). Although first stated in the context of surgical procedures, the individual's right to free choice and self-determination has evolved over the years into a requirement that physicians obtain their patients' informed consent to any medical treatment. When a patient refuses treatment, the doctor lacks legal authority to impose it — even if that intervention is necessary to save the patient's life (*Thor v. Superior Court*, 1993).

These general principles have specific application to the practice of psychiatry. In essence, a person with a mental disorder who is noncompliant with psychotropic medication is only one example of any ill person who is noncompliant with medical treatment. A patient, even a mental patient, retains the right to make his or her own decisions, however good or bad they are, unless and until a court declares the person incompetent. Although autonomous decision making is negated by incompetence, incompetence is not established solely by proof of mental disorder or proof that treatment is clinically indicated (Stone, 1981).

In most states, the decision to civilly commit a person does not, of itself, extinguish his or her right to refuse treatment. Courts have ruled that civil commitment deprives the person of his or her liberty, but absent an adjudication of incompetency, the patient retains other rights. As one judge noted, "Although committed patients do suffer at least some impairment of their relationship to reality, most are able to appreciate the benefits, risks, and discomfort that may reasonably be expected from receiving psychotropic medication. This is particularly true for patients who have experienced such medication and, therefore, have some basis for assessing comparative advantages and disadvantages." (*Rogers v. Okin*, 1979).

Although courts have recognized that competent, though civilly committed, mental patients have a right to refuse treatment, they have not ruled consistently on the question of who determines the patient's competence. Some courts have allowed a staff psychiatrist or a hospital committee to make an informal determination; others have required that the patient's competence be assessed in a hearing before a judge or other law-trained decision maker.

In 1990, for the first time, the Supreme Court directly addressed the issue of whether competent mental patients have a right to refuse treatment and who determines their competence (*Washington v. Harper*, 1990). In the *Harper* case, a psychiatrist evaluated a prison inmate and found him to be both mentally disordered and dangerous. The psychiatrist ordered psychotropic medication, which the prisoner refused. The prisoner asserted that the prison should not be permitted to override his treatment refusal decision unless a judge first determined that the prisoner was incompetent.

The Supreme Court ruled that the prisoner does indeed have a significant liberty interest in avoiding the unwanted administration of psychotropic medication. However, the Court rejected the prisoner's argument that this liberty interest requires a judge to determine the prisoner's incompetence before medically appropriate treatment can be administered. Rather, the court upheld a prison regulation that authorized involuntary treatment when a committee consisting of a psychiatrist, psychologist, and the facility's associate superintendent review the treating psychiatrist's decision and agree that the prisoner suffers from a mental disorder and is dangerous. The state's legitimate interest in prison safety and security warranted involuntary treatment without a full court hearing. At this time, it is unclear whether the *Harper* decision will be applied in nonprison settings involving nonprisoners.

In 1992, the Supreme Court decided another case involving medication refusal (*Riggins v. Nevada*, 1992). The *Riggins* case involved a criminal defendant who was forced to take psychotropic medication during his trial. The Supreme Court reversed the defendant's conviction because the forced medication may have violated the defendant's right to a fair trial. In ordering the defendant to take medication during his trial, the judge had not made any finding that medication was necessary to accomplish an essential state interest. *Harper*'s twin requirements of overriding justification and medical appropriateness, which allow the forced medication of convicted prisoners, are also required for criminal defendants.

Because criminal defendants are not confined in prison unless and until they are convicted, the law may even require more deference to their liberty interest in avoiding unwanted medication than is required for sentence-serving prisoners. In *Riggins*, the Supreme Court suggested that alternatives to involuntary treatment that are less intrusive to the individual's liberty must be considered before treatment — even medically appropriate treatment — is imposed. As worded, the *Riggins*' standard requires a consideration of whether the forced administration of psychotropic medication is necessary to accomplish an essential state policy. This issue is not within the expertise of psychiatrists; it is a question for the courts.

The Supreme Court has not yet decided whether civilly committed patients can be treated involuntarily without a judge's determination of incompetence. Such a determination may well be required. The state cannot claim that forced treatment of civilly committed patients without any court hearing is necessary to maintain prison safety and security. Unlike the prison inmate in *Harper*, civilly committed patients are not subject to punishment in a prison. The state cannot claim that forced treatment of civilly committed patients without any court hearing is necessary to determine their guilt or innocence. Unlike the criminal defendant in *Riggins*, civilly committed patients are not on trial.

Mentally disordered persons who are incapable of living in society or are dangerous to themselves or others are subject to civil commitment. The state's legitimate interest in protecting them, and in protecting others from them, is satisfied by the confinement itself — without coercing treatment. Although the state does have a legitimate interest in protecting other patients and staff from dangerous civilly-committed patients, the danger is far less in a mental hospital than it is in a prison. When emergencies arise, authority is needed to medicate dangerous patients temporarily. In non-emergency situations, greater deference to the civilly-committed patient's liberty interests in refusing treatment seems appropriate.

Regardless of whether the Supreme Court requires court hearings on mental patients' competence, the Court will only be deciding the minimum required by the United States Constitution. States may require more. Many state courts have relied upon their own state constitutions, statutes, and the doctrine of informed consent to uphold the civilly committed patient's right to refuse psychotropic medications unless a judge has found the patient incompetent.

SOLUTION: ATTITUDINAL ADJUSTMENT FOR PSYCHIATRISTS

The law imposes upon psychiatrists the duty to disclose to their patients the risks and benefits of, and alternatives to, the psychotropic medications they prescribe. This requirement of informed consent is viewed by many psychiatrists as an interference with medical practice. From the law's perspective, however, informed consent is not an interference with medical practice; it is a prerequisite to it. If a patient is competent to refuse medication, the law will no longer tolerate coerced compliance.

What is needed is a change in attitude. Psychiatrists do not treat mental disorders; they treat people with mental disorders. Those people are entitled to make their own decisions. When patients refuse treatment, psychiatrists must resist the urge to pressure them into complying "for their own good." Medical paternalism — doctor knows best — must be replaced by acceptance of patient autonomy — patient knows best.

Psychiatrists should not merely defer to competent decisions of their patients, they should actively promote competent decision making by their patients. Psychiatrists do so when they fully disclose information on the risks of, and alternatives to, the medication they prescribe. Patient empowerment is not only socially desirable, it is therapeutically desirable (Winick, 1994). Patient choice increases the patient's satisfaction and confidence in treatment. Patient choice promotes the patient's trust of, and confidence in, the therapist. A therapeutic alliance can be better achieved if therapeutic compliance is not coerced.

In a recent study, Lucksted and Coursey (1995) found that 30% of the mental patients in their sample population reported being pressured or forced to take psychotropic medications. Of those, 43% expressed feelings of fear or anger. Patients stated that coerced treatment had a negative effect on their relationship with the person who pressured or forced them into treatment. Although 81% of those who had not experienced coerced treatment expressed a belief that coercion may be permissible, 69% of those who had experienced coercion expressed a belief that it is not.

An American Psychiatric Association Resource Document, approved by the Association's Board of Trustees, urges psychiatrists, as a matter of good medical practice, "to maximize the patient's participation in the treatment decision making process; and, if the patient registers objections, to try to understand the basis for these objections and take them into account in formulating a treatment plan." (American Psychiatric Association, 1989). If patient participation becomes the standard of medical practice, informed consent will no longer be a burden that the law imposes on psychiatrists, but rather, an opportunity for a true therapeutic alliance that psychiatrists willingly offer their patients.

REFERENCES

American Psychiatric Association (1989). Right to refuse treatment resource document (p. 3).

Birnbaum, M. (1960). The right to treatment. *American Bar Association Journal, 46,* 499–505.

Cobbs v. Grant, 502 P.2d 1 (Cal. 1972).

Council of the American Psychiatric Association (1967). Position statement on the question of adequacy of treatment. *American Journal of Psychiatry, 123,* 1458–1460.

Griswold v. Connecticut, 381 U.S. 479 (1965).

Lucksted, A., & Coursey, R. D. (1995). Consumer perceptions of pressure and force in psychiatric treatments. *Psychiatric Services, 46,* 146–152.

Perlin, M. L. (1994). *Law and mental disability* (p. 191). Charlottesville, VA: Michie.

Rest, J. R. (1994). Background: Theory and research. In J. A. Rest, & D. Narváez (Eds.), *Moral development in the professions* (pp. 22–25). Hillsdale, NJ: Erlbaum.

Riggins v. Nevada, 504 U.S. 127 (1992).

Roe v. Wade, 410 U.S. 113 (1973).

Rogers v. Okin, 478 F. Supp. 1342, 1361 (D. Mass. 1979), *modified,* 634 F.2d 650 (1st Cir. 1980), *vacated and remanded,* 457 U.S. 291 (1982), *on remand,* 738 F.2d 1 (1st Cir. 1984).

Ross, J. W., & Halpern, J. (1995). Geriatric psychiatry — ethical issues. In H. I. Kaplan, & B. J. Sadock (Eds.), Comprehensive textbook of psychiatry, 6th ed. (pp. 2648–2649). Baltimore: Williams & Wilkins.

Roth, L., Lidz, C., Meisel, A., Soloff, P., Kaufman, F., Spiker, D., & Foster, R. (1982). Competency to decide about treatment or research: An overview of some empirical data. *International Journal of Law and Psychiatry, 5,* 29–50.

Roth, L., Meisel, A., & Lidz, C. (1977). Tests of competency to consent to treatment. *American Journal of Psychiatry, 134,* 279–284.

Rouse v. Cameron, 373 F.2d 451 (D.C. Cir. 1966).

Schloendorff v. Society of New York Hosp. 105 N.E. 92, 93 (N.Y. 1914).

Stone, A. A. (1975). *Mental health and law: A system in transition* (p. 94). Rockville, MD: NIMH.

Stone, A. A. (1981). The right to refuse treatment: Why psychiatrists should and can make it work. *Archives of General Psychiatry, 38,* 358–359.

Stromberg, C. D., & Stone, A. A. (1983). A model state law on civil commitment of the mentally ill. *Harvard Journal on Legislation, 20,* 330–335.

Thor v. Superior Court, 855 P.2d 375, 378 (Cal. 1993).

Washington v. Harper, 494 U.S. 210 (1990).

Weithorn, L. (1980). *Competency to render informed treatment decision: A comparison of certain minors and adults.* Unpublished doctoral dissertation, University of Pittsburgh.

Winick, B. J. (1994). The right to refuse mental health treatment: A therapeutic jurisprudence analysis. *International Journal of Law and Psychiatry, 17,* 99, 100–116.

Wyatt v. Stickney, 325 F. Supp. 781 (M.D. Ala. 1971), 334 F. Supp. 1341 (M.D. Ala.), 344 F. Supp. 373 (M.D. Ala.), 344 F. Supp. 387 (M.D. Ala. 1972), *aff'd sub. nom.* Wyatt v. Aderholt, 503 F.2d 1305 (5th Cir. 1974).

Youngberg v. Romeo, 457 U.S. 307 (1982).

6

Power and Coercion in Mental Health Practice

LAURIE C. CURTIS and RONALD DIAMOND

Power is a fundamental, however unspoken, dynamic in service design and delivery. It underpins our dialogue about the role and desired outcomes of the system, about approaches to treatment and support and who is qualified to provide these services, about risk management, about the guarantee and limits of rights, about motivation, recovery, and self-determination. It lies at the bottom of discussions about mandated treatment in community and institutional settings, about empowerment and opportunity, choice and responsibility. Perhaps one of the greatest ongoing challenges in mental health services is clarifying the use of power by an individual or an organized system to influence — or control — the actions of another for the purposes of healing and safety.

This chapter will provide an overview of ways in which power is exercised in the mental health service system, from paternalism and friendly persuasion to overtly coercive actions. It will discuss some of the ways that the use of power to influence or control behavior can impact on the process of healing, and how ethics can be used as a framework to guide the individual and collective use of power. Finally, guidelines for minimizing coercive interventions in mental health services will be identified.

EVOLVING CONTEXT OF PRACTICE

An important goal of mental health services is to help people to reach their own life goals. While bringing resources to the individual may be an important part of this process, a fundamental part of mental health services involves helping people to change. This change may entail helping the person develop new skills, change attitudes, control behaviors, or develop better understanding one's self and one's life.

97

The field has developed a number of ways to assist people to make these changes and often community support, rehabilitation, psychiatric treatment, and medication are a part of the process for individuals with disabling mental illnesses. Each of these interventions employs power in some form, whether through defining problems, imparting information, influencing attitudes, managing resources, teaching skills, coaching behaviors, or overt coercion to effect compliance or containment.

The practitioner has considerable control over this process and this power influences all aspects of the relationship with the client. How power is exercised within the relationship inevitably impacts on its course and often on its quality. In relationships between providers and consumers of mental health services, power is often used in direct and subtle ways to influence or control behavior. Such use of power may help individuals manage and even recover from the disabling impact of mental illness on their lives. It may also derail the best of intentions.

New approaches to mental health treatment also raise new questions about power, influence and ethics in practice (Curtis & Hodge, 1995). Respecting client's right to self-determination has been established as an important ethical principle (Darbyshire, 1991; NASW, 1992; IAPSRS, in press). There is also growing understanding about the relationship between self-determination and the process of rehabilitation and recovery (Anthony, 1993; Chamberlain, 1978; Rooney, 1992; Srebnick, 1992). At the same time, there are ongoing tensions about the relative balance between individual autonomy and other operant values in our culture. As practitioners, we struggle with our individual and collective power to both foster and restrict recipient choice and autonomy, and often find ourselves in the middle of swirling debates about whether we have too much or too little power — either as practitioners or as a service system.

These issues are congruent with other changes in mental health service delivery which have occurred over the past two decades. People with severe psychiatric disability are now living in the community who only a few years ago would have been confined to an institution. These individuals often require considerable support. At the same time that their need is great, some individuals refuse help, putting them at increased risk for rehospitalization, arrest, homelessness, and victimization. Their behavior may raise concern by community members who find them bothersome or frightening. Use of non-consensual or coercive interventions, particularly in community settings, highlights inherent conflicts between the treatment/ healing and social control functions of the mental health system, and spawns increasing questions about the power and "voluntariness" of mental health services (Blanch & Parrish, 1993; Diamond, 1995).

Against this backdrop, the mental health practitioner, whether professional or lay-person, must forge a working alliance with the individual receiving services. Most practitioners entered the mental health field out of a desire to be helpful, not as agents of social control. Consequently, a community mental health practitioner struggles daily with decisions about how to employ the power vested in the roles and how to reconcile this power with the values of self-determination which help guide our field (Surber, 1994). Hartman (1992, p. 484) points out,

> There is a painful paradox in being a professional and being committed to empowerment. A key part of the definition of a profession is the possession of knowledge and, in fact, the ownership of a specific area of knowledge. As professionals we are expected to be experts, but the power in our expertise can disempower our clients and thus subvert the goals of our profession.

ABOUT POWER

In its simplest form, power is our ability to control events around us. Power also measures the extent to which can we get what we want and consequently the extent to which we influence others to contribute to what we want. Power typically carries the potential for control, and continues to exist whether the control is actually used or not. The fact that this potential for control exists inevitably influences our relationship. Coercion may be considered the use of this power to actually control or influence events. There are many ways of using power to exert influence and control to achieve desired ends. These may be considered on a continuum from gentle persuasion and other informal ways of exerting influence, to control of consequences (such as the threat of being fired or having money withheld), to the threat and direct use force (such as physical restraint and involuntary commitment). Informal power is much more commonly used than formal control and can be just as effective as overt control in changing behavior.

The most common interpretation of power is "power over" a person or group of people. "Power over" may not actually be exercised in an authoritative or coercive way, but that potential exists whether or not it is used. Coercion is the application of this power to actually control or influence events. "Power over" is hierarchical and lends itself to struggles in which two or more individuals vie for the on-top position. However, there is increasing attention to "power with" or equity power as an effective approach to achieving the goal of getting what one wants. This redefinition of power within the mental health system is promulgated by many leaders and thinkers in the mental health consumer movement and reflects similar concerns in other aspects of our contemporary social debate.

Power in the mental health system, as in the rest of society, is derived from various sources, including formal position; special knowledge, expertise or information; personal charisma; and connections.

Position Power

Many roles and jobs are vested with degrees of power or authority, usually bounded by an identified purpose and limitations. This is known as position power. For example, a manager may have the power to hire or fire a staff person; a physician has the power to prescribe medications or involuntarily commit a person in crisis; the case manager may have the power to support or diminish a goal or dream presented by a client. The structure of the mental health system has historically sanctioned professionals to assume a considerable amount of power over the lives and resources of many persons with psychiatric disabilities.

> Many benevolent, humanistic clinicians see themselves as servants of the public, offering themselves and their services in a non-controlling fashion. They see their clients as free agents, free to accept of reject the offered services ... Yet this is where so many human service workers deceive themselves, because their roles are not only almost always societally sanctioned, but in an endless array of encounters between the server and the served, the server is the interpreter of and agent for the intents of society, and wields a truly amazing amount of power and control, even if he may not consciously perceive himself as so doing. (Wolfensburger, 1972, p. 1–2).

Position power in human services carries with it an assumption of fiduciary responsibility by the worker: the power of the professional is to be used for the client, not for the professional's gain (Lebacqz, 1985). Use of this power for humane, beneficent intent is viewed as ethical, while the use of this power for personal gain or purposes other than beneficence is considered unethical. To guide individuals in the use of "position power," professional associations establish and enforce ethical standards and service organizations institute conduct codes for employees. Since position power in human services is entrusted and externally sanctioned, it can be taken away.

Expertise and Information Power

People also gain influence and control the behavior of others based on their expertise and information. Information is power. A person's influence on others increases if they know how to work with someone who is angry or upset, how to organize a service plan which makes sense to all concerned, or how to fix a photocopy machine. Having access to information and persons in key positions also provides power — knowing who to call at Social Security to get a question answered, knowing who to contact for an emergency housing voucher. When the information is highly desired, the information holder attains a higher degree of status.

Not all expertise is valued equally. Society, including service users and providers, tend to value formal expertise such as knowing about medication or how to make a diagnostic assessment and develop a comprehensive service plan. The lives of persons with psychiatric disabilities may be heavily influenced by access to informal expertise. Knowing how to take a bus, where to get free food, or how to obtain subsidized housing may be critically important. These kinds of expertise are often held by consumers within the mental health system or by support workers. This expertise is typically less valued by both staff and consumers than more formal expertise. Part of empowerment is to acknowledge these various kinds of expertise and thereby enhance the role of people knowledgeable in these life survival skills.

Person Power

Another important base of power lies not with a particular position or role, but as part of the interpersonal process. Personal power is derived from cognitive abilities, personal commitment, credibility, and character. People tend to be more influential if they are seen as skilled, trustworthy, or committed to the goals of a group or organization. Style is an important determinate of personal power. Assertive people tend to have more power than those who are reticent.

Expression of person power is influenced by self-esteem and individual perceptions of power-fullness. There are also external forces which influence personal power. Attitudes about the relative power of different persons or types of persons can shape if and how person power is manifested. Historically, men have had more influence than women, people who are white have had more power in our culture that people of color, and people without labels of mental illness have had more power than people with labels. Perceptions about opportunity and oppression strongly influence the direction and intensity of person power. The enumeration and establishment of human, civil, and consumer rights helps establish and legitimize a base of personal power for individuals who are typically viewed as having less power within the system.

It is often naively assumed that the various sources of power are correlated — that the manager of a team is also the most skilled clinician as well as the most convincing. Often, reality is very different. A secretary low on a formal hierarchy of power and control may have influence based on having important information unavailable to anyone else. The psychiatrist with formal power to prescribe medication may not be the influential person in communicating with a client about the purpose of the medication or why it is important to take.

Empowerment

The concept of "empowerment" can be construed as the increase in exercise of personal power. There are many ways to facilitate empowerment. Decreasing negative perceptions and increasing self-esteem may help change interpersonal styles. Legitimizing the role and "voice" of persons with psychiatric disability may enhance the expression of both person and position power of an individual or group. Acknowledging the very real expertise of a person with a disability can influence their power from position and expertise, as well as increase their personal power within the group.

A consumer is the key expert about him or herself and holds information crucial to the success of any treatment or support intervention; the family is another important source of knowledge. However, these sources of expertise are often devalued by both service users and practitioners who tend to place a greater value on formal knowledge and expertise. Part of empowerment is to acknowledge, draw upon, and share these various kinds of expertise thereby enhancing the role of people as experts in their own lives. As a psychiatrist, part of my expertise is knowing about psychotropic medications. As a medication user, knowing how a medication makes me feel is part of my expertise. I also need information about the medications shared with me in order to make informed decisions and adequately communicate with my physician. Both bases of knowledge are imperative to developing an effective medication course.

Equity Power

Another kind of power comes from "power with" rather than "power over." "Power equity assumes mutual empowerment with everyone fully present, responsible, and valued for their diversity and resources" (Pierce, 1994, p. 6). This "power with" approach implies that power is not a finite resource which must be fought over. Increasing my power does not necessarily imply a decrease in your power. My power is actually enhanced because it has merged with yours for attainment of a common goal. Without you, my power is diminished; without me, your power is diminished.

Equity power is closely connected with some of the recent changes in mental health systems. While helping relationships in mental health programs have traditionally been seen as an interaction between a "knowledgeable expert" and a "subordinate client" there is an important shift in power occurring (Ayers, 1989). The fiduciary responsibility of the worker to use his/her position power in the best interest of the consumer remains intact, but the decision of what is in the best interest no longer rests entirely with the professional. Consumers and family members are becoming more active partners in service design and delivery, demanding and exercising voice in what had been primarily professional domains. As the balance of power shifts, the nature of helping relationships becomes less prescriptive and more collaborative (Kisthardt, 1992). Professionals are less likely to be entitled or empowered to make overarching treatment or lifestyle decisions which the staff person considers to be in the best interest of the client. While these changes may decrease the traditional power of the mental health professional, they may increase the mutual empowerment which allows shared goals to be accomplished.

ABOUT ETHICS

Ethics may be defined as a broad moral code outlining obligations and standards of conduct — personal, professional, spiritual

(Lebacqz, 1985). Ethics may constitute such subjective and unde-fined principles as: *Do no harm; Do the right thing; Be fair; Promote and ensure safety; Do nothing to diminish the dignity of any person or thing; Refrain from exploiting privileged position, power, or knowledge; Avoid unnecessary suffering; Optimize good consequences, and so forth.* All of these are derived from the principles of beneficence (do good); non-maleficence (do no harm), and autonomy (respect self-determination) (Rosenbluth, Kleinman & Lowy, 1995). Other ethical principles valued in mental health services include just distribution of resources, privacy/confidentiality, veracity, and informed con-sent (Curtis & Hodge, 1995).

Ethics within mental health services may be construed as a system for guiding the appropriate use of power for the greatest good. When we say something is ethical or unethical, we are passing judgement. While ethical standards may help shape our determination of what is "good," codes of ethical behavior also help define the ideal virtues of a group or society (Barker and Baldwin, 1991). Ethical standards are also a vehicle to pledge staff to high standards of care, to build uni-formity and identity within a profession, to minimize liability risk, and to outline expectations for professional etiquette. They may enun-ciate very broad standards for a profession and encompass a variety of theoretical approaches. However, codes of ethics cannot give pre-cisely what many people want — definitive rulings on highly com-plex and often personal moral issues. Vagueness and compromise exist precisely where the issues are most difficult.

When a mother says to a child, "Don't throw stones because you may hurt someone," she is also implicitly teaching the ethic, "Hurt-ing people is bad; helping people is good." While on the surface these seem to be simple decisions, there are many variables which impact on the "rightness" of any determination. Is it O.K. to throw stones at a cat, rather than a person? At the tree in the backyard? Into the pond when no one is swimming? What about if the stone is actually a soft ball? What if hitting someone was clearly an acci-dent? What if throwing the stone was the only way to get the per-son's attention and avoid a more serious accident?

Ethics imply choice and ethical dilemmas arise when there is a conflict between competing values (Abramson, 1985; Nash, 1990). Is it better to support the autonomy of a person to make his or her own decisions even if this will leave them homeless, or it is justified to be paternalistic and intervene to keep the person from being evicted from an apartment he/she likes? In mental health, some of the most complicated ethical dilemmas involve a conflict between what is best for the person and what is good for the system or community. For example, when does an individual's right to self-determination supersede the community's concern about deviance from local norms of dress or behavior? When does the community's responsi-bility to ensure the general safety of its citizens supersede the right of an individual to walk behind a school child? What is the responsi-bility of the mental health system when consumer choice results in reduction in safety for the consumer and possibly others? How is an

individual's preference reconciled with conflicting needs or desires
of a family group?

This tension is compounded by further debate about "Who decides?" — The person? The person's family? The doctor? The case
manager? The insurance company? The city council? The protocol
for making and enforcing these decisions is often unclear and rarely
guided by a clearly defined set of values.

ABOUT RIGHTS

When ethics are codified into law or established by litigation or
decree, they become rights. Individual rights are an important
counter-balance to the vested and statutory power of the mental
health system. Protection and advocacy organizations exist in
every state to help ensure and protect the rights of individuals with
disabilities. The use of influence or authority, particularly non-
consensual or coercive interventions, must be weighed against the
rights of the individual. At what point or under what circumstances
may individual rights be transgressed? Are there points at which
these rights *must* be superseded by other authority?

Human Rights

These are the common rights of any person and may not always be
specified in law. They are based on the highest moral standards or
ideals, and while different cultures may ascribe somewhat different
values to these rights, they are generally considered to transcend
political, social, cultural and economic boundaries. The United
Nations General Assembly *Universal Declaration of Human Rights*
(1948) outlines fundamental and basic rights of all persons which
include the right to a safe and humane environment, the right to
privacy, consensual intimacy, personal freedom, freedom from false
imprisonment, and so forth (McPheeters, 1980; World Federation for
Mental Health, 1989). Many advocates add a number of other human rights which include the right to decent housing, community
inclusion, a fair wage, and so forth.

Civil Rights

These rights apply to any citizen in our society and are guaranteed
by law. These include the right to vote, to self-determination and
self-expression, to buy and sell property, to marry, and so forth
(McPheeters, 1980). With few exceptions, these rights are to be upheld even when an individual is legally incarcerated or involuntarily committed — although this is not always the case in practice as
multiple class action suits have demonstrated (Sadoff, 1981; Weiner,
1981).

Statutory Consumer Rights

Consumer rights are based on legal doctrine, as well as to a set of implicit and explicit contracts between a provider and a recipient of services. Consumers have the right to know their rights, to confidentiality, to personal privacy, and to informed consent. Litigation has firmly established the right of an individual detained under a mental health commitment to receive treatment, the right to treatment in the least restrictive and most facilitative environment, and the right to refuse treatment (Weiner, 1981; McPheeters, 1980).

Every state has established laws and regulations pertaining to both voluntary and involuntary commitment which restrict and guarantee certain individual rights. While there are statutory variations, in most states involuntary commitment is based on evidence of mental illness and the indication of dangerousness to self or others. In some states, other factors may be considered as a basis for involuntary commitment to care. These include evidence of grave disability, refusal to consent, treatability, incapacity to decide treatment, and non-compliance with less restrictive options (Corey, Corey and Callanan, 1993).

Additional rights of persons with psychiatric disabilities have been delineated through various State statutes and Federal laws such as The Protection and Advocacy for Mentally Ill Individuals Act of 1986, Fair Housing Amendments Act of 1988, and Americans with Disabilities Act of 1992 which further delineate specific rights of persons with psychiatric disabilities in the United States. In 1991, the United Nations General Assembly amended the 1948 Universal Declaration of Human Rights by adopting a resolution on The Protection of Persons with Mental Illness and the Improvement of Mental Health Care. This resolution outlines important principles of human dignity and decency in treatment (United Nations General Assembly; 1992). There is a growing disability rights movement, encompassing individuals with psychiatric disabilities, which is organizing to help enforce these statutory, civil, and human rights (Carling, 1995).

PATERNALISM

Paternalism involves acting in what is believed to be the best interest of the person. Typically paternalism involves making decisions about or for an individual from a viewpoint external to the individual. For example, taking a friend's cigarettes to keep him or her from harming themself by smoking would be a paternalistic intervention. Paternalism in the mental health system is based on the assumption that, left to their own devices, persons with mental illness would be unable to ensure their own safety or welfare (Darbyshire, 1991). There are arguments that serious mental illness so profoundly impacts the judgment of some individuals that they are unable to make decisions (Jaffe, 1995).

Mental health services commonly use paternalism to justify coercive interventions. However, it is important to distinguish coercion justified by what is good for society from paternalism which is justified by what is good for the individual. At times, these can become confused. Community mandates to "control" the behavior of otherwise disruptive individuals can reinforce paternalistic justifications for the use of coercion. A practitioner may feel that hospitalization is in a person's best interest. This belief may be reinforced if the person is loudly disruptive and disturbing the mayor of the city. In the midst of calls from police, the mayor's office, and the person's family, it may become difficult to disentangle what part of the decision to use a hospital is for the person's own good, and what part is for the good of the mayor, the general community, and the treatment program that is facing the pressure to "do something."

There are often no clear set of rules about when we should intrude on someone who prefers to be left alone. "If we err in the direction of much intrusion, we risk alienating the client and the sins of commission. If we err in the direction of leaving alone, we risk neglect and the sins of omission" (Reamer, 1982, p. 268). Paternalistic attitudes may vary widely from gentle supervision to blanket assumptions that a person with mental illness must be "taken care of" in the same manner a parent would take care of a child — protectively overseeing virtually all aspects of the individual's general welfare. Because of the great potential for abuse of paternalism, Reamer (1982) argues that paternalism is justified only when an individual threatens or engages in potentially fatal self-destructive behavior. Clearly, the strongest situational justifications for paternalistic intervention exist when non-intervention would result in irreversible harm or when there is an immediate need to rescue (Rooney, 1992).

While the use of paternalism in justifying extremely intrusive interventions such as involuntary commitment is fairly clear, practitioners face daily the question of whether and how to use less coercive, non-consensual interventions. Most paternalistic interventions have a much weaker justification than life threatening behavior. Practitioners often justify intrusion into a person's life by asking themselves whether the proposed restriction on the client is likely to prevent more severe restrictions in the future. For example, assuming control of money may result in an individual avoiding a more restrictive hospitalization. This paternalism must be balanced by the client's own views on how to maximize autonomy and retain control of their life. Some individuals may feel that forced medications are more restrictive and invasive than prolonged hospitalization.

Use of interventions that apply varying degrees of pressure for a person to comply with a treatment plan are part and parcel of day-to-day community mental health treatment and support. For example, an individual in crisis may have the choice of being "voluntarily" hospitalized or an alternative which has an attached contingency such as taking medications as prescribed, allowing family to be contacted, or agreeing to a follow-up visit from an outreach worker. Should an individual not choose voluntary hospitalization or a less restrictive alternative, commitment proceedings for court-mandated treatment could be initiated.

Paternalism is not always bad, nor should it be entirely dismissed. Beneficence, doing good, has its foundation in kindness, charity, and consequently in paternalism. Outreach services to persons with a psychiatric disability, for example, are typically based on a paternalistic premise. Overt and sometimes very tenacious efforts are made to reach out to individuals who are in apparent need of services but may not desire them. The goal of these services is to engage individuals for their own best interest. The alternative to such paternalism is abandonment. In the name of choice and self-determination, some individuals with psychiatric disabilities have been abandoned to poor, incompetent, and even abusive situations – usually without the information necessary to make truly informed decisions.

Surles (1994) argues that individual choice is strongly linked with the process of recovery and that at the same time, there is a strong societal interest in preventing an individual from engaging in an activity which endangers his/her life or health. The decision for or against paternalistic intervention must be balanced against several factors: (1) the imminence and degree of danger; (2) the ability of the individual to understand the imminence and degree of danger; (3) whether the activity exposes others to danger; (4) the resources and limitations of the setting (e.g. hospital, community street, family home); (5) the risk of intervening on long term recovery outcome. The potential long term negative consequences of paternalism are most difficult to assess and most commonly ignored in decision-making.

An important issue in influence and coercion is the balance between short term risk and long term benefit. The frequent use of coercive intervention, particularly court ordered treatments, is the result of a crisis oriented system of care, rather than one based on providing long term treatment and support (Diamond, 1995). Practitioners are often under considerable pressure to rapidly solve an immediate problem. Forcing someone into a hospital, pressuring them to take medications, or placing them in a supervised residential facility often decreases immediate risk, and provide staff and community with a sense of control. Within the context of a crisis, coercive approaches are often applied without adequate identification and exploration of less intrusive methods.

It is much more complicated to assess the long term outcomes of coercive interventions. Many individuals report that their experience with involuntary intervention was not only harmful rather than helpful, but undermined personal recovery and continued to affect their lives in negative ways (Blanch & Parrish, 1993; Schwartz, Vigiano, Bezirganian, 1988). Mental illness is often persistent and the need for support ongoing. The issue is less whether an individual is taking medication in a week, but whether that individual is taking medication in a year (Diamond, 1995). Many consumers report that the use of coercion reduces the quality of the practitioner-consumer relationship. The more an individual perceives the mental health system as controlling and invasive, the less likely that individual is to voluntarily engage in services. This can increase the likelihood that coercive methods would be needed to engage that individual in the future, reinforcing a cycle that is destructive for the person, mental health system, and community. While coercion may ensure a resistant individual takes medication for a short time, a more collaborative approach increases the likelihood of the individual using the medication over the long haul.

There is growing concern about how paternalism may negatively impact on the ability or motivation of an individual to move naturally through stages of adult maturation or engage in a recovery process (Darbyshire, 1991; Deegan, 1992). The degree of paternalism exhibited directly impacts on the options of an individual to exercise autonomy or choice, and consequently may directly or indirectly shape an individual's perception of his/her abilities and potential. For many persons, this becomes a self-reinforcing cycle in which an individual begins to believe and then fulfill diminished expectations (Deegan, 1992). Risk-taking behavior is also restricted which limits the opportunity of individuals to learn and grow from mistakes (Chamberlain, 1994). Paternalism may also result in anger by an individual and an avoidance of treatment or support services, minimizing any potential benefit (Unzicker, 1989).

THE CONTINUUM OF COERCION FROM INFLUENCE TO OVERT CONTROL

Whether conscious or not, practitioners are engaged in an ongoing process of influencing, changing, and at times trying to control the attitudes, beliefs and behaviors of clients as part of day-to-day treatment and support activities. All of these activities exist on a continuum of coercion, from attempts to influence and convince that one regularly uses with friends and family, to overt control that depends on the imposition of power. Coercion encompasses a wide range of actions taken without the consent of the individual (Blanch and Parrish, 1993). These include not only the use of restraints and forced administration of medication, but also treatment planning conducted without consumer participation, and formal or informal rules linking access to service such as housing with treatment compliance. Mental health commitment and other court ordered treatment is at the extreme end of a spectrum of pressures or restrictions which make up influence and coercion in mental health services.

Methods of influencing the behaviors and attitudes of others range from strategic self-presentation, friendly persuasion, control of consequences and resources, to direct coercion, punishment, and court-ordered treatment. At exactly what point influence becomes coercion is difficult to determine. Similarly, it is difficult to determine when an attempt to influence or control becomes "excessive."

Strategic Self-Presentation

Strategic self-presentation is used by most people to manage the impressions others have of us in order to influence them (Rooney,

1992). Common self-presentation strategies include: (1) ingratiation — making one's self more attractive or likable through flattery, identification with the other, and agreement with opinions; (2) intimidation — direct and indirect efforts to elicit fear; (3) supplication — emphasizing ones inability and negative points in order to acquire sympathy and support; (4) facework — activities to diffuse blame or the impact of negative feedback; (5) self-promotion — making one's self appear more competent by emphasizing one's best qualities; and (6) exemplification — modeling and other efforts to emphasize integrity and moral worthiness.

These self-presentation strategies are employed to enhance power by both practitioners and clients. Consider the process of engaging an individual who is not voluntarily soliciting services. In this scenario, the consumer holds considerable power over the practitioner who, for whatever reason, needs to engage that person. The practitioner initiates a selling process, presenting the agency's capacity to help and the potential value of assistance in the best possible light. In addition to genuine empathy and concrete services, ingratiation, self-promotion, exemplification and other strategic self-presentation strategies are commonly employed to influence the individual to engage in the process proffered.

Strategic self-presentation is an important facet of building rapport in helping alliances. However well intended, when mis-employed they can be seen by consumers as disingenuous and manipulating (Unzicker, 1989). Rooney (1992) also suggests that strategic self-presentation strategies may be commonly employed by clients as an effort to retain or regain power in a clinical relationship and may also offer normalizing explanations for irritating behavior that has been labeled as a personality deficit. Consumers refer to these kinds of approaches when talking about how to "survive" or "work" the mental health system (Unzicker, 1989; Chamberlain, 1978; Estroff, 1981).

Persuasion

Persuasion is intended to influence attitudes and behavior through provision of information and rationales for making choices. Research suggests that individuals are more responsive to persuasion when (1) there is incongruence between a behavior and a deeply held belief; (2) when individuals can explain a change as contributing to their self-defined best interest (as opposed to hope of gaining a reward or avoiding a punishment); and (3) the person presenting the information is liked, trusted, and viewed as expert (Rooney, 1992). These dynamics are evident in the use of persuasion in many mental health practices.

With friendly persuasion there is little restriction of an individual's self-determination nor does the practitioner or service system attempt to manipulate or control the consequences of the process. In community support services, there has been increasing attention to making sure that clients have access to a wide range of information about resources and options in order to make personal decisions. The legal and ethical principle of informed consent requires that individuals have access to information which will permit informed choice. Persuasion can assist decision-making by increasing an individual's knowledge about alternatives and exploring their potential benefits and costs.

Persuasion can also be indirect. An important aspect of the effectiveness of many community support programs is their ability to coordinate all parts of an individual's treatment and support system. For example, a case manager may be in direct contact with a person's family, housemates, landlord, employer, other service providers, family physician, and even minister. This communication, even with the client's permission, has enormous potential to increase the pressure to take medications, to stay in a treatment program, to live in a particular setting, and generally to comply with "the plan." Consistency in messages and continuity of caring support are aspects of ideal network involvement. However, such pressure may also be over-encompassing and leave little latitude for individual autonomy or decision-making, except for massive defiance and rejection of the whole scenario. Persuasion, itself on a continuum, can become more coercive when administered by someone with a larger power differential, who gives the individual less permission to consider alternatives, and where there is a perception that other kinds of coercion could be applied if "persuasion" is not effective.

Medication compliance is an area in which persuasion is frequently used. Information about medications, their benefits and side-effects is increasingly available to consumers. Practitioners frequently help individuals identify the advantages and disadvantages of medication use, typically emphasizing the positive impact of symptom reduction in an individual's life, as well as the negative impact of uncontrolled symptomology. Unless the benefits of medication are congruent with the self-interest, values and goals of the individual, compliance to a medication regimen is likely to be inconsistent without utilization of more coercive approaches (Diamond 1983).

Persuasion is not value-neutral. It is difficult to engage in the process without communicating the attendant biases, preferences, and expectations of the practitioner through subtle as well as direct means (e.g. voice inflection, non-verbal expressions, how information is framed or discussed). It is also important for practitioners to acknowledge and present their personal or professional perspectives. Finally, and perhaps most importantly, a practitioner must listen to the perspectives and concerns of others, retaining an open mind and willingness to be influenced by new viewpoints and information.

Control of Resources

Practitioners have power to control resources in order to influence behavior. Control of resources, like persuasion, is on a continuum from pressure to complete control. Resources may range from luxuries to those that are essential. In general, controlling resources is more intrusive and coercive than persuasion. Control of resources may range from free rides or bus tokens as a reward for appropriate behavior, to extra time with the practitioner, to access to low income housing or the person's own entitlement money (Wertheimer, 1993). Similarly, control of resources also implies the practitioner has power to withhold or remove such resources contingent upon inappropriate behavior.

Controlling behavior by controlling resources is commonly used in community services. Fundamental resources such as housing, affiliation, support, and money are frequently controlled or made contingent upon appropriate behavior. For example, access to an emergency shelter or other residential settings may be contingent on medication compliance and signing a contract agreeing to attend a day program. Individuals may be evicted from housing or discharged from a program with little due process. A high-reward activity such as simply sharing a cup of coffee may be held contingent on engaging in a low-reward activity such as doing the dishes. A practitioner may opt to not provide increased contact to an individual who repeatedly engages in "attention-seeking" activities and may even reduce contact to effectively punish a person for undesired behavior.

Money is frequently used to manage behavior. So important is this tool that some programs routinely require control of an individual's funds. Others apply for control of personal funds only after an individual has repeatedly made financial decisions which negatively impact on their welfare. Persons who receive SSI or SSDI may be assigned a payee by the Social Security Administration with little due process protection. While a number of non-coercive steps should be taken first, such as voluntary assistance with budgeting and other forms of collaborative problem solving, these interventions can be time consuming and occasionally involve significant risk. When a financial payee is assigned, the payee controls not only the individual's entitlement money, but also effectively controls the process for returning financial control to the individual. Not infrequently, an individual is required by the payee or others to demonstrate ability to make choices or perform behaviors which have little to do with making sound financial decisions.

This "hook" can be extremely effective in helping to engage a person in a treatment program. If funds are only accessible through the service program, the individual is more likely to appear and provide staff with an opportunity to engage around other issues such as medication. The use of a payee can ensure that rent and utilities are paid and guarantee that an individual has adequate food and clothing. Some clients value the structure imposed by this kind of external control, but others resent the restriction so deeply that it significantly decreases the potential for helping alliances based on anything but coercion.

The enormous control of resources can lead to a significant potential for abuse. Practitioners control a wide range of resources from transportation vouchers to access to services with little chance for due process protection by an outside monitor such as a court of formal protection and advocacy mechanism. Attention to consumer rights and practitioner vigilance for ways to protect autonomy and promote empowerment are crucial. While there are typically efforts to employ less invasive or coercive approaches first, practitioners often use "more of the same" compliance strategies, increasing their intensity if they fail to yield the desired results (Rooney, 1992). Developing appeal procedures involving outside panels of consumers and practitioners may be one way to address the power imbalance inherent in the treatment relationship.

Court-Ordered Intervention

Court-ordered intervention refers to legal sanctions mandating compliance to community-based treatment or involuntary hospitalization. Such restriction of autonomy, whether for the purpose of treatment, protection or containment, is the ultimate use of the societally sanctioned power of the mental health system (Blanch & Parrish, 1993). It has been termed by the U.S. Supreme Court as a "massive curtailment of liberty" (cited in Levy, 1994). There is active debate about the ultimate value of non-consensual treatment in the course of serious mental illness and about the system of checks and balances necessary to safeguard both society and individual rights (Jaffe, 1995; Griffen-Fancell, 1995; Blanch & Parrish, 1993).

There are two primary sources of power for court-ordered intervention: (1) parens patriae — a legal form of paternalism which authorizes the state to care for people who are determined unable to care for themselves; and (2) police power — the authority to protect society from potential harm (Levy, 1994). Parens patriae forms the basis for restricting the autonomy of persons identified as "dangerous to self." There are many discrepant definitions of "capability to care for self." Mental illness may affect only limited areas of functioning and there have been some highly controversial attempts to broaden this standard to include persons whose lifestyles are neither esthetically pleasing or socially acceptable. At times, people are judged to be incapable of caring for themselves because necessary resources such as housing are unavailable, or because they make seemingly irrational choices such as deciding to live on the street rather than go into a homeless shelter that is perceived as more demeaning and dangerous. Police power forms the basis for commitments based on "dangerous to others." This standard also challenges, with the definition of "dangerousness" one of the most elusive concepts in mental health law.

Short of involuntary hospitalization itself, the threat of psychiatric hospitalization is one of the most powerful ways to influence compliance behavior in community services. The practitioner power to initiate commitment proceedings is recognized by both the practitioner and the client. This intrusion of commitment into the treatment relationship is psychologically present even in situations where both the practitioner and consumer are clear that the legal grounds for involuntary hospitalization are not met. Too often, the psychiatric hospital functions as either an implied or real punishment for non-compliance to other treatment.

Because of the massive curtailment of liberties involved in civil commitment, a number of states have instituted community-based court-ordered treatment statutes which provide an intermediary process between full autonomy in the community and full incarceration at a psychiatric facility. The intent of these court-mandated interventions is treatment, rather than protection, with medications being the most commonly ordered treatment method. Community-based court-mandated treatment may be used to divert individuals from more restrictive hospitalizations or as a conditional release from a psychiatric hospital. These approaches still typically involve standard civil commitment procedures and continue to be highly controversial (Levy, 1994; Rooney, 1992; Blanch & Parrish, 1993; Geller, 1990).

While there is a nationwide interest in reducing the overall utilization of psychiatric hospital beds, there is little data about the frequency of court-ordered community or hospital treatment. Even in communities known to be developing client-centered approaches with alternatives to coercive interventions, court-mandated treatment is still in use (Diamond, 1995). What distinguishes these communities from most others is the clear effort to explore alternatives to involuntary intervention prior to initiating the legal process, although this raises new concerns about the ethics of delaying treatment. Blanch and Parrish (1993) report that the frequent and continuing use of involuntary interventions is supported by a number of political, cultural/social and fiscal factors and reflects a number of demographic disparities in application. Oppressed groups are disproportionately represented in involuntary clients (Rooney, 1992).

Clinically, the use of court-ordered treatment has both advantages and disadvantages. A court mandate for community services may help some clients to escape a "revolving door" by allowing a period of stability and opportunity to develop more effective solutions to stressful situations (Hiday & Scheid-Cook, 1989; Tavolaro, 1992). It may also provide an opportunity for an individual to experience potential benefits of medications and to develop a working alliance with community mental health practitioners which would continue beyond the time period of the court order (Schwartz, Vigiano, Bezirganian, 1988). Research on court-ordered treatment for alcoholism suggests that coercion can be as effective as voluntary treatment when court orders are long-lasting and enforced. However, the effect diminishes over time and relapse is prevalent in both mandated and voluntary treatment (Rooney, 1992).

The use of court-mandated treatment does not always assure a successful outcome (Geller, 1990). Levy (1994) suggests that civil commitment may result in a lasting stigma that can impair the consumer's ability to obtain employment, housing, education, and other opportunities. There is a poor relationship between the use of involuntary hospitalization and the guarantee that individuals will voluntarily seek continued care (Griffen-Fancell, 1995). When services are inadequate, coercion to use those services will not improve outcomes (Zusman, 1985). Use of governmental or therapeutic power to enforce compliance is also seen as a sign of a totalitarian approach to society and raises the specter of incarceration for political purposes (Blanch & Parrish, 1993). There is no research support for the assumption that violence in a community will be diminished by increasing the capacity of the mental health system to perform civil commitments (Catalano & McConnell, 1993).

Overuse is also a concern. Commitment laws are couched with the understanding that they will be applied only to those few individuals who absolutely need treatment coercion or containment for the good of themselves or the community. However, practice shows that when commitment laws are available, they will be used (Durham, 1985; Hasbe & McRae, 1987). There are a great many people with and without mental illness who are potentially dangerous. It is both impossible and unethical to contain all individuals in this group, and it is impossible to accurately predict who among this group will actually engage in dangerous behavior. In efforts to preserve hard-won stability, there is often pressure from family, practitioners, and the community to continue someone on community-commitment status once it has been initiated (Wood & Swanson, 1985).

While there are arguments to support increasing coercion in mental health services, there are also equally strong arguments against it (Griffen-Fancell, 1995; Blanch & Parrish, 1993). "Any involuntary intervention, practiced in the name of treatment, may be a cruel violation of substantive due process of law. This means we may have to conclude there is no way this behavior can ever be justified as the practice of medicine, or consistent with the Hippocratic Oath" (Thompson, quoted in Blanch & Parrish, 1993, p. 19). Surles (1994) points out the trade off between autonomy and safety. "We cannot at the same time be more libertarian and more paternalistic. We cannot demand that the public mental health system ensure recipient choice and still guarantee recipient safety. It's not possible. If we are to promote choice, we have to be prepared to accept consequences. And if we give priority to patient safety, we should give up the pretense of defending patient choice" (p. 21).

REDUCING THE USE OF COERCION IN PRACTICE

While accepting that power and influence are fundamental aspects of all human relationships and inherent in all service systems, the use of coercive interventions raises concerns for multiple reasons: power, ethics, rights, and clinical outcomes. Many states are considering statutory changes which would make court-ordered treatment more readily available and there are strong advocates for and against this trend (Jaffe, 1995; Griffin-Francell, 1995). Yet it is clear that getting an individual into the treatment system earlier or forcing compliance to treatment or a support service program will not work if the system is either inadequate or ineffective. Often many of those labeled "treatment resistant" or "non-compliant" would accept help if the system was designed to meet their real needs in a helpful and respectful manner.

Ethical principles call for the minimization of coercion through the maximization of autonomy. There are multiple ways in which the mental health service system can reduce the use of coercive interventions and our knowledge in this area is increasing (Blanch & Parrish, 1993; Diamond, 1995; Carling, 1994). These strategies and our understanding of them derive from the basic awareness that (1) power within the mental health system is manifest in many ways, with different intensities and for divergent purposes; (2) the power is not inherently bad or misapplied, but there is enormous potential for abuse; (3) the power is not held exclusively by practitioners; and most importantly, (4) the power of individuals with psychiatric disabilities must be acknowledged, supported, and fostered in personal, programmatic, and systemic arenas.

Develop Helping Alliances Characterized by Respect and Dignity

The use of compliance-oriented interventions are minimized when helping relationships are based on respect for the experience base of the individual and congruence between what the individual desires and what the practitioner provides. This includes basing the relationship on the individual's own goals, clarifying core values, negotiating differences and maintaining alliances even when the individual refuses treatment. Most treatment systems have not traditionally encouraged the development of long-term, trusting and respectful relationships (Kanter, 1989). Yet, the kind of listening which is necessary to build these relationships, particularly with people who find it difficult to connect with others, takes time.

Respect and dignity in relationships goes beyond listening. It also requires mutuality — both giving and receiving within the relationship. In the process of validating another, we must also let ourselves be challenged, influenced and changed. "We have been mistaken before and we will be mistaken again. But we are only wrong when we continue to cling to our mistaken truths" (Hartman, 1992).

Integrity, demonstrating honesty and trustworthiness over time, is another important aspect of respectful relationships. Promises made should be kept; options should be identified and openly explored. Integrity demands that the practitioner be direct about his/her role, the degree of authority vested in it, and about the use and limits of that authority. Such parameters must be communicated clearly at the outset of the relationship. Integrity in relationships also requires that when a practitioner does countervene an individual's wishes, the practitioner has an obligation to discuss the action with the individual, providing opportunity to dialogue about reactions, feelings, and alternatives (Surber, 1994).

Ensure that Persons with Psychiatric Disability have a Chance for a Decent Quality of Life

Hope is the belief that things will be better. Hope is important for all of us, but is core to the process of rehabilitation and recovery for persons with psychiatric disabilities. Giving up hope locks people into the cycle of helplessness and victimization which has characterized chronicity of mental illness. People find they are better able to manage their illness or overcome their disability when they have something worth keeping — an apartment, a job, friends, or other elements of life which make it worth living.

The doctrine of informed consent suggests that an individual has understood and evaluated a full range of options before making a decision which might infringe on a personal right. There are both legal and ethical requirements for informed consent. Unfortunately, the principle is often violated in spirit, as well as in actuality. For example, a narrow set of options may be presented, while information about a wider range of options may be withheld, discarded, or ignored. Rooney (1992) suggests that "rather than treating informed consent as pro forma, it should be an opportunity to engage in a collaborative relationship consistent with a therapeutic philosophy of basic respect for all people" (p. 42).

Be Aware of Treatment System Values and How Decisions about Paternalism and Coercion Impact on these Values

We often confuse our means with the ends. Compliance is not the primary intent of the mental health system, but compliance is often taken as evidence of good adjustment or judgment. Taking medication is not an end; it is but one of many means to symptom management, personal growth, recovery, and enhanced quality of life. Sometimes our best intentions are undermined by our means of achieving them. If we feel that medication is an important part of helping an individual achieve a better quality of life over the next few years, then the issue is developing the kind of collaborative relationship which will help the individual discover personal benefits of medication use, or find satisfactory alternatives.

Be Clear About the Purpose and Alternatives to Coercion

It is important to be thoughtful about goals. Any intervention which employs compliance-oriented or court-mandated interventions requires even greater clarity and scrutiny. Too often, compliance-oriented or other coercive interventions are used with little thought to exactly how the intervention will help or its long term implications (Diamond, 1995). It is important to identify and explore alternatives before resorting to more coercive strategies. For example, using reminders such as placing medications next to the coffee jar or other less invasive approaches should be employed before making receipt of personal money contingent upon taking medications. In addition, the time limits on the intervention, the process for review of both the ethics and effectiveness of the intervention, and follow-up interventions should be identified. Reliance on compliance-oriented and coercion strategies precludes the development of more creative, voluntary approaches to meet the same goals (Blanch & Parrish, 1993).

Sundaram (1994) considers choice, compliance and coercion from the perspective of imminent and non-imminent risks of serious harm. In situations with imminent risks of serious harm immediate action should be taken to prevent harm and preserve the situation until other alternatives can be considered. Strategies may include: increase in supervision; protective orders; temporary restraint; involuntary interventions; and surrogate decision-making. If the risk of harm is not imminent, other methods of intervention should be employed, such as: educational efforts about risks and consequences, exploration of alternatives, or development of safeguards.

Develop a Continuous Range of Service Options

Most treatment systems are not designed to proactively help individuals avoid crisis or prevent a hospitalization. The greater the range of options available to a person before, during and after a crisis, the greater the likelihood the individual will be willing to accept one or more of them. Such services should emphasize individually tailored crisis prevention activities and provide flexible, diverse, and "user-friendly" early intervention options (Biss & Curtis, 1993; Blanch & Parrish, 1993; Blanch, 1988). Recognize that what one individual finds coercive or "restrictive" may be not see as such by another. For example, some individuals find long-term hospitalization less coercive than forced medications which may insult bodily integrity.

Consider Advance Directives

There is increasing interest in the concept of advance directives for mental health treatment, sometimes called "health care proxies" or "psychiatric living wills," as a strategy to help balance the concerns of autonomy and paternalism (Hopfensperger, 1992; Lefley, 1992; Rogers & Centifanti, 1991; Rosenson & Kasten, 1991; Levy, 1994). Prearranged at a time of relative stability, these documents are similar to living wills and establish an individual's wishes regarding treatment should their capacity to make these decisions be compromised at a later date. These decisions may include acceptance of, as well as rejection of, specific treatment interventions (including medications), preferences for treatment settings, or consent to notify particular individuals. There are a number of theoretical as well as technical issues involved in advance directives, but more states, consumers, family members, and practitioners are recognizing the potential utility of this approach to help individuals participate meaningfully in their own treatment.

A less formal approach to the psychiatric living will is a crisis plan which can be developed by an individual and practitioner

(Curtis, 1993). The crisis plan may specify individual stressors or "triggers," self-initiated coping strategies and supports, as well as points of intervention and an agreed upon plan of action.

CONCLUSION

Historically, mental health practitioners have assumed that they know what is best for the persons receiving their services. This assumption has been societally sanctioned by their assigned roles as treatment and care giver as well as protector of client and community welfare. Practitioners have held considerable power to influence and even control the lives of the people they serve. This kind of paternalism limits the autonomy of individuals receiving services and implicitly encourages them to settle for stability, rather than growth, by confusing compliance with success.

There are increasing tensions between the value of beneficence which is derived from paternalism and the value of autonomy and self-determination in the mental health system. An individual's right to effective treatment and to refuse treatment can be in conflict with concerns about the ability of the individual to weigh these decisions, particularly during times of psychiatric crisis. The benefits and costs of compliance-oriented and coercive interventions will continue to be argued from various perspectives. The mental health system is confronted by a new set of accountabilities to consumers and the community and our dialogue around these issues increasingly includes discussions about individual rights and personal responsibility.

There is growing recognition of the importance of individual self-determination and autonomy in community service outcomes. Community mental health practice is changing to support greater self-determination and voice by persons with psychiatric disabilities, but these changes are not without difficulties and challenge. Basic questions are being raised about the fundamental balance of power within the mental health system by consumers and practitioners alike. Ethical standards have traditionally provided guidance to practitioners about the use of power in the helping relationships and continue to provide a strong foundation to the field. However, there are many ways in which power is employed in mental health services, ranging from benign and unsolicited support to court-ordered intervention. While the ethics of many aspects of friendly persuasion and self-presentation may be discussed, these approaches are intrinsic aspects of all helping relationships and raise few ethical concerns unless applied in an extreme fashion.

While it is inevitable that influence and overtly coercive intervention will remain part of the mental health system in the foreseeable future, there is increasing knowledge about alternatives to non-consensual treatment. Are non-consensual interventions and coercion fundamentally antithetical to the helping relationship? Can we create new ways of both protecting society and individuals which do not undermine the process of recovery? Consumers and family members are crucial partners in developing these new understandings with the professional community of mental health, medical, and legal practitioners.

With this new knowledge comes the ethical obligation of the system to develop and implement approaches to mental health treatment and support which minimize non-consensual interventions and to forge collaborative treatment alliances which preserve and foster individual self-determination.

REFERENCES

Abramson, M. (1985). The autonomy-paternalism dilemma in social work practice. *Social Casework, 66,* 387–393.

Anthony, W. A. (1993). Recovery from mental illness: the guiding vision of the mental health service system. *Psychosocial Rehabilitation Journal, 16*(4), 11–24.

Ayers, T. D. (1989). Dimensions and characteristics of lay helping. *American Journal of Orthopsychiatry, 59*(2), 215–225.

Barker, P. J., & Baldwin, S. (Eds.) (1991). *Ethical Issues in Mental Health.* New York: Chapman and Hall.

Biss, S. M., & Curtis, L. C. (1993). Crisis services systems: beyond the emergency room. *In Community,* 3:2, 1–4.

Blanch, A-K. (1988). *Final Report of the Vermont Task Force on Community Crisis Options.* Burlington, VT: Trinity College of Vermont, Center for Community Change through Housing and Support.

Blanch, A. K., & Parrish, J. (1993). Reports of three roundtable discussions on involuntary interventions. *Psychiatric Rehabilitation and Community Support Monograph, 1,* 1–42.

Boulding, K. E. (1990). *Three Faces of Power.* Newbury Park, CA: Sage Publications, Inc.

Carling, P. J. (1995). *Return to Community: Building Support Systems for People with Psychiatric Disabilities.* New York: Guildford Press.

Catalano, R., & McConnell, W. (1993). *Do Civil Commitments Reduce Violence in the Community? A Time Series Test.* Berkely, CA: Institute for Mental Health Services Research.

Corey, G., Corey, M. S., & Callanan, P. (1993). *Issues and Ethics in the Helping Professions.* Pacific Grove, CA: Brooks/Cole Publishing.

Chamberlain, J. (1994). The right to be wrong. In Sundaram, C. J. (Ed.) *Choice and Responsibility: Legal and Ethical Dilemmas in Services for Persons with Mental Disabilities.* Albany, NY: New York State Commission on Quality of Care for the Mentally Disabled.

Chamberlain, J. (1978). *On Our Own: Patient controlled alternatives to the mental health System.* New York: McGraw-Hill.

Curtis, L. C. (1993). Crisis prevention: the cornerstone of crisis response. *In Community,* 3:2, 2.

Curtis, L. C., & Hodge, M. (1995). Ethics and boundaries community support services: new challenges. In Stein, L. I., & Hollingsworth, E. J. (Eds.) *New Directions in Mental Health Series. Maturing Mental Health Systems: New Challenges and Opportunities,* San Francisco: Jossey-Bass, 66, 43–61.

Darbyshire, P. (1991). Working with people with a mental handicap. Harker
    P. J., & Baldwin, S. (Eds.) *Ethical Issues in Mental Health*. New York:
    Chapman and Hall.
Deegan, P. E. (1992). The independent living movement and people with
    psychiatric disabilities: taking back control over our own lives. *Psy-
    chosocial Rehabilitation Journal* 15:3, 3–19.
Diamond, R. J. (1983). Enhancing medication use in schizophrenic patients.
    Journal of Clinical Psychiatry, 44:2, 7.
Diamond, R. J. (1995). Coercion and Tenacious Treatment in the Commu-
    nity: applications to the real world. In Stein, L. I., & Hollingsworth,
    E. J. (Eds.) *New Directions in Mental Health Series. Maturing Mental
    Health Systems: New Challenges and Opportunities*, San Francisco:
    Jossey-Bass, 66, 3–18.
Durham, M. L. (1985). Implications of need-for-treatment laws: a study of
    Washington State's involuntary treatment act. *Hospital and Commu-
    nity Psychiatry*, 36:9, 975–977.
Estroff, S. E. (1981). *Making it Crazy: An ethnography of psychiatric clients
    in an American community*. Berkeley, CA: University of California
    Press.
Geller, J. L. (1990). Clinical guidelines for the use of involuntary outpatient
    treatment. *Hospital and Community Psychiatry*, 41:7, 749–755.
Griffin-Francell, C. (1995). Changing the involuntary commitment laws is
    not the answer. *NAMI Advocate*, January/February, 17.
Hartman, A. (1992). In search of subjugated knowledge. *Social Work*, 37:6,
    483–484.
Hasbe T., & McRae, J. (1987). A ten-year study of civil commitments in
    Washington State. *Hospital and Community Psychiatry*, 38:9, 983–987.
Hiday V. A., & Scheid-Cook, T. L. (1989). A follow up of chronic patients
    committed to out-patient treatment. *Hospital and Community Psychia-
    try*, 40, 52–59.
Hopfensperger, J. (1992). Minnesota enacts psychiatric living will. *Counter-
    point*, 8:2, 10.
International Association of Psychosocial Rehabilitation Services (IAPSRS),
    (in press). *Code of Ethics of the International Association of Psychosocial
    Rehabilitation Services*. Columbia, MD: International Association of
    Psychosocial Rehabilitation Services.
Jaffe, D. J. (1995). Change involuntary treatment laws. *NAMI Advocate*,
    January/February, 16.
Kanter, J. (1989). Clinical case management: definition, principles, and
    components. *Hospital and Community Psychiatric*, 40:4, 361–368.
Kisthardt, W. (1992). A strengths model of case management. In Saleeby,
    D. (Ed.) *The Strengths Perspective in Social Work Practice*. New York:
    Longman.
Lebacqz, K. (1985). *Professional Ethics: Power and Paradox*. Nashville, TX:
    Abingdon Press.
Lefley, H. P. (1992). Developing living wills for the seriously mentally ill: an
    important aide when addressing psychiatric emergencies. *The Psychi-
    atric Times, Medicine and Behavior*, May, 7–9.
Levy, R. M. (1994). Involuntary treatment: walking the tightrope between
    freedom and paternalism. In Sundaram, C. J. (Ed.) *Choice and Respon-
    sibility: Legal and Ethical Dilemmas in Services for Persons with Men-
    tal Disabilities*. Albany, NY: New York State Commission on Quality of
    Care for the Mentally Disabled.

McPheeters, H. L. (Ed.) (1980). *Implementing Standards to Assure the Rights of Mental Patients.* DHHS Publication no. (ADM) 80-860. Rockville, MD: National Institute of Mental Health.

Nash, L. (1990). *Good Intentions Aside: A Manager's Guide to Resolving Problems.* Boston, Harvard Business School Press.

National Association of Social Workers (NASW) (1992). *NASW Standards for Social Work Case Management.* Washington, DC: National Association of Social Workers.

Pierce, C. (1994). *Power Equity and Groups or The Group is Loose, Now What Do We Do: A manual for understanding equity and acknowledging diversity.* Lanconia, NH: New Dynamics Publications.

Reamer, F. G. (1982). Paternalism in social work. In Loewenberg F., & Dolgoff, R. *Ethical Decisions for Social Work Practice.* Itasca, IL: F. E. Peacock. 254–268.

Rogers, J. A., & Centifanti, J. B. (1991). Beyond "self-paternalism": response to Rosenson and Kasten. *Schizophrenia Bulletin,* 17:1, 9–14.

Rooney, R. H. (1992). *Strategies for Work with Involuntary Clients.* New York: Oxford University Press.

Rosenbluth, M., Kleinman, I., & Lowy, F. (1995). Suicide: the interaction of clinical and ethical issues. *Psychiatric Services,* 46:9, 919–921.

Rosenson, M. K, & Kasten, A. M. (1991). Another view of automony: arranging for consent in advance. *Schizophrenia Bulletin,* 17:1, 1–7.

Sadoff, R. (1981). Changes in the law have improved treatment of the mentally ill. *Hospitals,* 55:9, 27–32.

Schwartz, H. I., Vigiano, W., & Bezirganian, C. (1988). Autonomy and the right to refuse treatment: patient's attitudes after involuntary medicine. *Hospital and Community Psychiatry,* 39:10, 1049–1054.

Srebnick, D. S. (1992). *Perceived Choice and Success in Community Living for People with Psychiatric Disabilities.* Burlington, VT: Trinity College of Vermont, Center for Community Change through Housing and Support.

Surles, R. C. (1994). Free choice, informed choice, and dangerous choices. In Sundaram, C. J. (Ed.) *Choice and Responsibility: Legal and Ethical Dilemmas in Services for Persons with Mental Disabilities.* Albany, NY: New York State Commission on Quality of Care for the Mentally Disabled.

Sundaram, C. J. (1994). A framework for thinking about choice and responsibility. In Sundaram, C. J. (Ed.) *Choice and Responsibility: Legal and Ethical Dilemmas in Services for Persons with Mental Disabilities.* Albany, NY: New York State Commission on Quality of Care for the Mentally Disabled.

Surber, R. W. (1994). Resolving value conflicts. In Surber, R. W. (Ed.) *Clinical Case Management: A Guide to Comprehensive Treatment of Serious Mental Illness.* Thousand Oaks, CA: Sage Publications.

Tavolaro, K. (1992). Preventative outpatient civil commitment and the right to revuse treatment: can pragmatic realities and constitutional requirements be reconciled? *Med Law, 11,* 249–267.

United Nations Information Center (1948). *Universal Declaration of Human Rights.* Proclaimed by the United Nations General Assembly December 10, 1948. Washington DC: United Nations Information Center.

United Nations Information Center (1992). *Declaration of Principles for the Protection of Mentally Ill person and for the Improvement of Mental Health*

Care. Resolution 46-119, adopted by the United Nations General Assembly December 17, 1991. Washington DC: United Nations Information Center.

Unzicker, R. (1989). On my own: a personal journey through madness and re-emergence. *Psychosocial Rehabilitation Journal, 13*(1), 71–77.

Weiner, B. (1981). A decade of litigation has led to redefinition of patients' rights. *Hospital, 55*:9, 67–70.

Wertheimer, A. (1993). A philosophic examination of coercion for mental health issues. *Behavioral Sciences and the Law, 11,* 239–258.

Wolfensburger, W. (1972). *The Principle of Normalization in Human Services*. Toronto: National Institute.

Wood, W. D., & Swanson, D. A. (1985). Use of outpatient treatment during civil commitment: law and practice in Nebraska. *Journal of Clinical Psychology, 41,* 723–728.

World Federation for Mental Health (1989). *Declaration of Human Rights and Mental Health*. New York: World Health Organization, World Federation for Mental Health, Office of the Secretary General.

Zusman, J. (1985). APA's model commitment law and the need for better mental health services. *Health Services, 36*:9, 978–980.

7

Cultural Diversity in the Treatment Alliance

JAMES MASON

This chapter concerns the culturally competent treatment alliance. The focus includes an overview of terminology, an explanation of why culture is an important consideration in mental health treatment, descriptions of value differences between mainstream and diverse cultures that can breed potential conflict, and implications for providers working with culturally diverse groups. The norms, values, and beliefs manifested by culturally diverse groups that often confound or run counter to mainstream thinking, social learning, and our professional training will be pondered.

The increasing cultural diversity in America requires that greater attention be placed upon cultural differences as they affect the therapeutic process generally and the treatment alliance specifically. Simple client-clinician matches based on race or culture is perhaps a stopgap measure, but not a panacea. While race or culture can be taken into account, racial and cultural identities are not necessarily congruent. The race of the professional is not always reflective of his cultural identity which may still reflect mainstream values (Helms, 1986). There is an acute need to train, recruit, and hire minority workers in the mental health field (Woody, 1991). However, there is still the need for everyone to understand the role culture plays in utilization and delivery of mental health services.

Establishing meaningful treatment alliances is tied to how the clinician views cultural diversity, equity and justice, and how the dominant society can negatively affect the client's life. The clinician must assess the degree to which the client feels safe in discussing personal issues associated with culture or race. The clinician must also be prepared to assess their own knowledge of the client's culture, community and culturally-based strengths, and (real or imagined) cultural or racial barriers in this society. One interesting potential for creating a strong treatment alliance is tied to the mutual rewards of sharing cultural insights, experiences, and perspectives between client and practitioner.

DEFINING TERMS AND TARGET POPULATIONS

Theories and terms for discussing issues of race and culture have not been used consistently (Ponterotto & Casas, 1991; Stanfield & Dennis, 1993). Pinderhughes (1989) notes the term cannot be comprehended without *power* being considered. One classic situation involves women who are not minorities in the United States. However, because they are underrepresented in positions of power and influence they rate protected status. The lack of power proportionate to numbers often results in discriminatory treatment of minority groups (Atkinson & Hackett, 1988).

Dobbins & Skillings (1991) relate that minority often implies less than, smaller than, or inferior. Usage of the term trivializes differences between and within groups, while prompting the tendency to lump all minority populations into one category.

Race is another term that has been difficult to define. Erhlich & Feldman (1977) argue that races are not biologically-defined entities. Instead they are socially-defined; people are classified in an almost arbitrary grab-bag of attributes including (real and imagined) physical features of the individuals, their class, and their ancestors. Often these physical features are associated with social stereotypes that were used as rationale for Western expansion and colonialism, the slave trade, and the genocide of Native Americans (Edson, 1989). This early maligning of racial differences influences our conscious and unconscious thoughts. Dobbins & Skillings (1991) admonish that one should not assume that there is a high correlation between race and culturally specific behaviors. Pinderhughes (1989) notes that although the meaning of race is ambiguous in people's minds, it is understood as a measure of cultural differences.

The most commonly used characteristics to distinguish races of people include pigmentation, head form, nasal index, lip form, facial index, stature, and the color distribution and texture of body hair (Simpson & Yinger, 1985). However, it has been suggested that there are many more similarities than differences among races (Binkley, 1989) and more differences within the existing categories than between them (Atkinson, Morten, & Sue; 1979). Unfortunately, much of the historic and even contemporary racial research has served to uphold the status quo, leading d'Ardenne and Mahtani (1990) to suggest that in everyday terminology *race* usually refers to skin color and is typically a negative term. Race in the context of this discussion refers specifically to four major groups of color in the United States, namely: African Americans, Asian and Pacific Islander Americans, Hispanic or Latino-Americans, and Native Americans or American Indians.

Race is still a very emotionally-laden concept in the United States. One critical consideration in establishing a culturally competent treatment alliance concerns the clinician's understanding of the history of racial dynamics in this country. Greater awareness in understanding the social histories and experiences of diverse racial groups in both American and global contexts will promote a healthy alliance because the clinician is more in touch with the barriers and frustrations encountered by clients.

Culture is easier to define if not harder to measure. Often used as a euphemism for race, culture refers to a social group's institutions, language, values, religious beliefs, patterns and styles of thought, artistic products, and patterns of social and interpersonal relationships. Green (1982) explains culture as a person's history, traditions, values, and social organizations that affect all human interactions and encounters.

Cultures arguably grow out of a social group's *world view.* World views impact how a cultural group generally behaves (Sue & Sue, 1990). Ibrahim (1985) describes world view as a "philosophy of life" that influences social, cultural, environmental, philosophical, and psychological dimensions. People of color have experienced racism and other forms of oppression which pervade their views of the world, but generally their world views emanate from the more traditional, less modern (i.e., non-urban), sociocentric societal ethic. While world views are hard to assess, clinicians should take time to note how the European perspective differs from the non-European perspective. This will simplify an understanding that may prevent unmanageable value conflicts. Being more aware of the world views of the four groups of color will help in making determinations between which aspects of behavior are adaptive in a normative manner and those that are culturally maladaptive.

Ethnicity is the connection between a group of people based on commonalities (such as religion, nationality, region, etc.) where specific cultural patterns are shared and transmitted to create a common history (Pinderhughes, 1989). Race takes on an ethnic dimension when and if members of a group have evolved specific ways of living. Ultimately, ethnic values and practices uphold the survival of the group while contributing to its cohesiveness.

While focusing on the four *cultural groups of color* in the United States one must not overlook other diverse groups. *Non-ethnic cultural groups* must also be acknowledged and include women, people with disabilities, elders, and gays and lesbians (Atkinson & Hackett, 1988). Non-ethnic cultural groups may also include groups such as the homeless, street youth and gang members, religious minorities, the poor, and even lefthanders.

Recent efforts to promote what is loosely described as cultural diversity in human services can culminate in a blending of cultural groups of color and non-ethnic cultural groups. This is done to create an all encompassing service delivery specifically, and to promote equity and justice generally. While this is noble, it blurs understanding about common areas of vulnerability and does not promote understanding the differences between cultural groups.

Emphasis must be placed upon how individuals representing cultural groups are vulnerable in the American context. It is important to remember that groups of color are not at risk in society in the same ways as non-ethnic minorities. For example, a non-ethnic minority when white can still benefit from or buy into white privilege or other prevailing paradigms (Hacker, 1992). Sensitivity to or even probing group-specific vulnerabilities should aid in establishing a strong treatment alliance.

INATTENTION TO CULTURE AS A BARRIER

In the rush to meet the demand for services, culture is often taken for granted, avoided, or overlooked in relation to establishing a strong treatment alliance. Because American society is rapidly increasing in cultural and racial diversity, taking the time to explore cultural issues has never been more important. Culture is a predominant factor in shaping how people view the world, their history and destiny, and their relationship to all that they know (Green, 1982; Cross, Bazron, Dennis, & Isaacs, 1989; Sue & Sue, 1990). Pinderhughes (1989) describes how culture shapes a group's perspectives about: relationships among individuals, the family, and the social system; the value orientations of the individual, family, subgroup, and social system; the geographical setting; and the interpenetration of all these systems and processes that operate in a reverberating and reciprocal manner.

Culture can often be obscure to many in the dominant culture. Dominant culture is propagated institutionally, therefore, members of the dominant society may feel as if they have no culture. Yet, the dominant culture is alive and well despite reports to the contrary. It is widely reflected in this society's views of time, nature, family, art, food and food preparation, holidays, clothing, language, laws, traditions, and social protocol. When culture is *institutionalized*, it is pervasive (i.e., mainstream), less openly visible, and self-sustaining. It is not important for mainstream people to convey culture, nor is necessary for them to actively oppress other cultures — this can occur institutionally as well. Inactivity by default perpetuates the status quo.

Jones (1988) argues that when bias is institutional its elimination is more complicated and its impact more pernicious. Institutions can create discriminatory outcomes whether they do so intentionally or not. In relating this view to the cultural oppression of African Americans, Jones (1988) points out how the dominant culture has the power to define difference as deficient, and to reinforce conformity to prevailing standards as essential aspects of cultural racism. In essence bias becomes endemic to a society and needs no conscious effort on the part of individuals to sustain. Two basic yet important admonitions emerge from this notion: (1) clinicians should not view diverse culture as deficient, and (2) clinicians should expect diverse clients to conform to the dominant culture.

Jones (1988) lists four recommendations for addressing cultural racism that have application to the development of culturally competent treatment alliances and enhancing cross-cultural interactions. First, one needs to examine diverse cultures evolving and adapting to discrimination and disadvantage; the strengths and ultimate coping skills therein may reflect a wider range of capabilities. Second, learn what culturally diverse communities have and can contribute to society with respect to commonly held problems and goals. Third, identify or develop opportunities in which majority and non-majority perspectives can be shared in order to develop a broader sense of cultural awareness and sensitivity. And, fourth, develop a perspective that does not stigmatize minority populations in relation to the dominant community. Ignoring culture can represent cultural oppression for the client and ultimately preclude a (strong) treatment alliance.

GENERAL AWARENESS OF CULTURE AND CULTURAL DIVERSITY

Limited awareness about one's own culture puts professionals at risk when working across cultures. It is hard to consider one's own culturally-based beliefs and behaviors in a vacuum. Professionals who lack cultural self-awareness will have a hard time discerning culture in others and can easily adopt (knowingly or not) a *culturally absolutist* perspective (i.e., the professional views his or her own culture as universally-relevant). Cultural diversity is not valued when the eradication of culturally diverse beliefs and behaviors is the primary focus of the therapeutic interaction (Ho, 1992). In this scenario, despite multicultural rhetoric, difference is treated as a deficit (Green, 1982; Sue & Sue, 1990; Pinderhughes, 1989; Lum, 1992).

Professionals must resist viewing diverse cultural groups solely in terms of the attributed stereotypes and cultural deficits. To do so, clinicians must be able to discern culturally- and community-based strengths when working with culturally diverse clients and communities. For example, professionals should look for coping and problem solving abilities, interpersonal skills, and other positive attributes in clients (Lum, 1992). Within diverse communities, strengths might include: natural helpers and helping networks of support, extended families, spirituality, group esteem and survival, as well as other culturally-affirming characteristics. This helps remind practitioners that some problematic behaviors are the client's or community's attempt to deal with the complexities of minority status. The ability to identify these and other strategies that people use to cope with low cultural group status and other harsh conditions are a way of respecting the diverse client and community.

Ultimately there are numerous frictions between cultures that continually tug at the treatment alliance. Practitioners must explicitly empower the client to speak out at inadvertent slights or clinician behaviors that they view as culturally or racially offensive. Following are several barriers to better understanding of cultural differences which can threaten a positive treatment alliance. This short list is not exhaustive, but represents a few of the areas where cultural differences exist that can cause conflict.

SERVICE HISTORY AS A BARRIER

People of color have faced historic and contemporary discrimination in social services beginning as early as the colonial days (Lum, 1992) continuing to the present (Knitzer, 1982; Cross et al., 1989; Green, 1982). There have been dubious medical and social experiments using people of color (Edson, 1989) which have made many communities skeptical of trusting social and human service professionals. Such research resulted in few (if any) improvements to the quality of life of the subjects. This prompts a reticence on the part of diverse populations to access services willingly. This hesitance can be viewed as paranoid behavior on the part of groups of color. Sue & Sue (1990) coin the term *paranorm*, which they perceive as adaptive and healthy rather than dysfunctional and pathological, suggesting its absence is more indicative of pathology than its presence. Certainly it is ιιι the best interest of both the client and the treatment alliance to help consumers of color to be better self-advocates around service delivery.

SOCIAL LEARNING AS A BARRIER

Few professionals have been specifically trained to consider cultural differences in treating mental health disorders and much of our social learning has negatively predisposed us to diversity. Metaphorically speaking, the intellectual hard drives of many professionals (as with most Americans) have been configured in ways that cause us to view racial and cultural diversity through a negative lens. Formal training and social learning creates much of the distrust, animosity, and even xenophobia. Typically this form of learning emanates from parents, teachers, clergy, story books, movies, jokes, and myths, making our exposure to such stimuli almost ubiquitous. Thus, reconfiguring our intellectual and emotional hard drives may be difficult. The myths, pseudo-scientific findings, contemporary media images, and even the lexicon regarding people of color, the poor, women, and other protected groups have hardened our psyches. Bias awareness, anti-discrimination, and other cultural awareness and diversity training models which are becoming widely available may be requisites for working cross culturally.

EMERGENCE OF THE PATHOLOGY PERSPECTIVE

Many people who have undergone a social science education have been exposed to subtle forms of bias. Coining the phrase *scientific racism* Thomas & Sillen (1972) point out how evidence used to support conclusions of inferiority were often fabricated to support white norms and standards. Erhlich & Feldman (1977) allude to early racial theory which asserted the genetic deficiencies in people of color. Examples include Darwin (1859) who posited the intellectual superiority of Europeans and genetic inferiority of non-European races; Galton (1869) viewed Africans as half-wits who made simple, childish mistakes, and Jews as physically and mentally inferior and designed as parasites on other nations; or, Gossett (1963) who attempted to show people of color as having more animalistic sensory systems which were less reflective and deliberate in thought than Europeans. These early theories influenced the social science knowledge base in a way that will take generations to overcome.

During the tumultuous civil rights and nationalistic movements of the 60's and the 70's such themes were revisited. Scientists asserted the intellectual inferiority of people of color (African Americans) in particular. Seemingly dead, this argument resurfaced in the 90's, implying helping groups of color was a losing proposition because their inherent problems were perhaps endemic. While the genetic model fell from grace, it was replaced by the cultural deficit model. The cultural deficit idea produced such terms as the *culture of poverty* (Banfield, 1974); *matriarchy of the black family* (Moynihan, 1965); and *the underclass*, (Wilson, 1978b). Although the assaults upon diverse cultures had early roots, it is reincarnated in various or sundry motifs today.

One backlash to increasing diversity that reduces anxiety when communicating cross culturally is *political correctness*. This approach to diversity is perhaps at best one of avoidance or at least minimization of conflict. In this scheme one is more interested in reducing what may be perceived as an intercultural offense, without any significant change in personal, professional, or organizational behavior. Thus, it is possible to be politically correct yet behaviorally bankrupt. In such a context, the treatment alliance may never be established or will only be superficial because the clinician may be respectful more out of anxiety than out of understanding for the individual. Worse, if the client finds out, he or she is being placated, the alliance might be doomed forever.

Another approach to diversity is to acknowledge cultural differences vis-a-vis mundane cultural manifestations (e.g., food, clothing, music, art). This approach pays very little attention to understanding culturally diverse belief systems and behaviors. While appreciating surface culture may be easier, more knowledge is needed with individual clients to include culturally-based views of human nature, technology, male-female relationships, humanity's relationship to nature, the nature of humanity, and other sublime foundations upon which cultural behavior is based (Sue & Sue, 1990).

INCREASING DIVERSITY AND PROFESSIONAL TRAINING

The American society is becoming increasingly more diverse. Between 1970 and 1980 the number of African Americans increased by 17.6% (22.6 million to 26.5 million), the Hispanic population grew 61% from 9.1 to 14.6 million, Asian Americans expanded by 126%, growing from 1.5 to 3.5 million, and Native Americans increased 71% from .8 million to 1.4 million (U.S. Bureau of the Census, 1987). Early in the next century people of color will not be a minority. As early as 2010, children of color may outnumber children of European descent. This is due to both natural increase (Ponterotto & Casas, 1991), and migration of people from foreign countries (Lum, 1992). Serving these populations effectively will be important. Ethics, economics, and politics aside, professionals will find it important to prepare for cultural competence.

The rationale for cultural competence training for mental health professionals can include the underutilization of services by culturally diverse populations (Lum, 1992); the training of mental health and other human service professionals which often ignores culture (Lefley & Pedersen, 1986); the lack of a diverse work force precluding a critical mass of key cultural informants; the premature termination of services (Flaskerud, 1986); and the fact that many non-mainstream racial and cultural groups are typically viewed in terms of stereotypes or pathologies.

Establishing cross cultural treatment alliances is not a requirement in many accredited programs (Pinderhughes, 1989). Training at the professional and graduate levels rarely take diverse cultures into account (Draguns, 1981; Green, 1982; Cross et al., 1989; Lum, 1992) and is based on the Western European social-cultural framework from which it arises (Sue & Sue, 1990). The issue is not so much that the client or professional must change their personal orientation to mental health treatment or the world, but that they be aware of and respect the views of each other. The inadvertent or unwitting imposition of dominant culture belief systems regarding psychopathology and psychotherapy is likely where much of the problem is based.

THE SOCIAL CLIMATE

One critical factor in any therapeutic encounter is the therapist-patient relationship. This relationship is best seen as an unconscious, unspoken commitment by both therapist and patient to stick together while forces against a positive union may be emerging. Racial and cultural tensions at the societal level are major threats to intercultural treatment alliances. While treatment may continue nicely, it can be stalled by something happening in the community, region, or nation that can strain or even dissolve the relationship.

Cultural values and beliefs must be comprehended in the context of a given community. For example, the historic patterns of ethnic and racial enclaves in America represent perhaps the cultural value of group welfare, but they must be also viewed in terms of the almost universal discrimination in real estate and lending practices. Similarly, the concentration of people of color with lower education attainment in lower paying jobs represents deficits (historic and contemporary) and is a legacy of longstanding biases in various American institutions. The death, infant mortality, and life expectancy rates for people of color suggest that health care institutions also reflect a pattern of discrimination. In the context of culturally competent treatment alliances the professional must be aware of how societal deficits (even when known) can create deep rifts between the client and the provider. Being unaware of such factors can preclude, retard, or truncate the progression of a strong treatment alliance.

WITHIN AND BETWEEN-GROUP DIFFERENCES

Any discussion of diversity must contain the caveat: pay attention to both between and within-group differences. In the rush to reconfigure our metaphoric intellectual and emotional hard drives pertaining to cultural diversity, we must be vigilant in recognizing that great variations exist within any culture. One must avoid trading old stereotypes for new ones. Culture can be seen as a starting point that should lead to more probing of individual differences among culturally diverse clients. Examining the various manifestations of within-group diversity provides many opportunities for the client and therapist to share views and develop the alliance.

Pinderhughes (1989) identifies several key dimensions within which individual differences may emerge: race, religion, ideology, nationality, ethnicity, appearance, body structure, behavior style, sex, age, size, family constellation, occupation, and socioeconomic class. Other factors include spatial differences (urban-rural), ethnoregional distinctions (from the South, Midwest, etc.), sexual orientation, language, cultural identity, and others. Professionals should not see the client as a demographic statistic or a cultural value but rather acknowledge traits or patterns and attempt to discern to what degree the client is affected (if at all). Assuming that someone grew up in poverty, did not speak (standard) English in the home, resided in a broken home, lived in an ethnic enclave, had low self-esteem, was on welfare, had few if any role models, or struggled in a culture of poverty will probably lead to trouble. Professionals must avoid falling into the deficit views of cultural and racial diversity, by having or developing some notion of group-specific strengths and related value orientations.

When encountering the client of diverse background, one must take the opportunity to assess the cultural orientation. Shirking from this responsibility may create more harm than harmony. Assessing cultural orientation is also good practice with the (mythical) mainstream population. White clients are often considered "culture-less". Perhaps this view may change with more East European migration to the United States. The point is that one must begin to routinize assessment of culture as a variable when establishing the treatment alliance and in the treatment process with all clients.

CULTURAL VALUES

Psychopathology is defined, diagnosed and assessed, and intervention approaches are based on European culture, values, norms, and beliefs. However new culturally-based theories are emerging regarding the definition and etiology of illness and health (Green, 1982; Lum, 1992; Ho, 1987, 1992) help-seeking behaviors (Green, 1982; Neighbors & Taylor, 1985), use of natural supports and the religious community (Cross et al., 1989; Gary, 1987), and what are relevant services (Zane, Sue, Castro & George, 1982).

It is important to assess the degree to which a client follows tradition in terms of adherence to cultural norms, their views of mental health and illness, their idea of relevant and timely treatment, and the value placed on cultural or racial identity. Occasionally, self-disclosure by the clinician is one way to expedite trust and promote the alliance. When comfortable and secure, clients will share their beliefs on cultural subtleties such as their view of human nature, technology, the environment, adult-child relations, ties to their racial/cultural community, extent and use of extended family, and other issues.

In establishing culturally competent treatment alliances it will be important for clinicians to become familiar with their own cultural perspectives and that of the organizations for whom they work. Examining culture in isolation is difficult. More important, cultural self-awareness helps the professional reign in their own beliefs and values so that they are not imposed upon or presumed to exist in others.

People and Nature Relationships

In the Western culture there is an emphasis on controlling nature. A person is seen as able to control his or her destiny. Therapists operating from this framework believe problems are solvable, and that both client and professional must take an active role in solving the problem through manipulation and control (Sue & Sue, 1990).

Ho (1987) viewed people of color as valuing harmony with nature or saw themselves as a part of nature. In this framework, life events are tied to fate, destiny, or the nature of world or life. The well-intended therapist operating on a Western notion of cause and effect who attempts to reorder the client's fate or karma may be viewed as inconsistent if not antagonistic with cultural beliefs. Potential strains to the alliance include unilateral, unexplained or non-consensual efforts to change family patterns, cultural or racial community ties, or relationships to mainstream norms. The goal is to help the client function better, but also function better within their own cultural and personal prerogatives. Modeling via cultural and racial heroes, or obtaining the support of relevant family members, cultually-sanctioned helpers and leaders should add credibility to the intervention.

Time Orientation

To many people around the world Western culture appears obsessed with time. Western beliefs emphasize the future (Katz, 1985; Ho, 1987; 1992). Time is viewed in the Western framework as a commodity that can be wasted. Ho (1987) posits that African Americans and Native Americans value a present time orientation, Asian Americans and Hispanic Americans value a present-past time orientation. This seemingly minor cultural difference between mainstream and non-mainstream values can create a conflict with respect to length of time for the intervention to produce change and the client's notion of being on time for appointments.

For some clinicians this will require breaking long term plans into incremental steps (or goals) so that the client's sense of time is operationalized. Otherwise, either the client or professional may feel things are going too slow or too fast. Thus, collaboration and reaching consensus about the pace of treatment and the concrete outcomes will prove important. Moreover, the therapist can share the values associated with mainstream perspective of time (e.g., savings, long range planning, etc.) with diverse clients as an added tool or resource, or even as an insight to mainstream culture.

Another potential conflict related to time orientation is manifest with respect to meeting appointment times. When the client shows up late, the professional can easily construe this tardiness as disrespect or insincerity when often no such slight was intended. The inevitable reprimand can cause a rift because the client does not understand why the professional is upset. In establishing a strong treatment alliance and providing treatment, it becomes important to share cultural views of time. This can be a safe entry point for establishing ground rules, the initial relationship, and the subsequent treatment alliance. For one, the professional can assess whether the client distinguishes when to use (or not) a mainstream or more traditional time orientation. One can begin to wonder with the client if they are aware of this duality. This is an important way of stressing to the client the importance of developing bicultural skills.

Individualism

The Western culture value orientation holds high regard for individualism and competition (Katz, 1985; Lefley & Pedersen, 1986; Pedersen, 1988). The individual is the typical target of the intervention, has primary responsibility for his or her actions, is highly valued for their independence, and is internally controlled and directed. While this behavioral characteristic is viewed as culturally normative and as healthy in American society, this seemingly universal value is not so universal. How the client views such a seemingly mundane value as individualism is rarely considered. Sue and Sue (1990) argue that racial groups of color in the United States value interdependence and stress cooperation over competition in their relationships with people.

Within the Western framework the family is defined as nuclear. In communities of color the family can have extended, intergenerational, and even fictive components. The family or group take precedent over the individual (Green, 1982; Sue & Sue, 1990; Ho, 1987, 1992; Pinderhughes, 1989; Lum, 1992; Hines & Boyd-Franklin, 1982; Inclan, 1985). Traditional Asian culture emphasizes the importance of the family even with regard to cherished ancestors. Traditional African culture stresses the collective over the singular person, which combined with the universal experience of racism and oppression has resulted in kinship bonds within the African American community that have generated extensive informal networks of support. In many Hispanic families the individual is obligated first to the family, preferences are afforded to family members over more objective criteria. Among Native Americans the tribe or clan can take precedence.

What seem normative family relations to many cultural groups of color can appear as enmeshed to the mainstream. In cultural groups of color the individual often comes second to the collective (e.g., the family, community, clan, or tribe). Establishing a better treatment alliance and empowering the client of color requires determining how the client views him or herself in the context of his or her social group. To suggest behaviors that inadvertently estrange the client from their social collective may be initially well-received but can result in cultural isolation or estrangement from potential or existing natural networks of support.

Communication Styles and Languages

Another area that jeopardizes establishing a sound treatment alliance concerns communication. One obvious issue being the language barrier. Even when English is the client's primary language there may still be issues of dialect, communication style, and variations in language. For example, the dialect and affect let alone the words and phrases used in traditional African American communities can confuse the clinician. Communication is often marked by affect, gestures, humor, and passion. What is credible communication in some communities will be questioned in others. The conflicts that can arise around appropriate expression of anger, happiness, disappointment, or other emotions can vary by group. Imposing meaning or snap inferences are to be avoided.

Forcing people who do not use mainstream English as their primary language to use standard language can be offensive. It may also cause a loss of esteem, generate a sense of shame or loss of face, have them appear as slow or dull-witted, or make them less comfortable while not necessarily making them a more effective speaker. Prompting the client to pursue standard English as a useful survival tool, and the appropriate contexts of its use (or not) is more appropriate in preparing the client for a multicultural world. Having them share the language or teach you a different language or dialect is probably more respectful and builds on or promotes the client's sense of mastery.

Intercultural communication skills are critical because many therapeutic interventions rely on verbal interaction to build rapport, collect information, and negotiate treatment planning and service delivery. Often a person's intelligence is judged by his ability to communicate using standard English. Therefore, it may be easier to view people of color as inferior, lacking in cognitive skills, or having blunted affect when they feel compelled to speak in an unnatural or foreign dialect (standard English). If the client tries to save face with clipped or shortened responses, the therapist can infer resistance or noncompliance on the patient's behalf. Sue & Sue (1990) suggest that effective therapy relies on the ability of both the client and clinician to send and receive both verbal and nonverbal messages accurately and correctly. The temptation to discern meaning based on use of language or communication style is dangerous. For example, the black dialect is often described as animated, affective, interpersonal, even confrontational. One dominant stereotype, of which many African Americans are well aware, describes the angry, hostile, black male. The assertion that black males are angry is often based on the language (style and content) that black males use. The treatment alliance is jeopardized when African Americans speaking frankly, in the traditional dialect and style are perceived as a threat. Another example is Asians' indirect style of communication, lack of direct eye contact, deference to authority, and restraint in voicing problems which may invoke erroneous notions of the sneaky or deceitful Asian.

In Western culture the client is expected to openly reveal their feelings and problems, this is less likely among traditional Asian Americans who may feel silence is virtue, or other groups who do not share personal information unless a relationship exists. Native Americans, utilizing turns at talk, indirect eye contact, and much longer pauses between sentences can be viewed in a negative light. Communication is the key to creating a strong therapeutic alliance; insight as to what is culturally normative communication within a given culture is required.

Sue & Sue (1990) admonish that professionals reared in a white middle-class society may assume that certain behaviors or rules of communication are universal. This cultural imposition may threaten the alliance. Therefore an important agreement to make is that if either party is unaware of what is being conveyed, insulted by what has been said, or is otherwise confused about the conversation, then this should be addressed immediately.

Since effective communication is a key component of an effective treatment alliance, therapists must have the ability to understand diverse cultural lexicons. Therapists often feign comprehension in the hope that the culturally diverse client will continue to communicate even though the therapist lacks real understanding. Green (1982) advocates a method in which the client is a cultural guide for the therapist. In this scheme, the patient guides the clinician through a variety of experiences that would otherwise be misconstrued. He suggests that the clinician should inquire about cover terms (i.e., vernacular and concepts alien to the interviewer) that can appear in every sentence. Thus, when slang, idioms, colloquialisms, and phrases (*cover terms*) emerge that elude the clinician, there exists a mechanisim to aid the clinincian in making the client's lexicon comprehensible. For example, an African American male client refers to his *homeys, the crib, the hood,* or *one-time* and the therapist's eyes glaze over. In this instance, if the professional pretends to understand and the client senses this the treatment alliance is ultimately jeopardized. It is also important in this process to inform the client that he or she is in essence a cultural guide, implying that the client has mastery and leadership in at least this respect. Moreover, it reveals to the client that the nature of the relationship is mutually beneficial and that the client has some strengths upon which others may be built. Equally important, the clinician should explore in depth with the consumer, the "covered" meanings of cover terms and their subsequent *attributions* (i.e., characteristics attached to the cover terms). Often due to mainstream professionals' newness to culturally diverse lexicons and continued negative portrayals of many diverse racial and cultural groups, attributions associated with cover terms and other slang may appear negative. Another approach to decoding cover terms which may be less conspicuous is by noting cover terms and then in natural pauses in the conversation revisiting the term to clarify its meaning. This approach to intensive interviewing helps to assure honest communication. Green also suggests that, "carefully prepared information on client values, behaviors, and preferences — information that is continuously checked and rechecked in client encounters — is basic to effective service delivery. Anything less means the workers function in ignorance of what is really happening in the lives of their clients" (p. 81)

CONCLUSIONS

There is simply too much to learn in a lifetime to think that one will be impervious to cross-cultural mistakes. There are many areas where conflicting values may clash. The evolution of culture is affected by the larger scheme of events and because it is generally dynamic, one never gets a total and permanent grasp. Therefore, one must be prepared to make mistakes, apologize and learn so that cultural errors are less likely to be committed in future relationships.

Ultimately culture will become more manifest in times to come. Cultural competence is generally defined as the ability to work in the context of cultural differences. Various models will emerge to facilitate cross cultural service delivery. One recent iteration is the cultural competence model (Cross, et. al, 1989). This model acknowledges culture as a factor in how people define health and illness, perceive and utilize relevant services and credible providers, and identify or solve problems. One goal inherent in the cultural competence model is to begin taking culture into consideration when providing social, human, and health services. Another important feature of the cultural competence model is that it is developmental. This implies that cultural competence is a process and not a product. One can become more competent over time with training and commitment.

Several principles of the cultural competence model that can be applied to the notion of cross cultural treatment alliances are described:

Valuing of Diversity

This principle implies that one must begin to develop positive ways to view diversity. One must be able to discern the inherent assets associated with the notion itself, as well as be able to identify and value the cultural strengths inherent in each group. This is important for two basic reasons: (1) to find something positive in the client's life and affect upon which other positives can be anchored; and (2) to offset much of the negative imagery propagated that influence how groups are defined in American society.

Valuing diversity can be manifested in various ways. One way may be via bias-awareness or anti-bias training activities. Activities such as identifying cultural and racial predispositions, identifying areas of conflicting cultural values, or illuminating the societal and cultural barriers one's clients are likely to encounter are important steps to valuing diversity. The goal is to set a foundation for positively viewing diverse groups. Other ways include re-designing office or work spaces to reflect a value for diversity (e.g., art, artifacts, books), developing personal libraries and resource materials, and creating a list of cross-cultural resources and events that can be culturally informative. The idea is to learn about the diverse perspectives of the world without stigmatizing differences, and to offset residual stigma.

Conducting the Cultural Self-Assessment

This principle stresses the importance of knowing one's own culture, the culture of their organization, and the culture of the community at large. It is often suggested that one must know oneself as an entry point to understanding others. The emphasis is upon knowing what values are important in ones own life and how those may clash or mesh with other groups. For example, if one values independence it is important to know that this is not universal. One goal is to avoid imposing culture upon others. The organizational culture must also be examined. Examples would include how the organization: defines 'amily; perceives time; recruits, hires, and promotes diverse individuals; or even, views human nature. Or in many cases, simply if the organization acknowledges or ignores culture as a factor in people's lives.

Fortunately there are many self-assessment tools that deal with issues such as racial, gender, and cultural bias. These may facilitate understanding the cultural foundations, histories, and the evolutionary processes in cultures undergo in a multicultural society. These curriculum may enable individuals to more clearly distinguishing myth and stereotypes from accurate perspectives of diversity. The ability to be respectful of someone's culture is critical in establishing cross-cultural treatment alliances.

Understanding the Dynamics of Difference

This principle is concerned with comprehending what happens when people of diverse backgrounds come together. Trust issues in particular must be understood. Often consumers will presume of the professional and vice versa. One area of concern involves client-practitioner differences, including implied power differentials and professional lexicon-client jargon. Often unspoken, such differences can be headed off when better understood.

Race (color), culture, gender, educational attainment, income, age, physical ability, religion, professional affiliation, even political outlooks present other major differences between and within groups. Multiple affiliations often exist within both the client and the professional. Other factors include culturally-prescribed patterns concerning greeting protocol, physical space (proxemics), gesture and affect (kinesics), and experiences. These and other issues of difference might be probed as an aspect of therapy, but certainly have implication for building a sound treatment alliance.

ACCESS TO CULTURAL KNOWLEDGE

This principle regards the professional's access or opportunity to learn about cultural diversity as it applies to the helping process. Implicit in this principle is the notion that professionals may need insights into culturally-normed diagnostic and treatment approaches, culturally competent interviewing and treatment planning strategies, even issues of cultural awareness.

Publications are increasing that address cultural competence and cultural diversity. Thus one source of information will be the theoretical and research literature. There are also other media formats (typically audiotape and videotapes, and monographs) that may be helpful. Many local colleges and universities offer classes or lectures concerning diversity. Community- and culturally-based advocacy groups and organizations may be a resource, and ethnic and women's studies programs in systems of higher learning should be considered. Other resources may include neighborhood associations, community forums, and cultural holidays, ceremonies, and places of worship. Professionals may seek to develop a list of cultural key informants who can be consulted to help distinguish cultural issues and which behaviors are culturally normative and which behaviors are culturally maladaptive. Being able to pick up the phone and ask questions and get answers will prove extremely valuable. It is imperative that professionals inventory their professional and social networks to identify cultural groups that are not represented. While it may not be a simple matter to establish this community network (due to inherent divisions in American society) once it is operative, the professional will find that the benefits greatly outweigh the expense of not having accessible cultural informants.

ADAPTATION TO DIVERSITY

This represents the actual changes professionals and systems might make to enhance cross cultural service delivery and to build culturally competent treatment alliances. This implies that the professional will need to make benign distinctions between individuals as a means of identifying problems and potential solutions of both an intrapsychic and environmental nature. Such adaptations may include spending more time to develop a relationship, using self-disclosure or modeling as a way of eliciting certain behaviors from the client, adopting ethnographic or other humanistic approaches to interviewing and gathering data, providing transportation or other supports, even making allowances for family or significant others' involvement in the treatment and treatment planning process.

Changes may need to occur at the attitudinal, practice, policy, and structural levels. One size does not fit all. The objective is to individualize services by taking culture, race, and other characteristics into account in providing mental health services.

There is no single approach to working, providing therapy, or even establishing treatment alliances cross culturally. The professional will need to be flexible, eclectic, and ultimately open to learning, accepting, respecting, and positively using cultural differences. The professional must also assume no guilt in being less knowledgeable than he or she would like. The professional's education (formal and informal), American culture and experiences, and the media have played a large role in obscuring the understanding of difference.

Finally, one must prepare to make mistakes along the way and to learn from the errors. Professionals must also take advantage of numerous opportunities for learning about cultural differences. One vastly overlooked resource in this equation are the consumers. Particularly when consulted during exit interviews, focus groups, surveys or other means they can provide information that is quite revealing. Civic and community events, places of worship, and community celebrations and holidays provide great opportunities for learning. The lessons learned can be applied to establishing a treatment alliance.

Culture is a factor in the helping process. When overlooked, minimized, or disrespected the treatment alliance can be threatened. When culture is acknowledged and adapted in conjunction with ways that the consumer finds respectful, the development of the treatment alliance and consequently the delivery and impact of mental health treatment will be mutually beneficial.

REFERENCES

Atkinson, D. R., & Hackett, G. (Eds.). (1988). *Counseling non-ethnic American minorities.* Springfield, IL: Charles C. Thomas.

Atkinson, D. R., Morten G., & Sue, D. W. (1979). *Counseling American minorities: A cross-cultural perspective.* Dubuque, IA: William C. Brown.

Banfield, E. C. (1974). *The unheavenly city revisited.* Boston: Little Brown.

Binkley, K. M. (1989). *Racial traits of American blacks.* Springfield, IL: Charles C. Thomas.

Cross, T. L., Bazron, B. J., Dennis, K. W., & Isaacs, M. R. (1989). *Towards a culturally competent system of care.* Washington, DC: Georgetown University Child Development Center, CASSP Technical Assistance Center.

d'Ardenne, P., & Mahtani, A. (1990). *Transcultural counseling in action.* London: Sage Publications.

Darwin, C. (1859). *On the origin of species by natural selection.*

Dobbins, J. E., & Skillings, J. H. (1991). The utility of race labeling in understanding cultural identity. A conceptual tool for the social science practitioner. *Journal of Counseling and Development, 70,* 37–44.

Draguns, J. G. (1981). *Cross-cultural counseling and psychotherapy.* New York: Pergamon.

Edson, C. H. (1989). Barriers to multiculturalism: Historical perspectives on culture and character in American society. *Coalition Quarterly 6*(2&3), 3–9.

Ehrlich, P. R., & Feldman, S. S. (1977). *The race bomb. Skin color, prejudice and intelligence.* New York: Quandrangle/The New York Times Book Co.

Flaskerud, J. H. (1986). The effects of cultura-compatible intervention on the utilization of mental health services by minority clients. *Community Mental Health Journal, 22*(2), 127–141.

Galton, F. (1869). *Hereditary genius.* New York: MacMillan.

Gary, L. E. (1987). Religion and mental health in an urban Black commmunity. *Urban Research Review, 11*(2), 5–7.

Gibbs, J. T., & Huang, L. N. (1989). *Children of color. Psychological interventions with minority youth.* San Francisco: Jossey-Bass.

Gossett, T. F. (1963). *Race: The history of an idea in America.* Dallas: Southern Methodist University Press.

Green, J. W. (Ed.). (1982). *Cultural awareness in the human services.* Englewood Cliffs, NJ: Prentice-Hall, Inc.

Hacker, A. (1992). Two nations. Black and white, separate, hostile, unequal. New York: Ballantine Books.

Helms, J. E. (1986). Expanding racial identity theory to cover counseling process. *Journal of Counseling Psychology, 33,* 62–64.

Hines, P., & Boyd-Franklin, N. (1982). Black families. In M. McGoldrick (Ed.), *Ethnicity and family therapy.* New York: Guildford.

Ho, M. K. (1992). *Minority children and adolescents in therapy.* New York: Sage Publications.

Ho, M. K. (1987). *Family therapy with ethnic minorities.* New York: Sage Publications.

Ibrahim, F. A. (1985). Effective cross-cultural counseling and psychotherapy: A framework. *The Counseling Psychologist, 13,* 625–638.

Inclan, J. (1985). Variations in value orientations in mental health work with Puerto Ricans. *Psychotherapy, 22,* 324–334.

Jensen, A. (1969). How much can we boost IQ and school acheivement? *Harvard Educational Review, 39,* 1–123.

Jones, J. M. (1988). Racism in black and white. A bicultural model of reaction and evolution. In P. A. Katz & D. A. Taylor (Eds.), *Eliminating racism. Profiles in controversy* (pp. 117–135). New York: Plenum Press.

Katz, J. (1985). Psychotherapy with Native adolescents. *Canadian Journal of Psychiatry, 26,* 455–459.

Knitzer, J. (1982). *Unclaimed children.* Washington, DC: Children's Defense Fund.

Lefley, H. P., & Pedersen, P. B. (Eds.). (1986). *Cross-cultural training for mental health professionals.* Springfield, IL: Charles C. Thomas.

Lum, D. (1992). *Social work practice & people of color.* (2nd ed.). Pacific Grove, CA: Brooks/Cole Publishing Co.

Moynihan, D. P. (1965). *The Negro family: A case for national action.* Washington, DC.: U.S. Government Printing Office.

Neighbors, H. W., & Taylor, R. J. (1985). The use of social service agencies among black Americans. *Social Service Review, 59,* 258–268.

Pedersen, P. (1988). *A handbook for developing multicultural awareness.* Alexandria, VA: American Association for Counseling and Development.

Pinderhughes, E. (1989). *Understanding race, ethnicity, and power: The key to efficicay in clincal practice.* New York: The Free Press.

Ponterotto, J. G., & Casas, J. M. (1991). *Handbook of racial/ethnic minority counseling research.* Springfield, IL: Charles C. Thomas.

Shockley, W. (1972). *Journal of Criminal Law, 7,* 530–543.

Simpson, G., & Yinger, M. (1985). *Racial and cultural minorities.* New York: Plenum.

Stanfield, J. H., II, & Dennis, R. M. (1993). *Race and ethnicity in research methods.* Newbury Park, CA: Sage.

Sue, D. W., & Sue D. (1990). *Counseling the culturally different.* New York: John Wiley and Sons.

Thomas, A., & Sillen, S. (1972). *Racism and psychiatry.* New York: Brunner/Mazel.

U.S. Bureau of the Census. (1987). *Statistical abstract of the United States: 1986* (107th ed.). Washington, DC: U.S. Government Printing Office.

Wilson, W. J. (1978b). *The truly disadvantaged: The inner city, the underclass, and the public policy.* Chicago: University of Chicago Press.

Woody, D. L. (1991). *Recruitment and retention of minority workers in mental health programs.* Washington, D.C., National Institute of Mental Health, Human Resource Development Program.

Zane, N., Sue, D., Castro, F. G., & George. W. (1982). Service system models for ethnic minorities. In D. E. Biegel & A. J. Naparstek (Eds.), *Community Support Systems and Mental Health: Practice, Policy, and Research* (pp. 229–257). New York: Springer Publishing Co.

SECTION TWO

Participants in the Alliance

8

Community Mental Health Programs: An Administrator's Viewpoint

MARY ALICE BROWN

INTRODUCTION

During the past 40 years, deinstitutionalization has changed the public mental health system for people with severe and persistent mental illness. As the number of hospital beds dramatically decreased and the role of state hospitals changed, the center of the public mental health system has shifted from the hospital to the community. A system has emerged that is much more community oriented. No longer are community mental health programs considered to be "aftercare." The community is the place where most people with severe mental illness live their lives with varying levels of mental health support (Hollingsworth, 1995).

There have been two different deinstitutionalization efforts, and they can be conceptualized as distinct "waves." The first wave, during the late 1960s and early 1970s, was guided by the principle of "least restrictive environment." It was conceived with good intentions but was, in actuality, bad policy. It focused primarily on the medical treatment of the illness and neglected patients' psychosocial needs.

During the second wave of deinstitutionalization, the public mental health system has matured, benefitting from the knowledge and experience gained from the first wave. The second wave extended the focus beyond medical treatment and least restrictive environments. It also presented community mental health providers with new challenges and opportunities (Stein & Hollingsworth, 1995). Mental health providers think less about compliance with medical treatment and "least restrictive environments" and more in terms of building alliances and client empowerment. Communication between hospital and community program staff helps to ensure that patients are served most effectively. Hospital staff are able to identify patients who do not need long-term hospital care but will require more intensive community support. Community mental health programs develop special programs or services to meet the needs of these patients, and patients are often involved in selecting specific programs and locations.

This chapter focuses on the treatment alliance from the perspective of a community mental health administrator. To be effective, mental health services require an alliance — an understanding that staff and clients are working together toward goals that are important to the client. During the first wave of deinstitutionalization, the helping relationship was primarily focused on the patient/client's treatment compliance. During the second wave, community mental health services have been reconceptualized in terms of community support systems. Within this comprehensive system of community based services, the alliance between staff and clients has been enhanced.

FIRST WAVE OF DEINSTITUTIONALIZATION

The first wave of deinstitutionalization of people with severe and persistent mental illness was made possible in good part by the new psychotropic medications. Many of the symptoms of the illness that had been particularly alarming to the public could be reduced or eliminated. The principle of "least restrictive environment" guided the discharge of thousands of patients into the community, where they would be maintained with medication management.

Unfortunately, the treatment compliance that had been assumed to occur was limited. Attendance rates for the first appointment in an aftercare clinic ranged from only 36% to 58% (Axelrod & Wetzler, 1989). Of those patients who did go to the aftercare programs at the community mental health centers, 40% dropped out after one session (Sue, McKinney & Allen, 1976).

HISTORICAL BARRIERS TO COMPLIANCE

Inadequate Resources

Although community mental health programs had become the primary locus of treatment, the range of services was limited. The Community Mental Health Centers Act of 1963, which had mandated decentralized, local "community treatment" rather than "institutional care" for people with severe mental illness, had failed to provide the comprehensive services needed (Bassuk & Gerson, 1978). With inadequate funding and little social planning, deinstitutionalization left "patients adrift in a sea of underfunded services and unrealized plans" (Wintersteen & Rapp, 1986, p. 4).

There was a significant gap between client needs and resources for client survival in the community (Wintersteen & Rapp, 1986). Patients were ill-prepared for life in the community. They faced challenges that had not been a part of daily hospital routine. In the hospital, a patient's basic needs — for food, shelter, security, social contact — were met, at least on a minimal level. Medications were administered by staff. Once discharged, former patients faced the difficult tasks of locating housing, shopping for food, preparing meals and other activities of daily living, while learning to take medications as prescribed, and getting to their appointments at the mental health clinic. They struggled "with the demons of inadequate income, lack of meaningful and fulfilling activities, and an illness that isolates them even when they live in the community" (Bevilacqua, 1995, p. 27).

The medical treatment of mental illness with medications reduced positive symptoms such as delusions and hallucinations but had little or no impact on negative symptoms such as low self-esteem, poor relationships, social isolation, poor self-care, lack of vocational and living skills (Liberman et al., 1986). Inactivity and lack of involvement caused further and unnecessary deterioration (Mechanic, 1987).

Although state hospitals were used less frequently for long-term stays, many individuals were hospitalized repeatedly, resulting in the "revolving door" syndrome. Unrealistic cost savings had been projected for community treatment, and the lion's share of state mental health funds was still required to maintain the hospitals. Resources did not follow patients into the community.

Stigmatizing Attitudes and Beliefs

Clients faced significant attitudinal barriers about their capacity to define their own needs, to comprehend information, and to make decisions. They were often considered to be too unmotivated, unrealistic and ill to select constructive goals, and their concerns or values were often "dismissed as the products of an irrational, psychotic mind" (Diamond, 1985, p. 30).

While hospitalized, the patient's capacity for autonomy, responsibility, and self-direction had often diminished due to a lack of use since others were directing their lives (Goffman, 1961; Rose & Black, 1985). Once leaving the hospital, they struggled to find new roles other than patient or passive recipient (Hatfield, 1989). However, the more firmly an individual had accepted and been accepted in the impaired role, the more difficulty he or she faced to become functional and independent (McCrory, 1988).

As a result, mental health professionals greatly underestimated the ability of their clients to make choices for themselves (Srebnik, Livingston, Gordon & King, 1995). Instead of attributing diminished capacity to make reasonable decisions due to "learned helplessness" (Seligman, 1975) or institutionalization (Goffman, 1961), many believed that their poor judgment was primarily due to the mental illness. Clinicians discouraged clients from setting "unreasonable" goals, such as working, or taking other risks that might jeopardize their ability to remain in the community. A pessimistic view of mental illness as a chronic, deteriorative disease prevailed. Hope for improvement was guarded, and failures were expected (Harding, Zubin & Strauss, 1987). One consumer/provider describes the process as "spirit breaking," in which hopes are sacrificed and replaced with apathy and indifference (Deegan, 1990). Another reported that her dreams, hopes, and identity had been reduced to a three-letter acronym, "CMI ... chronically mentally ill" (Blaska, 1991).

Reliance on Traditional Solutions

Much of the knowledge guiding community treatment was based on the medical model. Professional standards concerning clinical distance, emotional detachment and expert authority guided interactions. Services were office-based. Mental health professionals did little or no follow-up if an appointment was missed. If follow-up occurred, it was by mail or telephone; rarely did it include outreach.

Staff decided what services were most appropriate and placed clients in services that often only partially met their needs. Most programs were designed for groups of people because it was less costly. Residential services combined housing and treatment. When clients' conditions either improved or deteriorated, they were required to move. The need for professionally delivered services was expected to continue throughout the client's lifespan.

Imperfect Medications

Once in the community, many former patients did not take their medications as prescribed. One review found noncompliance rates of nearly 50% for individuals who were prescribed phenothiazines, antianxiety, and antidepressant drugs and 32% for those who were prescribed lithium (Barofsky & Connelly, 1983).

For some, the side-effects caused discomfort or more serious problems that interfered with their ability to function, such as akathisia or akinesia. Van Putten (1974) found that 89% of the patients who chronically refused to take medications had experienced extra-pyramidal side-effects while only 20% of the patients who regularly took their medications reported them. Awad (1992) noted that "the patient who experiences a less favorable ... response and the non-compliant patient may be one and the same" (p. 264).

Two myths predominated. First, medication noncompliance was attributed to the psychiatric nature of the illness; and second, relapse was considered to be the result of noncompliance. However, Barofsky and Connelly (1983) noted that the psychiatric patient was no less compliant than patients with other types of chronic medical problems. Schooler and Severe (1984) found that increased medication compliance did not necessarily reduce a person's risk of relapse. Some took their medications faithfully, suffered the side-effects, and still decompensated (Francell, 1994).

Although the primary goal of community-based mental health services was to "maintain" the patient in the community and decrease use of the hospital, admissions soared. Individuals were rehospitalized, treated with medications, and returned to the community once their symptoms were reduced. Patients who refused to take medications when they were hospitalized, were involuntarily medicated. Physicians reasoned that long-term benefits outweighed any immediate concerns about coercion. The cycle was repeated time and time again. The "revolving door" of the state hospital was described as the symbol of mental health care in the 1980s (Torrey, 1988).

Medications alone did not solve the problems of people with serious and persistent mental illness. They were an often necessary but insufficient treatment (Anthony, Cohen, & Farkas, 1990).

SECOND WAVE OF DEINSTITUTIONALIZATION

The pattern of care in the first wave had evolved from long-term hospital stays to one "characterized by multiple admissions and discharges ... which translated into more fragmented care at greater expense" (Geller, 1992, p. 907). Treatment policies and practices in community mental health centers had over-emphasized the medical aspects of the illness and under-estimated the psychosocial aspects. There was discordance in communication between "professionals focusing on the illness" while their clients were focusing "on their entire lives" (Ragins, 1994, p. 8). It was in this turbulent environment that the second wave of deinstitutionalization began to crest.

Some communities had created programs to help individuals with severe and persistent mental illness meet the demands of everyday life. Psychiatric (or psychosocial) rehabilitation programs helped participants to regain their confidence and develop skills needed for working, socializing, and living in the community (Hughes, Woods, Brown, & Spaniol, 1994). The Program in Assertive Community Treatment (PACT), originating in Madison, Wisconsin, created outreach teams as an alternative to hospitalization (Stein and Test, 1980).

These innovative and effective services were included in the comprehensive Community Support System (CSS). Conceived in the mid 1970s by a work group at the National Institute of Mental Health, the CSS was envisioned as a "network of caring and responsible people committed to assisting a vulnerable population" (Turner & Schifren, 1979, p. 2). In addition to rehabilitation services (social and vocational) and client identification and outreach, other key elements were: mental health treatment, crisis response services, health and dental care, housing, income support and entitlements, peer support for clients, family and community support, protection and advocacy, and case management services (Turner and TenHoor, 1979).

The federal Community Support Program, and its underlying philosophy, has served as a beacon to guide community mental health policies and services since 1978. These guidelines, and the longitudinal research conducted in several countries, have shaped the field by presenting evidence that people can recover, improve functioning, and learn to manage symptoms (Bleuler, 1972/1978; Ciompi, 1980; Harding & Brooks, 1984; Huber, Gross, Schuttler & Linz, 1980; Strauss, Hafez, Lieberman & Harding, 1985.)

Recently, staff at the Center for Psychiatric Rehabilitation at Boston University reconceptualized CSS services in terms of outcome (see Table 8.1). Under the umbrella of recovery, each element of service is analyzed in terms of its capacity to lessen the impact of severe mental illness, including impairment, dysfunction, disability, or disadvantage. Emphasized is the importance of treating the consequences of illness (rather than just the illness) and the process of recovery.

Anthony (1993) noted that "recovery" is best described in the writings of consumers, where:

> Recovery is described as a deeply personal, unique process of changing one's attitudes, values, feelings, goals, skills, and/or roles. It is a way of living a satisfying, hopeful, and contributing life even with limitations caused by illness. Recovery involves the development of new meaning and purpose in one's life as one grows beyond the catastrophic effects of mental illness (p. 19).

CONTEMPORARY CHALLENGES TO AN ALLIANCE

While many of the historical barriers continue to exist, albeit to a lesser degree, administrators now face additional challenges, as they attempt to build toward a recovery-oriented system. These contemporary barriers to effective treatment alliances include the financing of community mental health services, staying focused on consumer-based outcomes, changing roles and responsibilities, and redefining helping relationships. Yet, while these are significant challenges, many opportunities also exist.

Financing

Community mental health programs have become deeply dependent on Medicaid funds — especially during the past five years. Although federal health care reform is a fading memory, health care reform is occurring on a state-by-state basis through Medicaid waivers. At the federal level, different plans are being considered for managing the Medicaid "crisis" created by dramatic increases in service and a rising federal deficit. More of the federal responsibilities will be shifted to the states with block grant funding.

It is evident that there will be limits on mental health services and that these limits will impact the treatment alliance in different ways, but many of the details are unknown. The distribution of limited resources raises many critical issues. Questions include: How will resources be managed and who will be responsible for managing them? What criteria will be used to determine what services a client may access? Will public and private mental health care systems merge in caring for people with severe and persistent mental illness? Will there be universal coverage, eliminating the two-tiered system that now exists (between those who have Medicaid insurance and those who don't)? Will Medicaid patients be placed in health maintenance organizations, and will managed care be quality care?

It is difficult to predict the future, but the direction is clear: services need to demonstrate efficiency and efficacy. Client outcome is the driving force for service delivery, and documentation should demonstrate progress toward goals. Staff must be flexible, willing and able to try other options if current services aren't effective. Programs need to develop an array of options that can be tailored individually to meet client needs.

Staying Focused on Outcome

In addition to treating the symptoms of mental illness, mental health programs and systems are charged with assisting clients to achieve successful outcomes. Unfortunately, many mental health systems emphasize service activity rather than client outcome. State mental health authorities require specific reports from community programs that usually include: demographic information on enrolled clients, service reporting by number and type of service units, date and type of termination. The act of gathering this information implies that it is important and useful: documentation requirements become a priority, subtly influencing thinking and action.

With this information, program managers can track staff activity levels — the number of "billable units" or units of service delivered. The primary outcome tracked by most community programs is "community tenure." With data about the client's hospitalization(s) and length of stay, programs can calculate the number or percentage of clients "maintained" in the community without requiring hospitalization. However, it is far more difficult to determine whether staff are helping their clients to achieve their goals, or even if clients were involved in setting them.

Effective treatment alliances help to ensure agreement about where to begin. When the agency philosophy, values, and mission are clearly stated and driven by valued client outcomes, clients can know what to expect so they can participate more actively in the process. For example, most clients (like other adults) want to work in satisfying jobs, have a decent, affordable place to live, and friendships. Services can be developed with these client outcomes in mind. Staff orientation and development can focus on obtaining these outcomes and translate philosophy into guidelines for practice (Anthony, Cohen & Farkas, 1990). Procedures can outline the goal-setting process and delineate how services are delivered and documented to maximize client participation and describe progress toward goals. Program evaluation measures of effectiveness, efficiency, and overall success can be tied to program goals. Quality

Assurance can ensure that service delivery adheres to both internal value standards and the external standards imposed by oversight agencies.

In Table 8.1, mental health services and outcomes are focused on reducing the impact of mental illness and facilitating recovery. Within this framework, agency services can be evaluated in terms of focus and function. Ragins (1994, pp. 9–10) has elaborated on the recovery process and has provided three broad categories which are helpful to staff and clients when establishing goals and priorities:

1) Functions to be recovered, including the ability to read, to sleep restfully, to work, and to have coherent conversations

2) External things that may be recovered, including an apartment, a job, friends, family relationships, and education

3) Internal states that can be recovered, including satisfaction, self-confidence, spiritual peace, and a self identity other than being mentally ill

Changing Roles & Responsibilities

Within community support programs, many staff now work in the community, rather than in the office. They may provide *in vivo* skills training or support in a client's apartment, at a job site, or in other normal community settings. They are more active in their clients lives (Brown, Ridgway, Anthony, & Rogers, 1991). They may assist clients in taking their medications as prescribed, help clients manage their money and meet their basic needs, help them to locate housing and access benefits such as food stamps, medical and dental care (Brown & Wheeler, 1990). Staff serve as advocates and may have contact with the client's apartment managers, neighbors, family, and other social services. They also help clients to become involved in community activities and to develop friendships with people outside of the mental health system.

In each of these responsibilities, staff can provide considerable support and assistance. However, many of these same activities can also become coercive (Diamond, 1995) when staff exercise control without the client's consent. When a client has increased symptoms, staff are often involved in making some decisions *for* rather than *with* the client. When an effective alliance exists, staff are more likely to make treatment decisions that are consistent with the client's wishes. An Advance Directive for Mental Health Treatment allows clients to plan for a time when their decision-making capacity is impaired, to ensure that their desires are followed (Backlar et al., 1994; Backlar, 1995).

Staff who work in the community face a variety of difficult situations that are not encountered in office-based services. They are often involved in managing a client's money (controlling access to client trust funds) and in overseeing medications. The work requires

Table 8.1. Comprehensive Mental Health Services

Recovery: Development of new meaning and purpose as one grows beyond the catastrophic effects of mental illness.

IMPACT OF SEVERE MENTAL ILLNESS

MENTAL HEALTH SERVICES (and Outcomes)	IMPAIRMENT (Disorder in Thought, Feelings, and Behavior)	DYSFUNCTION (Task Performance Limited)	DISABILITY (Role Performance Limited)	DISADVANTAGE (Opportunity Restrictions)
Treatment (Symptom Relief)	X			
Crisis Intervention (Safety)	X			
Case Management (Access)	X	X	X	X
Rehabilitation (Role Functioning)		X	X	X
Enrichment (Self-Development)		X	X	X
Rights Protection (Equal Opportunity)				X
Basic Support (Survival)				X
Self-Help (Empowerment)			X	X

Note. From "Recovery From Mental Illness: The Guiding Vision of the Mental Health Service System in the 1990s" by W. A. Anthony, 1993, *Psychosocial Rehabilitation Journal, 16*(4), p. 11–24. Copyright 1993 by the Trustees of Boston University and IAPSRS. Reprinted by permission.

"flexibility and individualization, and with these come a degree of ambiguity" (Curtis & Hodge, 1995, p. 54).

Staff may feel challenged by a client who is angry because he or she lacks money for a desired purchase. Power struggles may occur, and in these struggles, it is easy to lose sight of the client's goals and "use power as a tool to restrain behavior" rather than as a resource for "teaching self-management, risk-taking and decision-making skills" (Curtis & Hodge, 1995, p. 46). And because staff work independently in the community it may be difficult for staff to ask for help and for managers to know when help is needed.

Medication, more than any other area of treatment in the past, has often involved coercion. However, medication can also be used as a tool to help individuals increase their options and sense of control. If it is presented in terms of the practical benefits in areas of concern to the client — for example, help in controlling behavior that's leading to eviction from a desired apartment — rather than in medical terms — decreasing paranoia or disorganization — it's more likely to be accepted (Diamond, 1983).

"Decisions regarding changes in dose or type of medication can become opportunities for collaboration between the individuals and their doctors" (Fisher, 1994, p. 14). The physician has knowledge about the range of medications available and their effectiveness in treating different symptoms. Yet, the "patient is most familiar with his disease and has a valid point of view. We are perfectly capable of studying, understanding, accepting, and dealing with our illness and its symptoms" (Leete, 1988, p. 51). As more effective medications become available, these communication skills will become even more important (Francell, 1994).

Agency support staff also have new responsibilities. A fleet of agency vehicles becomes essential in delivering services in the community. Client loan funds are often needed for rent and utility deposits and other one-time-only expenses. Agencies may initially hold a lease on a house or apartment so that a client with a poor rental history can live there. Client trust fund programs may be established to manage a client's benefit checks when other skill training and supports have not been effective. When a client is hospitalized, agency funds may pay for his/her rent and utilities, or staff may care for houseplants or pets.

Redefining Relationships

The key to an effective treatment alliance is the helping relationship. A recent study (Solomon, Draine & Delaney, 1995) noted that successful outcomes of people with severe and persistent mental illness are related to the "establishment of an open, trusting, and collaborative relationship" (p. 133). Goering and Stylianos (1988) found that, to clients, the most helpful aspect of the relationship was having someone who cared, accepted and understood them. The process of building an alliance involves developing trust, learning what is important to clients in their lives, and how staff can help them achieve their goals. It also involves expressing hope for the future and belief in the client's ability to make constructive changes (McWhirter, 1991). "Increasingly, the service recipient is being viewed as an equal partner in the treatment process, not a passive service user" (McCabe & Unzicker, 1995, p. 61).

In order to help clients make decisions based on their value system and interests, staff must have adequate time to develop the helping relationship and skill in facilitating the exploration. Without the commitment of staff and program administrators, client-determined goals will be replaced by staff-generated goals, which are usually "doomed to failure ... [after] initial superficial compliance" (Mosher and Burti, 1994, p. 164).

> The people with whom we are working ... have lost so many opportunities, so many possibilities, and so many people along the way that they are often in a state of an inability to engage ... While they may have the same hopes and dreams that we do — for a decent place to live and some peace and quiet and security — they may be far removed from their ability to hope (Moorhead, 1993, pp. 135, 138).

The goal-setting process requires time, skill, and commitment (Brown & Basel, 1989). "Practitioners must be as committed to listening to the goals of persons with psychiatric disabilities as psycho-pharmacologists are to assessing their symptoms" (Anthony, Cohen & Farkas, 1990, p. 219).

Staff who work with clients are a valued resource and represent the largest single expense item in a budget. Unfortunately, many staff who have completed academic programs are knowledgeable about pathology but are relatively unskilled in recognizing client strengths, facilitating exploration leading to goal-setting, or teaching clients critical skills.

During the past decade, staff skill training technology has been developed by the Center for Psychiatric Rehabilitation at Boston University. Current training packages include: setting self-determined goals, functional assessment, direct skills teaching, and case management. However, in-service training designed for skill development is of limited value unless the administration is committed to skill utilization. An agency must be prepared to modify programs and documentation in order to support and incorporate new technology.

As mental health systems become more focused on recovery, a key element is support — but not necessarily professional support. Staff, who are providing skills training and support in their clients' own environments, will also need to help their clients develop natural or folk supports (supports that are unpaid and available in the natural environment). Natural supports are an important aspect of supported housing and supported employment programs. Staff also encourage their clients to participate in self-help groups and help them to access them. "Self-help is not a miracle nor a cure-all, but it is a powerful confirmation that people, despite problems and disabilities, can achieve more than others (or they themselves) may have ever thought possible" (Chamberlin, 1990, p. 331).

To each of us, in our lives, personal support is essential. Unfortunately, people with severe and persistent mental illness have had difficulty finding it. The challenge for all community mental health programs is to help their clients build networks of support and to share in the positive experience many other citizens enjoy (Carling, 1995).

Clients who are denied the opportunity to make decisions miss the experience of learning from successes as well as mistakes, a powerful experience that helps them become accountable for their actions.

> When individuals with mental illness have the power to make decisions, they can be expected to take responsibility for them ... Having control over aspects of one's life requires accountability for actions (Hatfield, 1994, p. 7).

Returning to clients the responsibility for choices about their lives and their lifestyles is the very core of empowerment (Carling, 1995). It is the contemporary program administrator's task to ensure that people, programs, and resources are available and aligned to achieve this fundamental goal. This is the essence of contemporary (second wave) community mental health programs.

REFERENCES

Anthony, W. A. (1993). Recovery from mental illness: The guiding vision of the mental health service system in the 1990s. *Psychosocial Rehabilitation Journal, 16*(4), 11–24.

Anthony, W. A., Cohen, M., & Farkas, M. (1990). *Psychiatric rehabilitation.* Boston: Center for Psychiatric Rehabilitation.

Awad, A. G. (1992). Quality of life of schizophrenic patients on medications and implications for new drug trials. *Hospital and Community Psychiatry, 43*(3), 262–265.

Axelrod, S., & Wetzler, S. (1989). Factors associated with better compliance with psychiatric aftercare. *Hospital and Community Psychiatry, 40*(4), 397–401.

Backlar, P. (1995). The longing for order: Oregon's medical advance directive for mental health treatment. *Community Mental Health Journal, 31*(2), 103–108.

Backlar, P., Asmann, B. D., Joondeph, R. C., Smith, G., et al. (1994). *Can I plan now for the mental health treatment I would want if I were in crisis? A guide to Oregon's declaration for mental health treatment.* State of Oregon: Office of Mental Health Services, Mental Health and Developmental Disability Services Division.

Barofsky, I., & Connelly, C. E. (1983). Problems in providing effective care for the chronic psychiatric patient. In I. Barofsky & R. D. Budson (Eds.), *The chronic psychiatric patient in the community: Principles of treatment* (pp. 83–136) New York: Spectrum Publications.

Bassuk, E. L., & Gerson, S. (1978). Deinstitutionalization and mental health services. *Scientific American, 238*(2), 46–53.

Bevilacqua, J. J. (1995). New paradigms, old pitfalls. In L. I. Stein & E. J. Hollingsworth (Eds.), *Maturing mental health systems: New challenges* and opportunities. *New directions for mental health services* No. 66. (pp. 19–30). San Francisco: Jossey-Bass.

Blaska, B. (1991). First person account: What it is like to be treated like a CMI. *Schizophrenia Bulletin, 17*(1), 173–176.

Bleuler, M. (1978). *The schizophrenic disorders: Long-term patient and family studies* (S. M. Clemens, Trans.). New Haven, CT: Yale University Press. (Original work published 1972)

Brown, M. A., & Basel, D. (1989). A five-stage vocational rehabilitation program: Laurel Hill Center, Eugene, Oregon. In M. D. Farkas & W. A. Anthony (Eds.), *Psychiatric rehabilitation programs: Putting theory into practice* (pp. 108–115). Baltimore: The Johns Hopkins University Press.

Brown, M. A., Ridgway, P., Anthony, W. A., & Rogers, E. S. (1991). Comparison of outcomes for clients seeking and assigned to supported housing services. *Hospital and Community Psychiatry, 42*(11), 1150–1153.

Brown, M. A., & Wheeler, T. (1990). Supported housing for the most disabled: Suggestions for providers. *Psychosocial Rehabilitation Journal, 13*(4), 59–68.

Carling, P. J. (1995). *Return to community: Building support systems for people with psychiatric disabilities.* New York: Guilford Press.

Chamberlin, J. (1990). The ex-patient movement. *Journal of Mind and Behavior, 11*(3–4), 328–338.

Ciompi, L. (1980). Catamnestic long-term study on the course of life and aging in schizophrenics. *Schizophrenia Bulletin, 6*(4), 606–618.

Curtis, L. C., & Hodge, M. (1995). Ethics and boundaries in community support services: New challenges. In L. I. Stein & E. J. Hollingsworth (Eds.), *Maturing mental health systems: New challenges and opportunities. New directions for mental health services* No. 66. (pp. 43–60). San Francisco: Jossey-Bass.

Deegan, P. E. (1990). Spirit Breaking: When the helping professions hurt. *The Humanistic Psychologist, 18*(3), 301–313.

Diamond, R. J. (1983). Enhancing medication use in schizophrenic patients. *Journal of Clinical Psychiatry, 44*(6), 7–14.

Diamond, R. J. (1985). Drugs and the quality of life: The patient's point of view. *Journal of Clinical Psychiatry, 46*(5), 29–35.

Diamond, R. J. (1995). Coercion in the community: Issues for mature treatment systems. In L.I. Stein & E.J. Hollingsworth (Eds.), *Maturing mental health systems: New challenges and opportunities. New directions for mental health services* No. 66. (pp. 3–18). San Francisco: Jossey-Bass.

Fisher, D. (1994). Hope, humanity and voice in recovery from psychiatric disability. *The Journal of the California Alliance for the Mentally Ill, 5*(3), 13–15.

Francell, E. G. (1994). Medication: The foundation of recovery. *Innovations and Research, 3*(4), 31–40.

Geller, J. L. (1992). A report on the "worst" state hospital recidivists in the U.S. *Hospital and Community Psychiatry, 43*(9), 904–908.

Goering, P., & Stylianos, S. (1988). Exploring the helping relationship between the schizophrenic client and rehabilitation therapist. *American Journal of Orthopsychiatry, 58*, 271–279.

Goffman, E. (1961). *Asylums: Essays on the social situation of mental patients and other inmates.* Garden City, New York: Doubleday Anchor

Harding, C., & Brooks, G. (1984). Life assessment of a cohort of chronic schizophrenics discharged twenty years ago. In S. Mednick, M. Harway,

& K. Finello (Eds.), *The handbook of longitudinal research* (Vol. 2, pp. 375–393). New York: Praeger Press.

Harding, C. M., Zubin, J., & Strauss, J. S. (1987). Chronicity in schizophrenia: Fact, partial fact, or artifact? *Hospital and Community Psychiatry, 38*(5), 477–491.

Hatfield, A. B. (1989). Patients' accounts of stress and coping in schizophrenia. *Hospital and Community Psychiatry, 40*(11), 1141–1145.

Hatfield, A. B. (1994). Recovery from mental illness. *The Journal of the California Alliance for the Mentally Ill, 5*(3), 6–7.

Hollingsworth, E. J. (1995). Issues of politics, boundaries, and technology choice. In L. I. Stein & E. J. Hollingsworth (Eds.), *Maturing mental health systems: New challenges and opportunities. New directions for mental health services* No. 66. (pp. 31–42). San Francisco: Jossey-Bass.

Huber, G., Gross, G., Schuttler, R., & Linz, M. (1980). Longitudinal studies of schizophrenic patients. *Schizophrenia Bulletin, 6*(4), 592–605.

Hughes, R., Woods, J., Brown, M. A., & Spaniol, L. (1994). Introduction. In L. Spaniol, M. A. Brown, L. Blankertz, D. J. Burnham, J. Dincin, K. Furlong-Norman, N. Nesbitt, P. Ottenstein, K. Prieve, I. Rutman, A. Zipple (Eds.), *An introduction to psychiatric rehabilitation* (pp. 1–2). Boston: IAPSRS.

Leete, E. (1988). A consumer perspective on psychosocial treatment. *Psychosocial Rehabilitation Journal, 12*(2), 45–52.

Liberman, R. P., Mueser, K. T., Wallace, C. J., Jacobs, H. E., Eckman, T., & Massel, H. K. (1986). Training skills in the psychiatrically disabled: Learning coping and competence. *Schizophrenia Bulletin, 12*(4), 631–647.

McCabe, S., & Unzicker, R. E. (1995). Changing roles of consumer/survivors in mature mental health systems. In L. I. Steen & E. J. Hollingsworth (Eds.), *Maturing mental health systems: New challenges and opportunities. New directions for mental health services* No. 66. (pp. 61–73). San Francisco: Jossey-Bass.

McCrory, D. J. (1988). The human dimension of the vocational rehabilitation process. In J. A. Ciardiello & M. D. Bell (Eds.), *Vocational rehabilitation of persons with prolonged psychiatric disorders* (pp. 208–218). Baltimore: The Johns Hopkins University Press.

McWhirter, E. H. (1991). Empowerment in counseling. *Journal of Counseling and Development, 69*, 222–227.

Mechanic, D. (1987). Evolution of mental health services and areas for change. *New Directions in Mental Health, 36*, 3–13.

Moorhead, M. (1993). Speaking out: Why pick up the racquet? Notes from the hospital. *Psychosocial Rehabilitation Journal, 16*(3), 135–139.

Mosher, L. R., & Burti, L. (1994). Relationships in rehabilitation: When technology fails. In W. Anthony & L. Spaniol (Eds.), *Readings in psychiatric rehabilitation* (pp. 162–171). Boston: Center for Psychiatric Rehabilitation.

Ragins, M. (1994). Changing from a medical model to a psychosocial rehabilitation model. *The Journal of the California Alliance of the Mentally Ill, 5*(3), 8–10.

Rose, S., & Black, B. (1985). *Advocacy and empowerment: Mental health care in the community.* Boston: Routledge & Kegan Paul.

Rutman, I. D. (1992). As Ben Franklin once said, Let's all hang together. *Psychosocial Rehabilitation Journal, 16*(1), 1–2.

Schooler, N. R., & Severe, J. B. (1984). Efficacy of drug treatment for chronic schizophrenic patients. In M. Mirabi (Ed.), *The chronically mentally ill: Research and services* (pp. 125–142). Jamaica, NY: Spectrum Publications.

Seligman, M. E. P. (1975). *Helplessness: On depression, development, and death.* San Francisco: Freeman.

Solomon, P., Draine, J., & Delaney, M. A. (1995). The working alliance and consumer case management. *The Journal of Mental Health Administration, 22*(2), 126–134.

Srebnik, D., Livingston, J., Gordon, L., & King, D. (1995). Housing choice and community success for individuals with serious and persistent mental illness. *Community Mental Health Journal, 31*(2), 139–152.

Stein, L. I., & Hollingsworth, E. J. (Eds.). (1995). *Maturing mental health systems: New challenges and opportunities. New directions for mental health services.* San Francisco: Jossey-Bass.

Stein, L. I., & Test, M. A. (1980). An alternative to mental hospital treatment. I: Conceptual model, treatment program, and clinical evaluation. *Archives of General Psychiatry, 37,* 392–397.

Strauss, J. S., Hafez, H., Lieberman, P., & Harding, C. (1985). The courses of psychiatric disorder: III. Longitudinal principles. *American Journal of Psychiatry, 142*(3), 289–296.

Sue, S., McKinney, H., & Allen, D. B. (1976). Predictors of the duration of therapy for clients in the community mental healthcenter system. *Community Mental Health Journal, 12,* 365–375.

Torrey, E. F. (1988). *Nowhere to go: The tragic odyssey of the homeless mentally ill.* New York: Harper & Row.

Turner, J. E., & Schifren, I. (1979). Community support system: How comprehensive? In L.I. Stein (Ed.), *Community support systems for the long-term patient. New directions for mental health services* No. 2. (pp. 1–14). San Francisco: Jossey-Bass.

Turner, J. E., & TenHoor, W. J. (1979). The NIMH community support program: Pilot approach to a needed social reform. *Schizophrenia Bulletin, 4*(3), 319–344.

Van Putten, T. (1974). Why do schizophrenic patients refuse to take their drugs? *Archives of General Psychiatry, 31,* 67–72.

Wintersteen, R. T., & Rapp, C. A. (1986). The young adult chronic patient: A dissenting view of an emerging concept. *Psychosocial Rehabilitation Journal, 9*(4), 3–13.

9

Informed Choice: The Importance of Personal Participation in the Healing Process

DANIEL FISHER

Healing from extreme emotional turmoil often involves the emergence of a whole person capable of choice and control. A great deal of that emergence is influenced by the quality of our personal bonds. I will focus here on the impact of relationships and the decision-making process on emotional healing. Compliance emphasizes a paternalistic relationship which objectifies the person helped and perpetuates a feeling of being damaged. On the other hand, informed choice encourages the active participation of the person helped in such a way as to facilitate their healing process. I will conclude with recommendations to assist clinicians in facilitating the active participation of people receiving mental health services.

THE ROLE OF CHOICE IN MY HEALING

In this article, I will explain the discomfort I and others healing from severe emotional states feel with the term compliance. In giving voice to the discomfort, I hope to open the eyes of clinicians and the rest of the community to the need for all of us to transform our relationships from an emphasis on compliance and external control to one of understanding and choice.

My journey of healing plays a large role in the thoughts I will share here about compliance and informed choice. In my childhood, I was convinced that all emotions could be controlled by rational thought. Along with Descartes, my motto was "I think therefore I am". I also developed a conviction that the mind was a product of the chemical machinery of the brain. It was a time of unmitigated optimism about the possibilities of science to improve every dimension of human life. I obtained my Ph.D. in biochemistry at U. of Wisconsin and then made some fundamental discoveries regarding the neurochemistry of the brain during my five years as a researcher at NIMH. I believed that if we could discover the factors in the body which controlled the enzymes producing neurotransmitters, we could design drugs which would repair the chemical imbalance which lay at the heart of schizophrenia and the other major mental illnesses. As I explored more deeply the mysteries of these enzymes, I made other discoveries which altered my life. My first discovery was that rather than a few discrete determinants there were a myriad of conditions each of which individually and in combination played an important role in the regulation of those enzymes. These were pervasive conditions such as temperature, salts, oxygen, iron, etc., which affected each other as well as many other systems in the body. Regulation of these enzymes required a large scale coordination and control of the body and mind by the person themselves. I lost faith that mental illness could be cured by a single magic drug. My second discovery came through a year of psychoanalysis. That experience taught me I was personally unhappy and seeking direction on how to run my own life. I had led an emotionally remote life so it was difficult to know where to turn. After two months in daily analysis, I recall thinking that I had told my therapist all that had gone wrong in my life; now it was time for him to make the interpretations which would solve my problems and fix the broken machinery of my mind. My analyst frustrated my wish to have him answer these needs with statements like, "what is this need you have to know what I think you should do?" I started to see that I had to find answers in my deeper self. My inability to resolve the conflict between these humanistic discoveries and my mechanistic views led to my delusion that I was human but all other people were literally machines. I was hospitalized at the Navy Hospital across the road from NIMH and given Thorazine and other antipsychotic medications. I wish there could be alternatives to such treatments. Taking medications in a psychiatric hospital is almost always a question of compliance. Even when you take medication on a voluntary basis, it is based on fear that if you don't take the medication you might never leave.

During my last hospitalization, I became convinced I had a fundamental organic deficit causing my unhappiness. I asked my psychiatrist (my second) if I had brain damage which was a cause of my problems. He replied that I was basically whole. This view fit with his earlier statements that I had the capacity to heal; that he provided the setting but I did the healing myself. These views helped me to see that there was more to me than a collection of chemicals and helped that part of me which was capable of taking control of my life of doing so more actively. This shift in my sense of control over my life has allowed me to more actively enter into the dialogue needed for integrating new information. I can not only maintain a sense of self in relationships but in addition feel that my existence is enhanced in relationships. I have been able to take in information from people in positions of authority in a more considered fashion. Before, I felt either compelled to slavishly carry out their mandate (i.e. comply) or refuse altogether. I am now able to choose what makes sense and disregard other information. I no longer try to swallow final answers from totally outside of me but nurture the growth of concepts gradually through a process of conversation and dialogue. During times of turmoil, I was fearful of taking in new information. Though unaware then, I think I feared my thoughts would be overly controlled by new information. I now have a process view of information which has helped me considerably in this struggle. I emphasize to myself that: information is literally *in* formation, it is not the final word, it is a suggestion to build on, subject to interpretation. Now that I see that the information is always subject to interpretation, I can get to know more by getting to know a person who can interpret the information. Then there is the possibility of entering into true dialogue where information flows in both directions and where the deeper humanity of the persons involved is more important than any isolated bit of information. This points to the need for a process view of informed consent. Information about medications, coping, and healing is better shared as part of the ongoing dialogue of the helping relationship rather than as an isolated, unidirectional event.

HISTORY OF PSYCHIATRIST-PATIENT RELATIONSHIP

The doctor dresses the wound, but God heals the wound

We are told of the dramatic moment, during the French Revolution, when citizen Phillipe Pinel released those who were insane from the chains of the prisons of Paris. We are not told that in place of prison those people judged insane were transferred to a new institution, the asylum, where the chains of physician authority took the place of the metal ones. The asylum, the prototype of the modern psychiatric hospital, was based on a paternalistic model of patient-doctor relating. The basis of treatment in the asylum was moral, with the patient learning to follow the instructions of a father figure. Samuel Tuke, in England, had patients periodically share tea with the doctor and his family as a means of social skills training. (Foucault, 1965). Psychiatric authority in asylums was reinforced by the position of authority which the physician occupied in society during the 19th century. In the late 19th century there were considerable challenges to medical authority by other practitioners, many of whom were women. These challenges were reversed by the release of the AMA sponsored Flexner Report in 1910. The Flexner Report stated that only the scientifically-based curriculum of regular medical schools could accomplish the training needed to practice medicine (Derbyshire, 1969). Since then, the license to practice medicine and psychiatry, has depended on the completion of a course of education whose basic curriculum has changed little. This report laid the foundation of medical authority in the 20th century on the cornerstone of modern science.

As the authority of psychiatry was challenged by patients, other professionals, and communities in the 60's, we have seen psychiatry again appeal to science to legitimize its authority. Thus the majority of heads of departments of psychiatry are biological psychiatrists. In addition, we are in the decade of the brain and mental illness is now described as a broken brain. History points to a consistent theme of the doctor in a paternal role based on expert scientific knowledge and status in society. Friedson points out that a means of doctors maintaining status is by not sharing medical information (Friedson, 1960.)

PROBLEMS WITH THE CONCEPT OF COMPLIANCE

Power like a desolating pestilence
pollutes whatever it touches; and obedience
bane of all genius, virtue, freedom, truth
makes slaves of men and of the human frame,
a mechanized automaton.
                              by Percy Bysshe Shelley (Queen Mab, 1813)

An emphasis on compliance undermines empowerment and self-determination which are vital to recovery and healing. Compliance means following orders and regulations in an uncritical fashion. We all agree to laws and regulations to cooperate in society, but when obedience becomes the central focus of our interaction with a health professional, the healing powers within us are stifled. We become a "mechanized automaton." If there is a period when compliance is the main goal due to a court order or an emergency condition, I suggest that the medication be described as chemical restraint rather than treatment. There is some evidence in the medical field that constructive noncompliance may be a pathway to healing (P. Steinglass, personal communication, 1985; Thorne, 1990.)

Esso Leete has ably connected my earlier theme of the importance of having control and the problem with compliance when she states, "I find that my vulnerability to stress, anxiety and accompanying symptoms decreases the more I am in control of my own life. Unfortunately, our progress continues to be measured by professionals with concepts like "consent" and "cooperate" and "comply" instead of "choose," insinuating that we are incapable of taking an active role as partners in our own recovery. Indeed recovery is never even mentioned as a possibility."(Leete, 1994.)

FROM COMPLIANCE TO CHOICE

These words each have very different meanings. Each describes a relationship in terms of power dynamics. In psychiatry, people avoid discussing the power imbalances which exist between the person providing services and the person receiving them. The consumer/survivor movement has brought these issues to the forefront because we have found that a fundamental element in our recovery is the ability to take more control over our own healing and our own lives. A major part of that is making explicit the context of any given relationship. Consent is a little better than compliance, but it still implies major asymmetry in power in that the instructions and information come from the doctor and the patient consents or agrees to the recommendation. For many years Dr. Tom Gutheil has contended that informed consent should not be a single event which is documented once by a form in a chart, but should take place over time. I agree with this analysis, but I think that the concept and the name for it need to change in order for practice to change. Consent is still too one directional to allow for the unfolding process of dialogue and discussion. Instead I would use the term informed choice or choosing. Then the process and evolution would be documented over a period of time.

FROM PATIENT TO ACTIVE PARTICIPANT

In the classical medical relationship, the person receiving help is the patient and the person making the decisions is the doctor. The patient is expected to comply with those decisions. Parsons (1951) has described this role of doctor in terms of the social control function. The doctor is needed in society to certify when someone is not capable of work by the doctor's note or a disability determination. The doctor defines who is in a sick role. The sick role relieves the person of responsibilities but in return they must assume a child-like position relative to the doctor. The doctor also decides when a person no longer is in the sick role and can assume a fully responsible position in society. In addition, the doctor plays a supportive nurturing role. This allows the person to rely on the doctor and trust they will be taken care of. There are some correlations between age and educational level and the nature of the relationship. The higher the social class, the greater the education, and younger the adult being helped, the less likely the patient will want a paternal relationship. The biggest determinant however appears to be the severity of the illness. Nearly all groups show a strong preference for a paternal doctor at times of suffering a severe illness. (Ende, Kazis, Ash, & Moskowitz, 1989). The paternal relationship characterizes the biomedical model of relieving distress in which the doctor decides on the definition of the problem, defines the diagnosis, and designs the treatment plan. Modern technology with its MRI's, heart transplants, and drugs has increasingly reinforced the biomedical, paternal model of health care.

More recently, the person receiving help has been described as a consumer and the person providing help a provider. Implicit in the consumer description is a shift in power such that the consumer is making decisions about which provider to see and which treatment option to pursue based on cost and quality of care. There is evidence from research and personal accounts that recovery from a medical or psychiatric disability is greatly aided by the person being able to play an active role in their recovery. This point is well illustrated in Norman Cousin's account of his recovery from a connective tissue disorder. Mr. Cousins had tried various medical treatments, all of which failed. He decided that he needed to design his own treatment plan, and he found a doctor who respected his wish to do so. He stated that, "I was incredibly fortunate to have as my doctor a man who knew that his biggest job was to encourage to the fullest the patient's will to live and to mobilize all the natural resources of body and mind to combat disease. (Cousins, 1979, p. 44)"

Brody (1980) has pointed to the importance of the consumer being involved in decisions. Brody's group found that persons who played a more active role in their health decisions had less discomfort, fewer symptoms, a greater sense of control over their illness, and better medical condition than passive patients (Brody, Miller, Lennan, Smith, & Caputo, 1989). Greenfield and colleagues have reported similar findings in which they prepared patients for a doctor's visit to improve their verbal participation. They found a positive correlation between the active verbal participation by the patient, their blood sugar and blood pressure control, functional status, and quality of life (Greenfield, Kaplan, & Ware, 1985: Greenfield, Kaplan, Ware, Yano, & Frank, 1988).

Dr. John Sarno has described a very successful self-help approach to back pain which also encourages the sufferer to take an active role in their recovery. He emphasizes the close relationship between back pain and repressed emotions. He has developed a set of daily reminders some of which I am going to paraphrase. I have personally experienced remarkable relief by repeating them at times of severe back pain:

1. My back is basically normal and there is nothing to fear

2. The pain is due to muscle tension and repressed emotions

3. Physical activity is not dangerous and I should resume it

4. I intend to be in control

He also advocates that you talk to your brain and assert that you will not put up with the back pain. "What one is doing is consciously taking charge instead of feeling the helpless, intimidated victim," (Sarno, 1991, p. 73). As a final example I would like to describe an exciting collection of coping strategies for dealing with voices. Each of these strategies depends on the person seeing themselves and being seen by others as a whole person capable of finding ways to live with their voices. (Watkins, 1993; Romme & Escher, 1993). At the heart of these approaches is a common theme that the person must reach inside and find the part that can take charge. They need to recognize that each of them is a person who is greater than their voices. Romme and Escher (1993, p. 16) write that, "These comparisons have led us to an important conclusion: the crucial advantage enjoyed by those who succeed in coping well is their greater strength with regard to both their voices and their environment ..."

The closer we get to severe psychological states the more critical the question of control becomes. In fact, one of the hallmarks of acute trauma is the loss of control. Conversely one of the primary avenues to recovery from any trauma is the ability to reassert control in one's life. People healing from extreme emotional states have focused on the language of mental health because the self-labeling plays a major role in the perception of power and control within the helping relationship. The move from patient to consumer was seen as a useful step at first, but there are limitations in the term. It has a passive ring. Other terms we have used are: client, recipient, user, ex-patient. The independent living movement prefers the people-first language" a person who ..." I also prefer this longer version because it is more specific and it is a constant reminder that we are full human beings, a point we all tend to forget. When pressed to describe a group of us we will now use the multiple description consumer/survivor/ex-patient whose shortened form is c/s/x.

HOW CLINICIANS CAN FACILITATE ACTIVE PARTICIPATION BY THOSE THEY HELP

People have the right and duty to participate individually and collectively in the planning and implementation of their health care.
(World Health Organization, 1978, p. 3)

We live in a culture looking for magical cures and technical fixes as the following example illustrates. I had seen Mr. M for many years. He was sure that if I could find exactly the right medication, he would be cured. He would say, "There is a pill out there with my name on it." I attempted to go along with his belief and we tried a variety of pills. After many medications, he felt a little better, but was still dissatisfied. Finally, I said as directly to his inner most self as I could, that there was no medication which could cure him. I said medications could reduce his symptoms but he needed to heal himself and I felt that he could do so. He looked straight at my deeper self. His eyes widened. "You really think so," he replied in disbelief. I repeated that I thought he could do it. He started to smile a full encompassing smile and has made significant progress in his recovery since then with no major change in his medication.

Michael White and David Epston, the developers of the narrative approach, have come to similar conclusions regarding factors promoting recovery. They look for the "unique outcomes in people's lives and the counterplots associated with them. Seemingly ephemeral often forgotten experiences that contradict the dominant story of abnormality. 'There is always a history of struggle and protest-always,' says White. He finds the tiny, hidden spark of resistance within the heart of a person trapped in a socially sanctioned psychiatric diagnosis 'Schizophrenia ...' that tends to consume all other claims to identity. White liberates little pockets of non-cooperation, moments of personal courage and autonomy, self-respect and emotional vitality beneath the iron grid of lived misery and assigned pathology."(Wylie, 1994, p. 43).

The most fundamental step any helping person can take in facilitating an active role by a person helped is to undergo a shift in their attitude toward people who are labeled mentally ill. That label suggests the person will not heal. Yet helpers need to believe in the capacity of the person before them to grow in order for healing to occur. As Senge points out, personal change requires a change in beliefs:

> "For most of us, beliefs change gradually as we accumulate new experiences — as we develop our personal mastery. But if mastery will not develop so long as we hold unempowering beliefs, and the beliefs will change only as we experience our mastery, how may we begin to alter the deeper structures of our lives?"
>
> (Senge, 1990. p. 159)

In answer to Senge's question, one can break the cycle of disempowering beliefs/lack of mastery through a relationship of trust in which a helper is able to supply enough added emotional safety to allow exploration of an expanded view of oneself in the world. Very frequently belief in one's potential is the first step in growth. That is why the negativity of so much of society towards people with severe emotional problems is so damaging. Carl Rogers also highlights the importance of moving from compliance to choice in becoming a person: "from living only to satisfy the expectations of others, and living only in their eyes and in their opinions, toward becoming a person in his own right, with feelings, aims, ideas of his own: from being driven and compelled [to comply] he moves towards the making of responsible choices." (Rogers, 1959, p. 334)

Table 9.1 gives a summary of the change in roles people need to undergo in order to shift from a medical to an empowerment model of healing:

Table 9.1.

	Medical Model	Empowerment Model
Helper	Expert with scientific information most of which is too complex to explain to the patient a basis of their diagnosis and treatment	Educator who shares perspective and validates the importance of subjective information
Helpee	To receive information about their disease from the expert and to follow directions in the act of treatment	To be an active participant in the definition and healing

The following suggestions (Table 9.2) are common in working with people with minor emotional distress yet are neglected for people in more extreme states. Therefore, the fundamental shift in attitudes needed to facilitate recovery is to regard the person you work with as a full human being capable of all the activities of the "less disturbed" clients you see.

Table 9.2.

PHRASE	APPROACH
"the person I help is a person like me"	through dialogue with people healing from extreme states who are not your clients; through workshops; readings; use of people first language
"tell me in your words how we can best work together"	the person before you is always intact despite severe problems; their Self is not defined by their condition
"how do you see your strong points and needs"	cocreating a narrative description of strengths and problems using their words as much as possible enhances a person's voice and credibility
"you are a person with the following diagnosis, which may change in time and could be described in your community as ..."	people's identity becomes defined by their diagnosis, they feel it is their destiny; revise diagnosis often and put it in that person's words and culture
"these are the goals I understand you want to work on ..."	treatment planning as a joint venture based on person's stated goals
"we have the following options available for you; which would you choose?"	informed choice (not just consent) of all options available
"what do you feel has helped and hurt in the service?"	there needs to be an ongoing mutual assessment of progress or lack of it
"you have the capacity to heal, I (we) provide the setting"	from the beginning if clinicians are humble and can recognize the limitation of their treatments
"other people have found a variety of self help approaches helpful for similar problems, such as ..."	alternative or holistic health self-help and self-care
"what do you feel is of most importance and meaning in your life ..."	this is the most important question; all others come from this

"Do no harm to anyone"

(from the Hippocratic Oath)

I will end with a description of ways of minimizing the damage done in the name of treatment. In the long run, there needs to be an uncoupling of the concepts coercion and treatment. As long as psychiatry is used as an agent of social control, the basic relationship of the psychiatrist to the person helped will be conditioned by the fear that the psychiatrist can at any time commit the person they are seeing. I was reminded of this problem several years ago when I proposed that I could enter as an ex-patient and start a peer-run acting group in the clubhouse in our area where I am also medical director of a mental health center. A member of the clubhouse quickly set me straight. "No, Dr. Fisher, that would not be possible. You are our psychiatrist. You hold great power over our lives. You could commit us at any time. We could not at the same time view you as our peer."

The best we can do is create as many voluntary alternatives to psychiatric hospitalization as possible and try to be honest about the context and guidelines we operate under. I am clear that if someone is at risk of harming themselves or someone else that they may be committed to a hospital, as a public safety measure. I know that when I was committed to a psychiatric hospital, I wish this had been told to me. I believe that the inevitable trauma of hospitalization would be reduced by a direct discussion with the consumer about the steps to be taken and the reason for them. After all, identification of the circumstances of trauma is a big part of recovery.

REFERENCES

Brody, D. S. (1980). The patient's role in clinical decision making. *Annals of Internal Medicine, 93*, 718–722.

Brody, D. S., Miller, S., Lennan, C., Smith, D., & Caputo, G. (1989). Patient perception of involvement in medical care: Relationship to illness attitudes and outcomes. *Journal of General Internal Medicine, 4*, 506–511.

Cousins, N. (1979). *Anatomy of an illness as perceived by the patient.* New York: Norton.

Derbyshire, R. C. (1969). *Medical licensure and discipline in the United States.* Baltimore: Johns Hopkins Press.

Ende, J., Kazis, L., Ash, A., & Moskowitz, M. A. (1989). Measuring patients' desire for autonomy, *J. of General Internal Medicine, 4*, 23–30.

Foucault, M. (1965). *Madness and civilization.* New York: Vintage Books.

Freidson, E. (1960). Client control and medical practice. *Amer. J. Sociology, 65*, 374–382.

Greenfield, S., Kaplan, S., & Ware, J. (1985). Expanding patient involvement in care: Effects on patient outcomes. *Annals of Internal Medicine, 103*, 520–528.

Greenfield, S., Kaplan, S., Ware, J., Yano, E., & Frank, H. (1988). Patient's participation in medical care: Effects on blood sugar control and quality of life in diabetes. *J. of General Internal Medicine, 3*, 448–457.

Leete, E. (1994). Stressor, symptom, or sequelae? remission, recovery, or cure? *The Journal of California Alliance for the Mentally Ill, 5*(3), 16–18.

Parsons, T. (1951). *The social system*. Glencoe, Ill.: Free Press.

Rogers, C. (1959). A theory of therapy, personality, and interpersonal relationships as developed in the client-centered framework. In S. Koch (Ed.), *Psychology: a Study of science: Vol. 3. Formulations of the person and the social context*. NY: McGraw-Hill.

Romme, M., & Escher, S. (1993). *Accepting voices*. London: Mind Publications.

Sarno, J. (1991). *Healing back pain*. New York: Warner Books.

Senge, P. M. (1990). *The fifth discipline*. New York: Doubleday.

Thorne, S. (1990). Constructive noncompliance in chronic illness. *Holistic Nursing Practice, 5*, 62–69.

Watkins, J. (1993). *Hearing voices: A self help guide and reference book*. Australia: Publication of the Richmond Fellowship of Victoria.

World Health Organization/UNICEF (1978). Article 4, Declaration of Alma-Ata.

Wylie, M. S. (1994, November/December). Panning for gold. *Networker*, pp. 40–49.

10

The Role of Families in Compliance with Treatment

DALE L. JOHNSON

Years ago when I was the director of a treatment program for psychiatric patients, I encouraged them to make their own choices. Recommendations were made, but individual autonomy was given high priority. Noncompliance with hospital rules or the treatment unit was a subject for therapeutic investigation, and the sessions seemed valuable to patients. However, very few had psychotic disorders and these people did not do well. Today I would be less permissive, certainly with patients who have psychotic symptoms.

This change in attitude began when my oldest child developed schizophrenia at age 19. Now, twenty-three years later, he is quite disabled, but has not had a relapse in twelve years and does fairly well with support. His illness has given our family a great deal of experience with compliance issues. This has been expanded by our membership in the National Alliance for the Mentally Ill and contacts with other families who have had similar experiences.

Our son was reared to be independent and competent. He was a remarkably able child and an adolescent with high social, academic and athletic competencies. Despite evidence of withdrawal and some possible confusion in late adolescence, he was admitted to Harvard. He was unable to study and took leave at the end of the first semester. Full symptoms appeared several months later. Whether at home or at hospital, the main problem was that he could not acknowledge that he had a mental illness, and although reluctantly compliant when grossly psychotic, he would stop taking medications as soon as he felt organized. He insisted medications made him feel bad. He would stop taking them and relapse in eight to ten days. Then the struggle would begin again.

171

My son's compliance with psychosocial treatments was not much better, but here the issue was complicated by the lack of meaningful activities. Psychodynamic therapies were tried with consistently disastrous results; day programs consisted of cake baking and braiding belts; vocational rehabilitation was an exercise in failure.

For twelve years my son has been fully compliant with his medication and has done well in a group home and in long visits with the family. He takes classes at the junior college and has succeeded; he is polite, considerate and at times quite sociable. Inattentiveness and hallucinations are his continuing problems.

My experiences with a son in treatment for schizophrenia leads me to believe that noncompliance is extraordinarily complex, but if the treatment is appropriate, absolutely essential.

FAMILIES HELPING THEMSELVES

While parents bear the main burden as caretakers of children with severe mental illness, spouses, siblings, children, grandparents and other relatives often play a role (Lefley & Johnson, 1990). Different relationships obviously modify role expectations, the degree of responsibility, and the powers of persuasion available to influence the compliance issue.

Overall the family role is ancillary to that of mental health professionals; we are family members first and aides to treatment second. Some people have reservations about any involvement, avoid contact with professionals and do not participate willingly in treatment (Atkinson, 1986). Others may be unable to participate because of age, infirmity or geographic separation imposed by our mobile society.

Family involvement is often made difficult by the nature of the illnesses themselves which involve lack of judgment and lack of insight to a greater degree than in most illness (Amador, Strauss, Yale, & Flaum, 1993; Walker & Rossiter, 1989; Lin, Spiga, & Fortsch, 1979). The afflicted person has changed, sometimes gradually, sometimes quite suddenly. Gradual change typically involves withdrawal, secretiveness, uncooperativeness, reduced interest and finally expression of strange ideas, anxiety and erratic behaviors. All of this is difficult for family members to understand. As one father wrote of his son who developed schizophrenia "his illness and the behaviors it evoked dumbfounded and frightened us ... we sensed something was wrong; something was missing" (Weisburd, 1990).

The very strangeness of the behaviors associated with mental illness bring ordinary coping skills to a stop. Furthermore, usual methods of influencing the relative become ineffective. Families have to cope with cognitive deficits that are present in many patients. Furthermore, the behavior changes take place in an insidious and ambiguous way. Much of the time the ill person's behavior may be quite normal so that the family believes their hypothesis about abnormal behavior may have been inappropriate (Anonymous, 1983; Slater, 1986). Eventually, often after a crisis involving some form of violence, the family realizes that major changes have taken place that are not normal and that professional help is needed.

Lastly, it is helpful to consider what is legally or socially required of families. This is rarely made explicit, and legal requirements do not exist in the United States as they do in some countries such as Japan. Nevertheless, implicit social expectations exist. For example, on release from hospital, staff routinely assume that the patient, even if an adult, will be released to the care of family members, who are not asked if this meets with their approval. Families just as typically assume that they have an obligation to accept the patient. While the family role is always marginal in an official sense, the principle expectations are moral and affectional; they are based on tacit assumptions of good and bad relationships and colored by the bonds of affection that exist within the family.

Whatever the difficulties or limitations of an individual member's involvement, many studies have found that clinical outcome is improved by family participation (Verghese, John, Rajkumar, Richard et al., 1989) and that family satisfaction with initial treatment recommendations is the best predictor of its outcome (Bulow, Sweeney, Shear, Friedman et al., 1987).

Family members play an important role both in explaining the importance of treatment and keeping track of it. Because these illnesses involve lack of judgment or insight that interferes with basic understanding of the need for treatment, families can play a significant role in repeated explanations which improve compliance (Ekman, Liberman, Phipps, Blair, 1990; Selzer, Sullivan, Carsky, & Terkelsen, 1989). Compliance with treatment is problematic for any patient, but for people with cognitive deficits involving memory or attention, remembering may be sporadic at best. Family members act as an extension of the patient's memory. Relatives can remind the ill person about taking medications, attending the psychosocial clubhouse, going to psychotherapy sessions, and so forth. Carrion and associates (Carrion, Swann, Kellert-Cecil, & Barber, 1993) found the main reason clients with schizophrenia said they missed clinic appointments was that they forgot or lacked transportation. Driving a car is hazardous for people with impaired attention and managing public transportation is difficult for the same reason. Relatives are sometimes able to meet these needs.

Impediments to Family Support

How Tough to Be? The greatest obstacle by far is that the sick family member will not cooperate with treatment. Some people state that treatment is unnecessary or harmful. Other comply superficially, but cheek the pills and run to the bathroom to be rid of them.

Relatives find after several unfortunate relapse experiences, that they have to monitor treatment closely and in doing so depart from the practice of encouraging autonomy. In addition to monitoring, they use persuasion, ruses, deceptions and threats to encourage compliance. For many families compliance with treatment is so important that ordinary family rules are suspended and anything goes that will be effective. For example, should they hide medication in liquid form in their relatives orange juice? Most relatives soon learn that ruses, deceptions and threats undercut the trust essential in family relationships. Families want to know of better ways of managing compliance.

Families do not understand why family members who are obviously severely mentally ill and in need of medication should be allowed by hospital staff to refuse. Families ask why the patient isn't simply forced to take the medication. When told that this might be a violation of civil rights (Geller, 1986) families are shocked: "How can a person who is psychotic, who lacks judgment, who endangers self and others, be assumed to have the competence to make such an important decision?" Families would probably agree with Paul and Lentz (1977) that treatment should be enforced if empirical evidence exists for the effectiveness of a treatment and if it is the judgment of experts that the patient would be likely to benefit.

Beliefs About Treatment Efficacy — One of the most common questions raised by families is how important the treatment really is for well-being. It is not uncommon, especially early in treatment, for families to go along with the patient who says, "These pills are destroying my mind. I feel better without them and won't take them." Neither the patient nor the family has grasped just how important medications are. At a time when holistic health is in the ascendancy some people do not believe in taking medications, which are seen as "chemicals" or "unnatural" and they prefer vitamins, exercise, massage, etc. Within psychiatry these proposals have received support from the orthomolecular movement (see commentary by Yudofsky, Hales, & Ferguson, 1991). A larger number of families do believe that medications are necessary but question other treatments. They dismiss psychotherapy as unimportant for illnesses that have a biological cause.

Confidentiality — Families often report that they are not told enough about their relatives condition because professionals evoke confidentiality. This is extremely irritating to families because it places them in a bind: They are expected to be caretakers, but are deprived of information.

Complexity of Compliance — A major obstacle to obtaining and maintaining adherence to prescribed treatments is their complexity. Taking medications is not easy under ideal circumstances; adding other treatments from the psychosocial arena makes the matter almost impossibly complex. Complexity increases even more with dual diagnosis whether it is a combination of serious mental illness with substance abuse or with developmental handicap.

FAMILIES HELPING FAMILIES

Families should know about the National Alliance for the Mentally Ill (NAMI), Depressive and Manic Depressive Association (DMDA) and the local and state organizations. NAMI is comprised of people with personal experience of mental illness as consumers, relatives or friends. These people have a vast collective experience with treatment and the issue of compliance.

Valuable information is also provided at local, regional and national meetings which include talks by mental health professionals on medication and other forms of treatment.

Although mutual support groups are typically viewed as important in offering an opportunity to express feelings related to the burden of mental illness, these groups also serve vital networking functions. In addition, information is provided through national media such as the *NAMI Advocate* and state and local newsletters.

There is little research on the effect of mutual support group participation and compliance. In one of the rare studies, members of DMDA were surveyed about their medication beliefs and practices. This study of consumers and their relatives (Kurtz, 1990) found the belief in the efficacy of medication improved after participation in DMDA groups.

An important form of family education that is being implemented nationwide by NAMI members is the "Journey of Hope." Twelve classes are held for family members with trainers who are members of NAMI, not necessarily mental health professionals. The goal is to provide families with the information they need to cope effectively with serious mental illness. These are described, a biological etiology is emphasized, coping methods are detailed and the importance of medication is stated.

PROFESSIONALS HELPING FAMILIES

There are a variety of ways in which professionals can assist families in coping with their sick family members (Bernheim & Lehman, 1985; Bernheim & Switalski, 1988). This includes psychiatrists (Diamond, 1986), nurses (Mulaik, 1992) social workers (Bentley, Rosenson, & Zito, 1990), and case managers (Mason & Siris, 1992).

Providing Information — Surveys indicate that families want information of all kinds about mental illness and complain that professionals do not provide enough. Families appreciate professionals who listen to the relatives and are willing to provide advice on coping and resources. At the very least professionals should suggest useful reading such as Torrey's *Surviving Schizophrenia: A Family Manual* (1988). This book is regarded as essential by most families.

Professionals should be aware of their restricted language code (Bernstein, 1971). Families may not know the terms used or standard treatment procedures. Assumptions about what families know should be clarified and communication tailored to assure understanding (Barroughclough, Tarrier, Watts, Vaughn, Bamrah, & Freeman, 1987). As a member of the National Alliance for the Mentally Ill (NAMI), I often hear complaints that professionals will not listen to family members who know through experience that a particular medication is not effective or causes severe side effects. Professionals then ignore the relative and prescribe the drug anyway. Discussion of treatment is essential and welcomed by families.

Families sometimes report that they are not invited to participate in treatment (Spaniol, Zipple, & Lockwood, 1992). Holden and Lewine (1982) found that only half of families were told why medications were prescribed and only a quarter were given information about side effects. In our multicultural society it is also important that professionals be aware of the different ways in which various cultures view the role of the family in the treatment alliance and the ways in which attitudes and beliefs may differ from traditional Western medicine (Ng, 1993; Kinzie, 1986).

In some states, professionals are required to provide information to families, spell out the treatment plan, the options for medications and psychosocial treatments including the benefits and side effects. Confidentiality should not be an issue if the patient agrees to sharing information. Very few patients refuse when they are told why the information should be shared. In those rare instances of continued refusal professionals can hold joint consultations with patient and family members so that what is said to one is heard by all.

Adequate Assessment of Compliance Problems — Physicians sometimes fail to identify the causes of noncompliance because they make assumptions about their patients that may not be warranted (Bartlett, Higginbotham, Cohen-Cole, & Bird, 1990). Open-ended questioning results in information that has more relevance for individual patients. Enquiry should include the following: 1) experience with past treatment. Has the patient received treatments before and what happened? 2) The patient and family beliefs about treatments and their efficacy. 3) Family communication and influence patterns. Is it likely the family will be able to modify compliance?

Appropriate Intervention Strategies — Professional suggestions about how to maximize compliance may include the following:

1) Keep a record of all medications taken. This should be a permanent log for future reference. It should note both the side effects and benefits of different medications.

2) List all medications taken at a given time and when scheduled.

3) Arrange medications by dose in plastic envelopes, boxes or some other convenient form. It should be possible to tell if a medication has been taken as prescribed.

4) Pairing medication taking with habitual activities, such as eating breakfast, brushing teeth, etc.

5) Asking family members to suggest other procedures that they think will help.

These suggestions help the family monitor medication compliance and forestall relapse. The procedures have another effect: by systematizing and routinizing medication procedures, emotionality surrounding compliance is reduced. It is no longer an issue of "you are trying to get me to do something I don't want to do" or "you are upsetting me by not following prescribed treatments."

Professionals should recognize that all interventions will be more effective if they are individualized, identify informational deficits, provide specific facts or training, and check to confirm learning has occurred (Brophy, 1986).

Family Consultation — The family consultation model was introduced by Bernheim (1982) and elaborated by Wynne and Associates (Wynne 1987; Wynne, McDaniel, & Weber, 1987). This model was developed as an alternative to family therapy which had been found to be inappropriate for severe mental illnesses (Terkelsen, 1983). In this model the professional serves as a consultant. The family declares what their concerns are and the professional is available as a source of information and support. The family may accept or reject the consultant's suggestions and the question of "resistance" does not arise. In carrying out the consultant role the professional must have expert knowledge about illness and resources available for treatment and rehabilitation. Consultants must have skills in understanding family systems and in making recommendations based on a systems analysis. Treatment compliance is a natural part of this work.

An attractive feature of the family consultation model is this great flexibility; it is easily tailored to meet the specific needs of individual families. The negative feature is that it does not provide for the support and information that can be obtained within a group of families working together.

Family Education — One form of education for family members is the Survival Skills Workshop, a full-day session on the causes, forms and treatment of illness and ways in which families may facilitate the recovery process (Anderson, Reiss, & Hogarty, 1986). The information is similar to the "Journey of Hope," but mental health professionals typically are the presenters.

Kelly and Scott (1990) developed two interventions to improve compliance and patient outcomes. One focused on engaging families in the rehabilitation process and the other trained patients to be consumers. Both interventions improved medication compliance.

Bipolar patients and their partners have been found to benefit from group education sessions (Goodwin & Jamison, 1990). According to Van Gent and Zwart (1991), these sessions resulted in increased knowledge of illness, medication and social strategies. It should be noted that Lam (1991) in his review of family education found that this approach did increase knowledge, but did not reduce relapse rates suggesting that it did not improve compliance. An exception to this, not reviewed by Lam, is the practice of having psychiatric nurses visit the home and provide information, counseling and support to the family and the ill relative (Pai & Kaipur, 1982).

Family Psychoeducation — Psychoeducation differs from family education because it includes the patient and the whole family; both receive training in coping with mental illness and managing stress. In his review, Lam (1991) concluded that psychoeducation is more effective than education alone in reducing relapse. Furthermore, it seems to offer an ideal context for promoting compliance in all its forms. Treatment, including medication compliance, is emphasized and families are trained to make changes gradually to reduce stress. The approach also involves an optimistic outlook with families encouraged not to expect rapid change, but to look at long-term outcomes.

Falloon (Falloon, Boyd, McGill, Razani, Moss, & Gilderman, 1982) found participants in a family psychoeducation program were more compliant in medication taking than the control group. In other family education programs (Leff, Kuipers, Berkowitz, Eberlein-Fries, 1982; Tarrier, Barroughclough, Vaughn, Bamrah, Porceddu, Watts, & Freeman, 1988) compliance has been excellent in both experimental and control groups, perhaps due to the nonspecific attention paid to participants in a research program (see Chapter 1).

The success of family psychoeducation has been attributed by Birchwood and Cochrane (1990) to the fact that advising relatives about changes in their coping styles is coupled with an understanding of the origins of the behavior of their mentally ill relatives.

CONCLUSION

Professionals and family members seem to agree that families play an important role in compliance with prescribed treatments. It is also clear that compliance can be enhanced using methods of working with families. Unfortunately, there is little evidence that mental health professionals have made concerted efforts to apply these methods, and there is little research about the most efficient and effective means of improving compliance with the aid of families.

REFERENCES

Amador, X. F., Strauss, D. H., Yale, S. A., & Flaum, M. M. (1993). Assessment of insight in psychosis. *American Journal of Psychiatry, 150,* 873–879.

Anderson, C. M., Reiss, D. J., & Hogarty, G. E. (1986). *Schizophrenia in the family: a practitioners guide to psychoeducation and management.* New York: Guilford.

Anonymous. (1983). First person account: a father's thoughts. *Schizophrenia Bulletin, 9,* 439–442.

Atkinson, J. M. (1986). *Schizophrenia at home: a guide to helping the family.* New York: New York University Press.

Barroughclough, C., Tarrier, N., Watts, S., Vaughn, C., Bamrah, J. S., & Freeman, L. (1987). Assessing the functional value of relative's knowledge about schizophrenia: a preliminary report. *British Journal of Psychiatry, 151,* 1–8.

Bartlett, E. E., Higginbotham, J. C., Cohen-Cole, S., & Bird, J. (1990). How do primary care residents manage patient nonadherence. *Patient Education and Counseling, 16,* 53–60.

Bentley, K. J., Rosenson, M. K., & Zito, J. M. (1990). Promoting mediation compliance: strategies for working with families of mentally ill people. *Social Work, 35,* 274–277.

Bernheim, K. F., (1982). Supportive family counseling. *Schizophrenia Bulletin, 8,* 634–641.

Bernheim, K. F., & Lehman, A. F. (1985). *Working with families of the mentally ill.* New York: Norton.

Bernheim, K. F., & Switalski, T. (1988). Mental health staff and patients' relatives: how they view each other. *Hospital and Community Psychiatry, 39,* 63–68.

Bernstein, B. (1971). *Class, codes and control: Volume One.* London: Routledge & Kegan Paul.

Birchwood, M., & Cochrane, R. (1990). Families coping with schizophrenia: coping styles, their origins and correlatives. *Psychological Medicine, 20,* 857–865.

Brophy, J. (1986). Teacher influences on student achievement. *American Psychologist, 41,* 1069–1072.

Buchanan, A. (1992). A two-year prospective study of treatment compliance in patients with schizophrenia. *Psychological Medicine, 22,* 787–797.

Bulow, B., Sweeney, J. A., Shear, M. K., Friedman, R., Plowe, C. (1987). Family satisfaction with psychiatric evaluations. *Health and Social Work, 12,* 290–295.

Carrion, P. G., Swann, A., Kellert-Cecil, H., & Barber, M. (1993). Compliance with clinic attendance by outpatients with schizophrenia. *Hospital and Community Psychiatry, 44,* 764–765.

Diamond, R. J. (1986). Strategies for medication compliance with resistant patients. *Psychiatric Annals, 16,* 664–666.

Ekman, T. A., Liberman, R. P., Phipps, C. C., & Blair, K. E. (1990). Teaching medication management skills to schizophrenic patients. *Journal of Clinical Psychopharmacology, 10,* 33–38.

Falloon, I. R. H., Boyd, J. L., McGill, C. W., Razani, J., Moss, H. B., & Gilderman, A. M. (1982). Family management in the prevention of exacerbation's of schizophrenia. *New England Journal of Medicine, 306,* 1437–1440.

Geller, J. (1986). Rights, wrongs, and the dilemma of coerced community treatment. *American Journal of Psychiatry, 143,* 1259–1264.

Goodwin, F. K., & Jamison, K. R. (1990). *Manic-depressive illness.* New York: Oxford.

Holden, D. F., & Lewine, R. R. J. (1982). How families evaluate mental health professionals, resources, and effects of illness. *Schizophrenia Bulletin, 8,* 628–633.

Kelly, G. R., & Scott, J. E. (1990). Medication compliance and health education among outpatients with chronic mental disorders. *Medical Care, 28,* 1181–1197.

Kinzie, J. D. (1986). Mental health treatment that transcends cultural barriers. *Hospital and Community Psychiatry, 37,* 1144–1147.

Kurtz, L. F. (1990). Use of lithium and other medications by members of a self-help group. *Lithium, 1,* 125–126.

Lam, D. H. (1991). Psychosocial family intervention in schizophrenia: a review of empirical studies. *Psychological Medicine, 21,* 423–441.

Leff, J. P., Kuipers, L., Berkowitz, R., Eberlein-Fries, R., & Sturgeon, D. (1982). A controlled trial of social intervention in the families of schizophrenic patients. *British Journal of Psychiatry, 141,* 121–134.

Lefley, H. P., & Johnson, D. L. (1990). *Families as allies in treatment of the mentally ill.* Washington: American Psychiatric Press.

Lin, I. F., Spiga, R., & Fortsch, W. (1979). Insight and adherence to medication in chronic schizophrenics. *Journal of Clinical Psychiatry, 40,* 430–432.

Mason, S. R., & Siris, G. (1992). Dual diagnosis: the case for case management. *American Journal on Addictions, 1,* 77–82.

Mulaik, J. S. (1992). Noncompliance with medication regimens in severely and persistently mentally ill schizophrenic patients. *Issues in Mental Health Nursing, 13,* 219–237.

Ng, M. L. (1993). Cultural factors in psychiatric rehabilitation in Hong Kong. *International Journal of Mental Health, 21,* 33–38.

Pai, S., & Kaipur, R. L. (1982). The burden on the family of a psychiatric patient: development of an interview schedule. *British Journal of Psychiatry, 138,* 332–335.

Paul, G. L., & Lentz, R. J. (1977). *Psychosocial treatment of chronic mental patients.* Cambridge, MA: Harvard University Press.

Selzer, M. A., Sullivan, T. B., Carsky, M., & Terkelsen, K. G. (1989). *Working with the person with schizophrenia: the treatment alliance.* New York: New York University Press.

Slater, E. (1986). First person account: a parent's view on enforcing medication. *Schizophrenia Bulletin, 12,* 291–292.

Spaniol, L., Zipple, A. F., & Lockwood, D. (1992). The role of the family in psychiatric rehabilitation. *Innovations and Research, 2,* 27–34.

Tarrier, N., Barroughclough, C., Vaughn, C., Bamrah, J.S., Porceddu, K., Watts, S., & Freeman, H. (1988). The community management of schizophrenia: a controlled trial of a behavioural intervention with families to reduce relapse. *British Journal of Psychiatry, 153,* 532–542.

Terkelsen, K. G. (1983). Schizophrenia and the family: adverse effects of family therapy. *Family Process, 22,* 191–200.

Torrey, E. F. (1988). *Surviving schizophrenia: a family manual.* New York: Harper & Row.

Van Gent, E. M., & Zwart, F. M. (1991). Psychoeducation of partners of bipolar-manic patients. *Journal of Affective Disorders, 21,* 15–18.

Verghese, A., John, J. K., Rajkumar, S., Richard, J. et al. (1989). Factors associated with the course and outcome of schizophrenia in India: results of a two-year multicentre follow-up study. *British Journal of Psychiatry, 154,* 499–503.

Walker, E. F., & Rossiter, J. (1989). Schizophrenic patients' self-perceptions: legal and clinical implications. *Journal of Psychiatry and Law, 17,* 55–73.

Weisburd, D. E. (1990). Planning a community-based mental health system: perspective of a family member. *American Psychologist, 45,* 1245–1248.

Wynne, L. C. (1987). The family consultant: a redefined role for collaborating with families of schizophrenics. Unpublished Mysell Lecture at Harvard University, January 15.

Wynne, L. C., McDaniel, S. M., Weber, T. T. (1987). Professional politics and the concepts of family therapy, family consultation, and systems consultation. *Family Process, 26,* 153–166.

Yudofsky, S., Hales, R. E., & Ferguson, T. (1991). *What you need to know about psychiatric drugs.* New York: Grove Weidenfeld.

11

Reactance and the Psychotherapeutic Alliance

THOMAS L. KUHLMAN

My interest in noncompliance began with a childhood beholden to the authoritarian precepts of pre-Vatican II Catholicism. Life thus proceeded through an adolescence that was rather predictably noncompliant of many otherwise legitimate authority figures. Doctors and nurses were not numbered among these — until they ran afoul of my deep love for playing basketball.

In my mid-twenties I sustained a whiplash injury in an automobile accident. After X-rays and consultations, two of three orthopedists recommended immediate spinal fusion surgery. A third conceded that I could put the surgery off until my pain grew worse, but in the meantime I would be at risk for becoming some kind of "-plegic" if I sustained another such blow to my head or neck. All three doctors were adamant that I should never ski or play contact sports again.

I declined surgery. When my neck pain receded I resumed playing full-court basketball, eventually returning to my pre-accident frequency and intensity. I played for another ten years, quitting only when my skills had eroded. Perhaps twice a year I would absorb a blow that would send a wave of numbness to reverberate through my body. After a brief time-out I would resume playing. I was never seriously injured. An X-ray taken twelve years after the accident did not show any residual damage from the whiplash.

Interestingly, I have yet to resume downhill skiing since the accident. This island of ongoing compliance with the orthopedists' recommendations has now lasted eight years beyond the negative X-ray findings.

181

When I reflect upon such inconsistent behavior by a presumably intelligent and well-educated patient, the concept of compliance-noncompliance seems absurdly misshapen as a dichotomous variable. I am also aware of the study by P. Ley (1986) which found that health care professionals were highly noncompliant as a group when they themselves were forced into the patient role by illness or injury.

In my professional life as a clinical psychologist I have gravitated to settings visited by dangerous, disturbed, and/or difficult people. This includes thousands of contacts with homeless persons during several years of providing direct service work in urban shelters and drop-in centers. In these kinds of settings, dire necessities grant one the freedom to be noncompliant with prevailing clinical wisdom and practices. One learns that non-compliance may be an addiction for some but that it is a Darwinian life force for others. It has proven worthy of my cautious respect even as I myself have been cast in the role of the authority figure who is opposed or defied.

The motivational spark for this chapter came from my recent literature review of the social-psychological construct known as reactance. Reactance theory loosens noncompliance from both its negative definition (i.e. as merely the absence of compliance) and its negative connotations.

A final note concerning my use of the term "patient." I believe that there are substantial implications for understanding compliance behaviors through the labels that we assign to "patients," "clients," "consumers," "recipients," and so forth. Since exploring these implications is beyond the scope of this chapter, I have selected the term "patient" for stylistic consistency. I do so in deference to the professional tradition which predominates among the book's sponsor, editor, chapter authors, and target audience.

Reactance motivation. Psychological reactance is a motivational construct which has emerged from the last twenty-five years of social psychological research on processes of persuasion and attitude change. The assumptions which underlie reactance theory place a premium upon an individual's perception of available personal freedoms. In its most basic form, the theory proposes that the loss of a freedom (or threat of same) will give rise to a motivational state propelling the individual to restore that freedom to its previous condition (Brehm & Brehm, 1981.) In this theory, "freedom" refers not to a global value or spiritual entity but rather to the moment-to-moment flow of specific behaviors and mundane events over which a person believes one has some control. Reactance motivation will be strongest when the threatened freedom is an important one (e.g. in the author's case, to play basketball) and when the person believes that personal effort can restore that freedom or remedy its threatened status. If attempts at the restoration of such a freedom prove futile and it comes to be perceived as permanently lost, reactance motivation dissolves into the amotivational state of learned helplessness, the cognitive aspect of clinical depression. Losses of or threats to unimportant freedoms (e.g. in the author's case, to go downhill skiing) do not arouse reactance motivation nor progress to learned helplessness. Whether a person deems a particular freedom to be important or not is a function of one's unique developmental history.

A number of parameters which govern the freedom-reactance relationship have been specified, and many testable hypotheses which flow from the theory have been confirmed in social-psychological experiments (see Brehm & Brehm, 1981.) For example, a recent study of reactance theory investigated alcohol consumption by underaged students across ten colleges (Allen, Sprenkel, & Vitale, 1994.) It was conducted in states which had recently raised the legal drinking age, thus restricting the freedom to drink of people who had previously exercised this freedom. The study authors found a pre-legislation to post-legislation increase in alcohol consumption among the newly underaged subjects, but not among control subjects who were of legal age both before and after the legislation. Across the same time period there was no corresponding increase in the rate of illicit drug use among the newly underaged drinkers. This too was consistent with reactance theory: because the laws in question entailed no new restrictions upon the freedom to engage in this activity, they engendered no reactance motivation to increase drug use behavior.

The present chapter explores the relevance of psychological reactance for understanding and ameliorating compliance problems in psychotherapy with patients who have severe mental impairments and/or are homeless. From the psychotherapist's perspective, patient compliance signifies a tacit interpersonal contract. Requests of the patient by the therapist are likely to be complied with to the extent that the patient freely chooses the patient role and freely concedes expert status to the therapist. Placebo effects are thus construed as heightened suggestibility triggered by a person's exercising the freedom to adopt the patient role.

It is submitted here that psychological reactance is a converse (but equally powerful) process relative to placebo. The degree of reactance motivation present is a barometer of the extent to which a person is a less-than-free participant in the working alliance. Reactance must be expected not only in involuntary treatments (as imposed by judges and court agents) but also in less-than-voluntary treatments (such as outreach work in which the person must be recruited to the patient role before treatment can begin.) The case vignettes which illustrate the chapter are drawn from the author's experiences in involuntary settings (locked impatient units for committed patients) and the less-than-voluntary context of street outreach work with homeless persons.

Semantics. A brief diversion to compare and contrast reactance with other compliance-related concepts is in order. The value of construing reactance as an interactional process (like placebo) rather than a patient characteristic (like "lack of insight" or "treatment resistant") will become apparent.

"Lack of insight" is a phrase which is commonly used to denote that some severely impaired patients do not seem to know that they are impaired. It refers to a presumed deficit in a patient's self-awareness or self-understanding, but it exists only by implicit comparison with a therapist's awareness and understanding. Certainly there are patients whose accurate self-perception is precluded by cognitive disruptions or positive symptoms. But in many cases it is wise to consider whether or not an apparent lack of insight reflects a patient who is reactant to the therapist and the patient role. Such a patient may perceive important cognitive and behavioral freedoms being restricted by the process of being assigned a diagnosis.

> A difficult woman with paranoid schizophrenia was encountered by a street outreach team. She insisted that she had been a victim of "submarine germ warfare" during her military experience. The team was ultimately successful in getting her to move from a cave on the Mississippi River into a supportive living facility. This success was achieved only after all team members adopted the phrase "submarine germ warfare" in their interactions and negotiations with her, and then were willing to write the phrase into professional reports which the patient insisted upon examining (Kuhlman, 1994, p. 65–66.)

This patient was conceded her private label; her compliance with placement and, later, with treatment reflected an implicit insight that she was in need of help. To acknowledge this at outreach would have restricted her freedom to see herself as a special case or a government victim. In this and other cultures, acceptance of the role "psychiatric patient" closes off many avenues of consciousness that normally uphold one's sense of self-respect.

Reactance motivation is a dynamism that cuts many ways. Some of the personal freedoms encumbered by the patient role will be discussed shortly. For present purposes it will suffice to note that viewing such patients as reactant invites a problem-solving orientation, i.e. "what important freedoms of this person are being threatened or restricted by meeting with me under these conditions?" In contrast, "lack of insight" is dismissive. It assigns blame to the patient for the failure to establish an alliance and may subtly undermine a therapist's efforts to get to know the patient. Who has not seen this phrase in a therapist's report without lowering one's expectations about the patient's prognosis?

Reactance is more readily confused with the term "resistance," which also has unfortunate connotations. As Kirmayer (1990) observed, it suggests willful opposition to the therapist is being attributed to the patient. Some behavioral and cognitive therapists have taken the opposite position and asserted that there is no such thing as a resistant patient (see Dowd, 1989.) They suggest that resistant behaviors are appropriate responses to ineffective therapists or ineffective techniques. The opposing positions converge in their assumptions that resistance means something is wrong with the alliance and that someone must be blamed.

A more normalizing view is to consider resistance as a potent variety of reactance motivation that arises under the following conditions: (1) the patient role has been accepted; (2) a working alliance has been established on grounds of mutual trust and agreed-upon goals and role expectations; and (3) reactance occurs when core aspects of the patient's pre-therapy world views are being challenged. Put another way, the patient resists when freedom to remain allied with the pre-therapy world views is threatened or restricted by the therapist's interventions. Whether the therapist construes these core world views in terms of unconscious conflicts (psychoanalysis), the sense of meaning to one's life (existentialism), or the ability to predict and control life events (cognitive-behaviorism) is of little relevance to resistance itself. It *is* relevant to expect a patient to safeguard the freedom to regress to world views that have served the patient so long (if inadequately) in the past. Resistance is thus a normal, even an encouraging marker of effective psychotherapy. The therapist is advised to reflect upon such episodes for patient freedoms being breached or threatened. This may prove more beneficial than awaiting new opportunities to "work through" the resistance by repeating the intervention or dismissing the intervention as ineffective.

Reactance as a state variable. Psychological reactance was originally studied as a situationally-induced motivational state rather than an ingrained character trait. It arises in the process of one party attempting to persuade or change the attitudes of another.

The present focus is on severely impaired persons who take less-than-voluntary stances toward the patient role. Accepting the patient role is not an all-or-nothing decision. The freedoms lost by choosing to become a patient will retain their attraction until effective treatment can create or expand cognitive and behavioral freedoms of its own to outweigh those given up. Until these benefits of treatment accrue, it will be half of the therapist's challenge to persuade the person of the value of treatment. The other half of the challenge is to verbalize and explore whatever personal freedoms the patient perceives to be lost or threatened by becoming a patient. Psychological reactance should dissipate as a person consents to abridging or surrendering personal freedoms — but only when such consent represents an exercise of cognitive or behavioral freedom. Such is the task that confronts the outreach therapist.

Minkoff (1987) was one of the first to argue that the challenges of deinstitutionalization in the 1990's are quite different from those encountered in the 1960's and 1970's. The original cohort of deinstitutionalized patients had been long-term residents of psychiatric hospitals. Many of them had endured so many years of restricted freedoms that reactance had given way to learned helplessness. They emerged from the state institutions as dependent, submissive, skill-deficient, and in need of considerable training and modeling to deal with their many newly-restored freedoms. In contrast, the "deinstitutionalized" homeless person of the 1990's is much less likely to have endured extended hospitalization during an era of relaxed commitment laws and economic disincentives. Many patients have successfully fought civil commitments or seen them dropped in response to their reactant opposition. Such escapes from the patient role are later recalled or recounted with pride. Even those who are actively psychotic are by no means as skilless as those of the first wave of deinstitutionalization. The outreach therapist must look beyond a person's symptoms and poverty to the meanings that the person associates with becoming a patient.

Some obvious freedoms restricted by the patient role are those imposed by treatment. Psychotropic medications or electro-convulsive therapy entail surrendering control of brain processes to an outside agent. Side effects may appear, dietary restrictions may be imposed, appointments need to be kept, perhaps blood tests will be required. Therapists tend to take for granted such mundane impositions of the patient role. Work with homeless persons throws them into sharper relief. Daily uncertainties about shelter, food, transportation, and child care render time-honored practices like the fixed appointment a serious imposition on an already difficult lifestyle.

The freedom to think of oneself as healthy is subtle and readily taken for granted. Suffering may render patients willing to surrender this belief, but they will also seek its reinstatement as soon as possible. Witness the fact that many patients stop taking medicines as soon as they feel better rather than finishing them as prescribed (Meichenbaum & Turk, 1987).

Many therapists find it difficult to fathom how people with psychosis cling to the illusion they are well. Some of these people are reactant to the prospect of a higher quality of life if they must label themselves as psychiatrically disabled (Kuhlman, 1994). Others pride themselves on mastering the difficult street culture and challenge therapists to prove that they can do it as well. And psychotic symptoms may have survival value (Koegel, 1992). The author has witnessed a psychotic woman rout a trio of male predators by conjuring a bizarrely psychotic state that she had never displayed before nor after (Kuhlman, 1994). Some homeless persons will acknowledge that medications reduce their symptoms and suffering, but side effects of sluggishness or longer reaction times render them at a disadvantage for defending themselves. Finally, advocates for homeless people have made many of them aware how the diagnosis of mental illness is used to blame the victim.

It is excellent therapy to help prospective patients voice such beliefs, and to empathize with them. The grounding for such empathy is the ubiquity of the phrase "in denial": it is human nature to cling to the belief that one is healthy even as evidence is mounting otherwise. Outreach therapists are trained to address the basic needs (food, shelter) of a homeless person first and treatment needs second. This may be sufficient to entice some into treatment, but others who must surrender their sense of psychological fitness (however illusory) will not be so easily persuaded. Therapists need to make at least a tacit or implicit connection with whatever beliefs such persons need to surrender in becoming a patient.

Beyond threats to the freedom to think of oneself as healthy are restrictions imposed by thinking of oneself as sick. The stigmatization of mental illness in the U.S. is widely acknowledged. There are homeless persons who will refuse to live in housing for mentally ill people. Many board-and-care facilities treat adults like children. There are curfews, mandatory group therapies and medications; patients are forbidden to indulge in alcohol or sexual activity. Violations of such rules may mean an appearance before a committee or some "Nurse Ratchett" authority figure. This allusion to One Flew Over the Cuckoo's Nest is not incidental. Many people with no treatment experience (and some with it) shape their concepts of what the patient role is like from such films.

Negative associations may have also been taught by parents. "Crazy" relatives may have been mocked or ridiculed at the supper table. Mother's visits to the hospital during depressive episodes may have been communicated in "don't ask" euphemisms to the children. Other potential patients may have been subjected to repeated verbal abuse by a parent who called them "crazy," "insane," or "out of your mind". Still others observe symptoms in themselves that they first saw in parents or relatives during episodes of mental illness. Any and all such experiences attach private, personalized aspects to the public stigmata of mental illness. It must be part of the outreach therapist's work to free a person's adoption of the patient role from as many of these negative associations as possible.

Some homeless persons who have insight into their impairments shun the mental health patient role, yet seek some treatment equivalent from paraprofessionals, ministers, or public health nurses. In the author's experience almost none of the well-intentioned referrals of such potential patients from their proxy therapists work out. It may be better to leave such persons in the counsel of a proxy therapist but remain available in the guise of a consultant or adviser.

This vignette concerns a man with schizophrenia in his fifties. He had been institutionalized for more than two decades after having committed several violent felonies during a psychotic episode. He was one of the first patient transfers to a new maximum security ward in a new forensic hospital where the author had been hired as the first "unit chief". The patient was court-ordered to take medications but religiously eschewed other forms of therapy. He drew his identity and self-esteem from being kept with the most dangerous (and otherwise much younger) patients.

A week after the unit's opening, he approached the author in the dayroom and brayed a sardonic challenge in front of several other patients: "So you're the unit chief, huh?" Consistent with the unit's gallows humor, the author responded that this title was not correct, that a ward of tough guys like this one needed a king rather than a mere unit chief. The patient was dumbstruck and the effect was reinforced when staff began to behave in accordance with this ludicrous premise. This patient turned to the other patients and mockingly exclaimed, "he thinks he's a king!" After that he would often address the author with a tongue-in-cheek, "your majesty." But, more importantly, in private he would abandon much of his tough guy persona. And he was compliant with all of the author's requests during the next year of his hospitalization. He ultimately complied with placement in a community-based supportive living facility, something that he had protested against in the past (Kuhlman, 1988.)

Another source of reactance motivation in the patient role is its implicit deference to external authority on innermost thoughts or feelings. In a maximum security setting this extends to such elemental freedoms as where one can walk or when one can use the bathroom. This patient was not freed from these constraints even when he opted to address the author as "your majesty." But once the author mocked his source of power over the patient, the patient became less motivated to mock that power himself according to prevailing maximum security custom. Nor was he the exceptional case: two years after the unit had opened, its dangerous patients with psychoses evidenced only infrequent episodes of aggression.

There are less dramatic ways to address reactance that is evoked by one's authority or expertise. I usually introduce myself as "Dr. Tom Kuhlman." This sometimes elicits hesitation or smiles from patients who are not sure whether to think of me as "doctor" or as "Tom." If I am queried about which I prefer, I cede the choice to the patient and most seem content. Many patients seem to want both formality and informality, the trappings of both authority and friend — these will address me as "Dr. Tom." If how to be addressed is not an important freedom to the therapist, why not cede that freedom to the patient? (I would note here that I have never introduced myself as "Tom" in any outreach contact. Not mentioning one's professional status and role can later be seen as deception or trickery, thereby dooming any alliance.)

Reactance as a trait variable. Some people experience reactance motivation to the slightest restriction on the least important freedom. Behavioral consistency across time and situation is the definition of a personality trait, and at least two tests have been developed to measure reactance this way (Dowd, Milne, & Wise, 1991; Hong & Page, 1989.) In Dowd's (1989) view, the unique developmental and learning histories of some individuals render all of their free behaviors to be of grave importance and all threats to freedoms of grave magnitude. He suggests that these people are the colloquial "control freaks" who do not see themselves as having enough mastery of their environments. They are hypervigilant to situations where others might be perceived as assuming control over them. In this vein reactance has been linked with the constellation of traits known as the Type A personality and advanced as an explanation for Type A individuals being non-compliant with medical treatments (Rhodewalt & Fairfield, 1991.)

It is seldom clear at a therapist's first contact with a patient whether reactance is a situational or a characterological response. However, situational reactance is often amenable to negotiation and education: "no, I will not recommend ECT or drugs;" "no, I cannot read your mind;" "no, I won't challenge your belief that the FBI is following you." To the extent that reactance is confined to one or few issues, and the patient seems comfortable with the deferential aspects of the patient role, then the therapist may address reactance with empathic listening, support, or education.

Those who are reactant by trait will show contrarian attitudes on a wide variety of subjects. Diagnostically, trait reactance is most closely associated with oppositional-defiant disorder in children and paranoid and passive-aggressive personality disorder in adults. But it is wrong to expect the characterological manifestations of reactance to be confined by diagnosis. This trait is prevalent among hard-to-reach, severely impaired homeless individuals. This is particularly true in communities which have relatively good public sector mental health services. In such communities where the needs of compliant, non-reactant patients are well met, there will be a greater concentration of reactant patients among those who are on the streets and not in treatment. Outreach therapists who believe that persons who are homeless and psychotic are merely underserved or unaccessed should expect some rude awakenings.

Inpatient therapists' worst nightmares involve the contrarian behaviors of patients who are diagnosed with borderline personality disorder. The struggles that emanate from attempts to control the suicidal behaviors of such patients are difficult to resolve. Psychoanalysts may construe such struggles in the language of projective identification and splitting, but reactance motivation proved to be a sufficient explanation in the case study which follows (Kuhlman, Green, & Sincaban, 1988.) Effective management did not occur until the treatment team surrendered their efforts to control the patient.

> Ms. B was a 26 year old single woman who was a four year resident of a locked state hospital unit. By that point in her hospitalization, a wide range of treatments (including ECT) and community placement attempts had failed. If she had changed at all it was in the direction of increased suicidal behavior. Two of her attempts had been life-threatening. In one, nursing staff had cut her down from an attempt at hanging. The residual effect on staff was that of a shared post-traumatic stress syndrome. Beyond being the centerpiece of the staff's work stress, Ms. B was bright, verbal, and adept at exploiting the limits of complicated treatment plans that were written and revised to minimize her opportunities to traumatize the staff. After these treatment plans were put into effect, Ms. B would behave in ways that would elicit inconsistent implementation by different staff and different shifts, and she would calmly explain these inconsistencies in exquisite detail at progress review meetings. Not surprisingly, many staff came to despise her, and after a four year siege there appeared to be an increasing risk that staff might passive-aggressively fail to intervene in one of her suicide attempts. She could not be transferred from the unit because there was no more secure setting available.
>
> The watershed intervention occurred when staff publicly acknowledged that she was more powerful than them, and that staff would cease efforts to treat her according to a traditional plan. Instead, staff formulated a plan with the goal of treating their own anxieties about having to deal with such a powerful patient. The plan was called dice therapy because Ms. B's behavioral freedoms (i.e. off-ward privileges, seclusion room for suicidality, etc.) for any eight-hour shift were to be determined by her roll of a die at the beginning of the shift. With her treatment pre-determined in this fashion, staff were relieved of interacting with her around suicide issues, privilege granting, and other freedom-granting and freedom-restricting issues. This unusual plan required Ms. B's informed consent and she consulted with a patients' rights advocate before signing it.
>
> Dice therapy lasted for two weeks. At that point Ms. B requested another chance at a community placement which she had previously sabotaged by suicide attempts (the advocate had explained to her that she could also end dice therapy by withdrawing her informed consent, but she did not do this.) The community placement worked out; a month later the unit received a letter in which she said she missed the staff but "I sure as hell don't miss those damned dice." A year later she was readmitted to the unit for stabilization in the face of significant life stressors. She did not revert to her previous persona

nor attempt suicide during this hospitalization, and the staff did not revert to dice therapy. She was discharged in less than two months after an unremarkable course (Kuhlman, Green, & Sincaban, 1988.)

This case had a good outcome insofar as the therapeutic alliance with the patient survived despite a paradoxical intervention. Successful paradoxical interventions with severely impaired patients have also been reported by Rosen (1953) and by the Palo-Alto group, of which Jay Haley's work is best known (Haley, 1963, 1976.) But there is no research support for recommending such approaches with severely impaired patients, and the change mechanisms underlying paradoxical interventions remain subject to debate. Most importantly, therapeutic alliances with severely impaired patients who require ongoing care may not survive the "archness or trickery" and "problematic moral status" of such strategic interventions (Kirmayer, 1990.) The goal of dice therapy was only to terminate a treatment alliance that had become iatrogenic. Ms. B subsequently established a treatment alliance with a therapist in the community who provided her the necessary ongoing care.

There are less controversial approaches which can be taken with characterologically reactant patients. Some who are genuinely unaware of their behavior may be responsive to a carefully timed and worded interpretation. Another approach is for the therapist to couch directives, recommendations, or between-sessions homework, in either probabilistic terms (e.g. "if you choose to do X you will have a Y% chance of a Z outcome") or in some other parlance which safeguards the patient's freedom of choice (e.g. "in the event you don't wish to follow my recommendations, you should know that X% of clinically depressed patients like yourself show spontaneous recovery within Y months.") This might be characterized as shifting from the role of therapist into the role of consultant.

Concluding Remarks. Given the premium it places upon a person's perception of freedoms and personal control, reactance theory may be peculiar to western, individualistic cultures (Dowd & Seibel, 1990.) Extrapolations from the theory to the behavior of people from collectivistic cultures are questionable in the absence of cross-cultural research support. People who are socialized to prize the welfare of the group over the individual may find the reactance construct foreign to their world views and experiences.

Reactance theory may be equally foreign to another group: doctors and therapists trained in the traditional health care culture wherein behavioral freedoms and treatment controls were ceded to the professional, and the patient was expected to be trusting, submissive, and compliant. For better or worse, that health care culture has changed. As noted in the Forward to this volume, the concept of compliance has come to acquire connotations of coercion and authoritarianism. The conceptual shift from treatment compliance to treatment alliance invites a corresponding shift from treatment resistance to reactance motivation. Collaboration problems between therapist and patient would then be seen as normal, even expectable developments in the course of resolving them. Continuing to blame one side of the dyad for such problems while exonerating the other perpetuates a true lack of insight.

REFERENCES

Allen, D. N., Sprenkel, D. G., & Vitale, P. A. (1994). Reactance theory and alcohol consumption laws: Further confirmation among collegiate alcohol consumers. *Journal of Studies on Alcohol, 55,* 34–40.

Brehm, S. S., & Brehm, J. W. (1981). *Psychological reactance: A theory of freedom and control.* Orlando, FL: Academic Press.

Dowd, E. T. (1989). Stasis and change in cognitive psychotherapy: Client resistance and reactance as mediating variables. In W. Dryden & P. Trower (Eds.), *Cognitive psychotherapy: Stasis and change.* New York, NY: Springer.

Dowd, E. T., Milne, C. R., & Wise, S. L. (1991). The therapeutic reactance scale: A measure of psychological reactance. *Journal of Counseling and Development, 69,* 541–545.

Dowd, E. T., & Seibel, C. A. (1990). A cognitive theory of resistance and reactance: Implications for treatment. *Journal of Mental Health Counseling, 12,* 458–469.

Haley, J. (1963). *Strategies of psychotherapy,* New York, NY: Grune & Stratton.

Haley, J. (1976). *Problem-solving therapy.* San Francisco, CA: Jossey-Bass.

Hong, S. M., & Page, S. (1989). A psychological reactance scale: Development, factor structure, and reliability. *Psychological Reports, 64,* 1323–1326.

Kirmayer, L. J. (1990). Resistance, reactance, and reluctance to change: A cognitive attributional approach to strategic interventions. *Journal of Cognitive Psychotherapy, 4,* 83–104.

Koegel, P. (1992). Through a different lens: An anthropological perspective on the homeless mentally ill. *Culture, Medicine, and Psychiatry, 16,* 1–22.

Kuhlman, T. L. (1988). Gallows humor for a scaffold setting: Managing aggressive behavior on a maximum security forensic unit. *Hospital and Community Psychiatry, 39,* 1085–1090.

Kuhlman, T. L. (1994). *Psychology on the streets: Mental health practice with homeless persons.* New York, NY: John Wiley & Sons.

Kuhlman, T. L., Green, J. A., & Sincaban, V. A. (1988). Dice therapy: Deterring suicidal behavior by a borderline patient. *Hospital and Community Psychiatry, 39,* 992–994.

Ley, P. (1986). Cognitive variables and noncompliance, *Journal of Compliance in Health Care, 1,* 171–178.

Meichenbaum, D., & Turk, D. C. (1987). *Facilitating treatment adherence: A practitioner's guidebook.* New York, NY: Plenum Press.

Minkoff, K. (1987). Beyond deinstitutionalization: A new ideology for the post-institutional era. *Hospital and Community Psychiatry, 38,* 945–950.

Rhodewalt, F., & Fairfield, M. (1991). An alternative approach to Type A behavior and health: Psychological reactance and medical noncompliance. In M. J. Strube (Ed.), *Type A Behavior.* Newbury Park, CA: Sage Publications.

Rosen, J. (1953). *Direct psychoanalysis.* New York, NY: Grune & Stratton.

12

The Physician Who Prescribes

BARRY BLACKWELL

To forge an effective treatment alliance requires knowledge of both the generic demands that illness imposes on physicians and patients as well as the specific issues associated with persistent mental illness, psychotropic medication, the treatment regimen, and the patient's support systems. Above all else alliance implies a deep level of intuitive understanding, acceptance and mutual respect.

THE PHYSICIAN

Attempts to understand "compliance" have focused almost exclusively on the attitudes, beliefs and behaviors of the patient and hardly at all on the physician. What is most taken for granted is least often questioned (Blackwell, 1982). From the time of the shaman and the medicine man it has been the unique prerogative of the physician to prescribe. While state legislation is slowly eroding this absolute on behalf of nurses, psychologists, and optometrists, the truly dangerous drugs remain the physician's domain. This is not a light burden. Some years ago I was asked to address a class of freshmen medical students on the topic of "being a physician" (Blackwell, 1984). Shortly before I was to deliver my address, I had a dream. In it I was treating a woman newly admitted to the hospital with a bleeding disorder. I decided to set up an infusion but was uncertain of which drug to use. The ward copy of the Physician's Desk Reference was missing so I was forced to conduct a fruitless search elsewhere. When I returned to the patient's bedside, still in doubt, I found that the intern had started an infusion. As I approached the bed, the patient began to bleed profusely from around the infusion

193

needle. The flow of blood grew rapidly from a trickle to a deluge. I grabbed at the sheets and bedclothes in a futile attempt to staunch the bleeding and at the same time was aware of the beseeching eyes of the intern, the recriminatory eyes of the nurse, and the terrified eyes of the patient. Then I awoke. The dream encapsulated the unique stresses of the physician's role: the necessity to make decisions in ambiguous situations, to take control in emergencies, to be responsible for finding a cure.

By the end of the internship year these awesome responsibilities are so taken for granted and the anxiety that underlies them is so effectively stifled, that physicians seldom if ever again question the correctness of their drug choices or the assumption that patients will accept them. Despite considerable evidence to the contrary, most doctors assume that most of their patients are compliant and that they can tell when they are not.

These ingrained assumptions of acute medicine are inappropriately carried into practice; "curing" preempts "caring" and "doing to" subordinates "working with". I first learned this distinction after my nine year old son fractured his ankle close to the epiphysis. Concerned about the possibility of a poor surgical outcome, we consulted two different orthopedic experts. One was brusque, matter-of-fact and presented a strong, unequivocal recommendation. The other was personable, showed my son the X-rays, and discussed choices. When asked which surgeon he would prefer, my son replied "I'd like the first one to operate on me and the second to care for me afterwards."

Over time and with experience, some psychiatrists come to realize that caring for patients with severe and intermittent mental illness requires much more mutual negotiation and participation if an effective treatment alliance is to occur. Ours is not a surgical subspecialty.

THE PATIENT

All long term illness, medical or psychiatric, imposes generic burdens on those who suffer. These challenge the core human needs to feel in control, autonomous, intact and connected to others. Severe illness arouses feelings of ambiguity, loss of integrity, dependence, and stigma or isolation. Irrespective of the specific disorder, each individual's way of dealing with these issues will reflect their coping capacity, personality structure, and previous experiences (Oldham, 1994).

As with physicians, patients possess a unique set of attitudes, beliefs, and experiences concerning their illness. These may include its cause, the appropriateness or otherwise of treatment, and its likely outcome. Patients with a strong belief in the psychological or spiritual origins of mental illness are likely to resist medication management. Patients seen in health care for homeless clinics have often had bruising experiences of uncaring or coercive traditional treatment which make them slow to accept advice or offers of help. Many people share an attitude that the body sometimes "deserves a rest" from continuous medication and as a result they take "drug holidays."

THE ILLNESS

The unique deficits of each major mental disorder are grafted onto generic burdens that the illness imposes on an individual's adaptation. Impaired concentration, poor memory or thought disorder, and anxiety all interfere with effective information exchange. Delusional (particularly paranoid or suspicious) ideas can erode the trust necessary for a working alliance. Depression, apathy and the negative symptoms of schizophrenia are barriers to the persistence and motivation necessary for long term treatment. Lack of awareness or acceptance of illness ("insight") has been discussed extensively in an earlier chapter but is a particular problem in bipolar patients where impulsivity and lack of social judgment create additional difficulties. Sometimes what appears to be rejection of disease may be a reaction to the indignity of being labelled and reflects more of a struggle to retain respect and feelings of self-worth than "absence of insight".

Not often mentioned but of great practical significance are the difficulties encountered by patients who have extreme forms of symptom sensitivity (somatization) or bodily concern (hypochondriasis) (Blackwell, 1992). These individuals may also suffer from panic disorders with episodic autonomic arousal that reaffirms fears that they are "allergic" or supersensitive to allopathic medications. As a consequence, they are often attracted to homeopathic remedies or alternative therapies which may be ineffectual but not necessarily harmful.

Added to these problems of the major disorders is co-morbidity with substance abuse. This is a general risk factor for all forms of non-compliance but is a special problem in psychiatric illness because the pharmacologic effects of alcohol or drugs may interfere with the therapeutic action of medication or may be used by the patient as a surrogate form of self-treatment to stifle psychotic symptoms or temporarily alleviate depression.

In contrast to this rather bleak litany, it is worth noting that major psychiatric disorders possess some characteristics that can facilitate compliance. Unlike hypertension, glaucoma and diabetes, they are not "silent" conditions — they manifest symptoms that the patient can feel motivated to suppress. Secondly, the course of illness is intermittent and recurrent. This creates an opportunity for the person to learn the linkage between medication taking and symptom relief. Finally, the prevalence of most major psychiatric disorders is in early to mid-life, when cognitive skills and social connections are better preserved than is the case with degenerative medical disorders associated with aging.

PSYCHOTROPIC MEDICATIONS

Psychotropic drugs and their target organ possess properties that complicate compliance. The brain is finely tuned but well protected. For drugs to penetrate the blood-brain barrier requires large amounts to be absorbed before they are metabolized or excreted. The receptors with which psychotropic drugs interact exist elsewhere in the body, often in the peripheral nervous system or in the gut (which develops from the same part of the embryo as the brain). These two factors ensure that unwanted effects are almost inevitable and are experienced as disturbances of cardiovascular, sexual or gastrointestinal function. The newer, more selective drugs are less prone to this drawback.

Secondly, changes in brain chemistry often occur slowly due to up or down regulation of receptors. As a result, most therapeutic effects are delayed while many side effects occur immediately. This asynchrony is an invitation to poor compliance partly because it is also counterintuitive. People are used to the immediate effects of alcohol, cocaine, nicotine and caffeine on mood or behavior and do not expect to wait for benefit.

The natural history of major psychiatric disorders also conflicts with commonsense lay models of disease and treatment. In acute illness people take medicine until they feel better and then stop. In severe psychiatric illness, treatment must continue beyond the restoration of normal function, often for many months. Because repeated episodes of illness generate their own likelihood of recurrence ("kindling"), long-term treatment or prophylaxis is often desirable but may be resisted by patients who fear unwanted dependence on medications.

THE TREATMENT REGIMEN

To be successful, treatment should be tailored to fit the convenience and lifestyle of the patient. Although pharmaceutical companies have gone to considerable trouble to develop medications that can be taken once daily, compliance is not usually compromised unless the patient is taking multiple medications or one medication more than three times a day (Blackwell, 1979). Turn of the century tonics or panaceas were used three times daily "after meals" and most patients still use mealtime as their principal cue to medication taking.

The inconvenience of taking medications must be traded off against the advantages — these often remain unclear unless the physician explains exactly what benefits can be expected in plain language. These can include restful sleep, increased energy, unmuddled thoughts, absence of voices or banishment of alien ideas.

Side effects are an obvious deterrent, particularly if they occur unexpectedly or when they interfere with sexual function, the ability to think clearly, or other activities of daily living.

The linkage between medication taking and relief can sometimes be demonstrated by having a person keep a daily checklist of symptoms, side effects, or expected benefits. This may be especially helpful in symptom sensitive patients since keeping records utilizes their compulsive skills and produces a feeling of being in control.

THE SUPPORT SYSTEM

The presence of another concerned person is among the most important facilitators of participation in treatment. This may be a relative, friend, health care provider, case manager, or payee. Unfortunately, many people with persistent mental illness are bereft of family or friends and the task of encouraging compliance falls to professionals. It is important to remember that critical or intrusive involvement may be counterproductive and can even provoke psychotic episodes in vulnerable individuals (Vaugh & Leff, 1977). At our health care for homeless clinic, the staff strive to create a nurturant and optimistic milieu in which encouragement is gentle but persistent. Failed appointments are followed by telephone calls and those who live in shelters or on the streets can attend daily or are given weekly supplies of medication in pill containers. At the clinic social, medical, and psychiatric needs are cared for simultaneously and people receive hot drinks, snacks, and sometimes clothes as well as pills (Blackwell, et al., 1990).

Communication with payees may be especially helpful since they encounter their clients on a regular basis and can monitor medication taking as well as keeping an eye open for the use of alcohol or drugs which may interfere with the taking or efficacy of medication.

THE ALLIANCE

Reflexive demands of the role that sickness imposes on both physician and patient present obstacles to an alliance. The doctor's need for total control and instantaneous cure may rub up against the patient's desire for autonomy and independence. If the physician evokes fear or uses coercion to obtain compliance, these tactics can arouse resistance or regression. By contrast, empowerment of the patient often produces an experience of personal control which reinforces belief in treatment efficacy.

Negotiating a productive alliance requires that the physician inquire about the patient's attitudes, beliefs and knowledge concerning their disorder and its treatment. These can often be accommodated without sacrificing the essential ingredients of successful treatment. If a person believes in megavitamin therapy, no harm is done provided they are willing to take traditional medication as well. Also essential is a sensitive awareness of the patient's dynamics so that developmental issues are not stirred up by an overly parental approach.

Not every patient seeks or is willing at first to accept complete responsibility for coping with the burden of illness; it is the physician's task to titrate the interaction, to explore resistance or regression, and to take steps that discourage passive adoption of the sick role. A patient's ability to assume control also depends on the phase and severity of illness. In acute episodes, psychotic symptoms, cognitive impairment and poor insight or impulse control are impediments. Later on apathy or negative symptoms may interfere. Moves towards autonomy must often be graduated so that an individual who starts out on parenteral monthly injections of decanoate may be slowly weaned onto daily or weekly attendance for oral medication.

When developing an alliance, physicians must be aware of their own need for control and be willing to relinquish it in appropriate circumstances. This may involve taking calculated risks, including the possibility of relapse and potential dangerousness to self or others. In work with persons who have mental illness we have learned that the short term benefits of coercion during acute exacerbations quickly dissipate over the management of long-term illnesses (Lucksted & Coursey, 1995). The patient must learn their own lessons of how medication modifies voices or impulses and calculate their personal cost benefit ratio between side effects and therapeutic change. The physician's advice and predictions are just that — inexact but hopefully well informed guesses. The more often these are correct, the stronger the patient's trust and the better likelihood they will follow later suggestions in the lifelong course of a relapsing and remitting illness. In doing so the patient develops a strong sense of self and personal responsibility reinforced by making their own decisions. The physician's tolerance for ambiguity and risk is bolstered when the patient has a strong attachment, not only personally, but to nursing and social work colleagues as well as to the clinic or shelter where help is sought.

The importance of the therapeutic alliance in effective treatment outcome is demonstrated by the following two illustrative vignettes.

Randolph is a 30 year old former intravenous drug abuser with a diagnosis of schizoaffective disorder who was recently informed that he had become positive with HIV. During a recent admission to hospital for medical treatment, the nursing staff felt he was paranoid and depressed. Randolph had previously rejected offers of medication or had grudgingly accepted but never taken it. On this admission his urine was positive for cocaine. When questioned at the bedside, he freely admitted using this to counter feelings of "disgust". Randolph also agreed that after each brief euphoric interlude he was back again in the real world, feeling even more suspicious and disgusted.

Our conversation began with a detailed analysis of why Randolph used cocaine, what it did for him, and how he thought it worked. Based on his experience, Randolph agreed that chemicals could alter mood and behavior but at some cost. I suggested he might consider an alternative in the form of prescribed medications. I pointed out that unlike cocaine these worked slowly, that benefit was gradual but that also unlike cocaine, the results persisted. If he was willing to attempt an experiment, chances were he would feel less suspicious and disgusted. As a bonus, he might no longer crave cocaine. Randolph agreed it was worth a try. After discharge, he came to our homeless clinic and was started on an antidepressant and an antipsychotic. Two weeks later he was pleased and surprised to report that his voices were fading slowly away, he was sleeping soundly and feeling much less disgusted with life. His urine was clean.

Agnes is a 42 year old single female well known throughout our city for frequent admissions to several hospitals over many years. She usually arrived accompanied by police in an acute manic episode, combative, provocative and totally lacking all capacity to view herself as ill or in need of treatment. Although highly intelligent, Agnes was unable to hold a job and received Social Security with Medicaid health benefits. She was unable to find a private psychiatrist willing to treat her and was unpopular with the inpatient staff who viewed her behavior as "borderline".

Our first several months were spent learning more about each other and during this time Agnes was admitted twice again to hospital. While Agnes was willing to take medication, she detested the way "mood stabilizers" stifled her creativity. As a result, she experimented continuously with various forms of meditation and marginal religious cults. In doing so, she gave herself frequent "drug holidays". In our initial dialogue, each of us attempted to convert the other. I quickly learned how sensitive Agnes was to control issues; her father had been a benevolent tyrant and her mother was critical and unloving. Agnes agreed that she found her experiences with the police and in hospital humiliating. I encouraged her ongoing search for spiritual meaning and nondrug methods of thought control but I also maintained that these could be compatible with medication if she was willing to explore the tradeoff between a benefit she valued (staying out of hospital) and side effects she didn't (slowing of thoughts). Together we agreed on a target — to persist with medication in a sustained way until Agnes had been out of hospital for longer than any previous interlude (about 11 months).

It is now two years since Agnes last suffered the humiliation of hospitalization; she has found a source of spiritual solace and she continues to complain bitterly about side effects. Together we are looking forward to a new generation of more specific psychotropic compounds that will stabilize moods without stifling creative thought.

These vignettes reflect the paradigm shift that has accompanied deinstitutionalization, the failure of the community mental health system and its replacement by evolving community support and outreach programs.

Psychiatrists who prescribe medications are now challenged to meet the needs of people striving to lead normal lives in the community despite sustained mental illness, homelessness or substance abuse.

To prescribe is often necessary but never sufficient. Coercion is ineffective and the concept of compliance is inadequate. Medications have become part of an alliance that embraces each person's beliefs, experience and lifestyle — not simply their diagnosis, chemistry or genes.

ACKNOWLEDGEMENT

I am grateful to Dan Fisher for his thoughtful comments and suggestions.

REFERENCES

Blackwell, B. (1979). The drug regimen and treatment compliance. In R. B. Haynes, D. W. Taylor, & D. L. Sackett (Eds.), *Compliance with Therapeutic and Preventive Regimens*. Baltimore: John Hopkins University Press.

Blackwell, B. (1982). Treatment Compliance. In J. H. Greist, J. W. Jefferson, & R. L. Spitzer (Eds.), *Treatment of Mental Disorders*. New York: Oxford University Press.

Blackwell, B. (1984). Dream doctor. *Archives of Internal Medicine, 144*, 806.

Blackwell, B., Breakey, W., Hammersley, D., Hammond, R., McMurray-Avila, M., & Seeger, C. (1990). Psychiatric and mental health services (pp. 184–203). In P. W. Brickner, L. K. Scharer, B. A. Conanan, M. Savarese, B. C. Scanlan (Eds.), *Under the Safety Net*. New York: WW Norton.

Blackwell, B. (1992). Sick role susceptibility. *Psychotherapy and Psychosomatics, 58*, 79–90.

Lucksted, A., & Coursey, R. D. (1995). Consumer perceptions of pressure and force in psychiatric treatments. *Psychiatric Services, 46*, 146–152.

Oldham, J. M. (1994). Personality disorders. *Journal of the American Medical Association, 272*, 1770–1776.

Vaughn, C. E., & Leff, J. P. The influence of family and social factors on the course of psychiatric illness. *British Journal of Psychiatry, 129*, 123–27.

13

Compliance and the Treatment Alliance in Serious Mental Illness: The Pharmacist' Role

JAYME C. TROTT and SHEILA R. BOTTS

INTRODUCTION

On Wednesday afternoons at 1:00PM our treatment team meets for "staffing". This initial team meeting with each new patient allows us to pool our individual assessments and design a rational treatment plan for that individual. This week, the first patient is well-known to me. She is a cherubic-looking 47 year old woman who seems a lot younger than her years. This is her twenty-third admission to our institution. When she left us about three months ago, her mood was "euthymic", she had stopped hearing the angels singing to her, and she understood that she was not pregnant with the baby Jesus. She says that she took her medications at home just like she was told to, but she ran out about the same time her husband left her and she just never got to the clinic to get them refilled. Now she believes she is the Virgin Mary again, talking incessantly and laughing at what the angels are telling her. The team decides that one of our interventions will be to assign her to the Clinical Pharmacists' Medication Education Group.

I am familiar with the second patient, as well. This is only her third time here, but Maria is very ill. This woman is dark and gaunt-looking, with vacant eyes and stringy hair. She refuses to speak or look up at anyone. Her collateral history indicates that her last admission lasted three months. When she left the hospital, she was smiling a little, and her speech was "logical and goal-directed." She still kept to herself most of the time, but her sister and mother assured us that she was "back to her old self." Recently, her family had lost track of who was making sure she received her medicine — the sister thought the mother was taking care of it, and the mother thought the sister was. It had been three weeks since Maria last received a dose. When the sheriff's deputy brought the patient here this time, she told the admitting physician that people were putting poison in her food. The team is unanimous in agreeing that Maria must be offered Medication Education Group as part of her psychosocial programming. But I wonder how much I can do. Who will educate her mother and sister? What other ways do we have to help Maria, and others like her, to remember to take their medications? For that matter, how can we motivate her to recognize a *need* to take them?

Pharmacists have been struggling to answer these questions for as long as the profession has existed. Our role has changed dramatically over the past two centuries, but the focus of care has always been the patient. From the apothecary who diagnosed ailments and dispensed carefully compounded medicinal products, to the modern-day clinician who may have little to do with the drug product itself, the pharmacist's goal always has been to ensure safe and appropriate medication use by patients.

Traditionally, the pharmacist has been the last person to handle the drug product before the consumer receives it. Once the medicine and information about that medication had been delivered to the patient, the pharmacist's responsibility for the transaction was complete. More recently, the profession of pharmacy has adopted the philosophy of providing *pharmaceutical care* to patients. As with providing medical care or nursing care, the provision of pharmaceutical care entails assumption of responsibility for patient outcome.

Pharmaceutical care, as originally defined by Hepler and Strand (1990), is "the responsible provision of drug therapy for the purpose of achieving definite outcomes that improve a patient's quality of life." Pharmacists, irrespective of their practice sites, work cooperatively with patients and other health care providers to develop, implement and monitor drug therapy plans that will result in positive patient outcomes. Within this framework, the three major functions of the pharmacist are "(1) identifying potential and actual drug-related problems, (2) resolving actual drug-related problems, and (3) preventing drug-related problems." Clearly, medication noncompliance is a major drug-related problem. This chapter discusses pharmacy's efforts to decrease medication noncompliance in the mentally ill.

MEDICATION EDUCATION GROUPS

The idea that educating patients would promote their adherence to a prescribed medication regimen became popular well over 20 years ago. It was reasonable to assume that if we educated our mentally ill patients about their illness' and medications this would naturally improve how well they would adhere to a given regimen. Education was designed to improve the patients knowledge and understanding of the illness and how the illness can be managed (with particular emphasis to the role of medications). While the attempt to educate patients has been employed by all health care professionals, the introduction of more organized interventions in the way of group education and individual counseling has been largely employed by nurses and pharmacists. This group format is usually offered to inpatients as part of their multi-disciplinary treatment program, as well as to outpatients at mental health clinics. Individual counseling is often used to assess and target specific problem areas for each patient (e.g. stigma of illness, family attitudes toward medication, difficulty completing activities of daily living) and also focus on patients who are unable to benefit maximally from group education alone (e.g. for those patients who are distracted, have poor attentive skills, or who have overall poor cognitive functioning).

Several models have been proposed to explain patients' behavior regarding taking medication. Ereshefsky (1981), proposed that compliant behavior is a result of cognitive, attitudinal and psychomotor influences. It follows then, that noncompliance with medication and treatment may result from problems in any of these domains. Medication education should not be limited to imparting information about mental illness and side effects of psychotropic medications. Patient and family attitudes toward mental illness, perceived benefits of treatment and physical or psychological impediments affecting compliance behavior must also be addressed. All of these factors can be targeted within the structure of a medication education group.

Groups offer advantages over individual counseling by fostering interactive discussion. This interaction allows patients to learn from each others' experiences and develop their own sense of expertise. The topics covered in group range from discussions of mental illness and the role of psychotropic medications to specific medication management strategies. The goal is to empower patients to be more active participants in the management of their drug therapy.

Medication Education groups are generally similar in content but differ in form. Information is delivered in lecture format, informal presentation or interactive non-structured discussion. Each of these provide advantages to certain patients. A lecture format may be less anxiety provoking for patients uncomfortable participating in groups, whereas interactive discussion may benefit the patient with poor attentive skills who needs to be continuously re-engaged. Innovative group formats, such as the "coffee group" designed by Olarte and Masnik (1981), encourage adherence to the treatment regimens by lessening the anxiety associated with follow-up care. Patients who attended the monthly coffee group, in lieu of individual sessions, demonstrated decreased hospitalization rates over an extended period of time. Hinkes, Morales-Llosent, & Sadowski (1993), have used a Jeopardy game at the end of each formal lecture to reinforce information presented to inpatients. The game served to motivate patients not only to attend but also participate as prizes were given to the winners.

Patients receive verbal and/or written information. Both mediums have shown to be successful in improving knowledge and neither is felt to be superior (Brown, Wright, & Christensen 1987). Many

patients with psychiatric disorders suffer from disorganized thinking, poor attention and poor interpersonal skills. Written information provided along with verbal information may benefit these
patients by serving as a repeated reinforcer and also a reference.
Management strategies may be put on an index card and carried
with the patient to serve as a motivating cue for problem solving.
For example, the card may tell a patient whether to take a missed
dose after a certain period of time, or to wait until the next dose.

Pharmacists with good communication skills are ideally trained
to plan and facilitate medication education groups. Their education
and experience gives them in-depth working knowledge of appropriate medication usage and potential for drug-related problems.
Clinical pharmacists who specialize in psychiatry have additional
didactic and experiential training in psychiatric drug therapy. This
training, usually in the form of a post-doctoral residency, emphasizes individualized patient assessment for drug therapy response
and ongoing monitoring for emergence of adverse effects ("ASHP,"
1994). Psychiatric pharmacy specialists utilize these skills during
medication groups in several ways. In addition to imparting essential information about psychiatric illness and medications, they also
identify and recommend strategies for managing drug-related problems individual patients may be experiencing.

Education programs have led to positive outcomes in several
studies of non-psychiatric patient cohorts. For instance, patients
with hypertension and heart disease have demonstrated increased
overall medication compliance. Additionally, they experience reduced hospital admissions, numbers of outpatient visits and dupli-
cate prescriptions. Results of studies measuring the impact of
medication education directed toward patients with chronic mental
illness are less robust. Impact on compliance and hospitalization
rates is modest at best (Boczkowski, Zeichner, & DeSanto 1985,
Kleinman, Schachter, Jeffries, & Goldhamer 1993). Although these
programs *can* increase patients' level of understanding, this increased knowledge has not been proven to translate into better long-
term compliance. Whether or not it is reasonable to use compliance
as the best outcome measure for assessing the value of medication
education is in question. The effects of medication education on the
quality of treatment and overall outcomes are difficult to measure.
Medication education cannot address all factors that influence compliance behavior and is likely to be most beneficial when combined
with other interventions, such as improving ADL's, creating a structured environment and increased supervision. To illustrate this
point, consider a patient with schizophrenia who may perceive the
illness much like a common cold — expecting the illness to resolve
on its own with time. This patient is also likely to have poor communication skills and difficulty with structure and planning.
Increased understanding of the illness and need for chronic medication may provide some benefit to this patient. However, unless social skills improve, and the home environment is adequately
structured, the person is unlikely to fully adhere to a medication
regimen, whatever the level of understanding.

Certainly other means of intervention, in addition to patient education, are needed to fully address noncompliance with medication. One such area pharmacists may target is educating family members about mental illness and psychotropic medications. Family members are the providers for many patients with chronic mental illness and often supervise medication use by the patient. It is important that family members have an adequate understanding of mental illness and medication treatment if they are to function as a support network for the patient. Corrigan, Liberman, and Engel (1990) describe several efforts that have been targeted at educating family members and making them a valuable component of the treatment alliance. These efforts include education groups similar to those described for the patient. Additionally, some groups focus on problem-solving and involve both the patient and family members. Educating families may minimize negative attitudes and stress associated with the stigma of mental illness. A more adequate understanding of the patient's illness and need for medication may allow family members to become more active participants in the patient's treatment plan. This in turn can help ensure adequate medication management by the patient.

INDIVIDUAL PATIENT COUNSELING

Pharmacists have been referred to often as the "front line" of health care. The public recognizes pharmacists as trusted professionals. Community pharmacists in particular, serve as readily accessible sources of accurate information on health-related matters. In addition to dispensing prescription drugs, pharmacists provide a number of cognitive services for which patients rarely have to pay. They answer consumers' questions about drugs and disease states, counsel patients on the appropriate use and storage of medications and help patients determine whether to self-medicate a condition with over-the-counter products or consider a visit to the physician's office.

Community pharmacists must have strong communication skills to effectively counsel patients. Perhaps the most important is that of being a good listener. Good listening skills are especially important when counseling patients with serious mental illnesses. Rather than instruct the patient about a new prescription by reciting a laundry list of precautions and warnings, a more effective technique is to use a series of open-ended questions. Answers can provide important information about the patient's attitudes and ability to self-manage his or her medication regimen. Questions the patient asks may give important clues as to the need for additional counseling. For example, a patient may express doubt that a prescribed drug will offer any benefit, and ask the opinion of the pharmacist. The pharmacist can use this opportunity to reinforce the potential positive effects which can be derived from following this drug regimen. Explaining factors such as expected delay to onset of therapeutic efficacy with antidepressants, anticipated development of tolerance to adverse effects and suggestions for counteracting minor adverse effects can be extremely important in reassuring the patient and increasing the likelihood of compliance.

Many of the requirements for counseling and review of patient records are no longer optional. Even those pharmacists who would prefer to remain "behind the counter" are now required by law to provide many of these services (Omnibus Budget Reconciliation Act of 1990).

When a patient's responses or behavior suggest early symptoms of illness relapse, the pharmacist is in an excellent position to intervene. Having established a good rapport, the pharmacist may be able to convince the patient to contact the psychiatrist for evaluation. If family members or caretakers are present, perhaps they can be engaged to provide support. Of course, the ideal situation for averting such drug-related problems exists when the pharmacist, psychiatrist and patient are all part of a therapeutic alliance.

DRUG THERAPY MONITORING

Developing a strong pharmacist-patient therapeutic alliance facilitates open dialog, builds trust, and encourages a sense of loyalty on the part of the patient to use a particular pharmacy (Kelly & Trott, 1979). Since the ability to monitor compliance is impeded when patients purchase prescriptions from more than one pharmacy, the "allegiance" of a patient to a particular pharmacy is very helpful.

In addition to patient counseling, pharmacists have other means at their disposal for recognizing and anticipating problems of medication noncompliance. Routine review of patient medication profiles, attention to medication refill records and simple observation of patient behaviors can help the pharmacist to identify potential compliance-related problems. Pharmacists are uniquely trained to recognize factors in a patient's drug regimen that may contribute to noncompliance. Their in-depth knowledge of drug-drug and drug-disease interactions and pharmacokinetics allows them to recognize potential problems when new medications are added to established therapeutic regimens. For example, if a patient's family practice doctor prescribes cimetidine for dyspepsia, the pharmacist is trained to recognize that addition of this drug to the antipsychotic regimen is likely to elevate serum concentrations of the antipsychotic and put the patient at risk for adverse effects. The physician and/or psychiatrist involved are alerted and the pharmacist can make suggestions for alternative therapies with equivalent therapeutic effects that lack drug interaction potential.

Prescription refill records provide pharmacists with valuable (though not always totally accurate) information about patient compliance. Increasingly, pharmacists are using innovative record-keeping systems and computers to pro-actively attempt to decrease noncompliance with chronic medication therapy. In some cases follow-up phone calls are made within a few days to two weeks after filling new prescriptions. Although post-card reminders are used by many community pharmacies, computer programs have eased the process of providing reminders to refill chronic medications. For example, the Med-Minder Compliance Module as described by Berg et al. (1993), is a voice-synthesized (may be the pharmacists voice) computer system which calls the patient and delivers a reminder message. Also with patient's drug profiles readily available on computer data bases, identifying those patients who are late in refilling their medications becomes relatively easy.

Pharmacists are likely to recognize other factors which may be preventing patients from refilling prescriptions. Financial concerns or inability to pay for medication may deter patients without prescription insurance or government funding from purchasing medications. Alternatively, they may decrease the frequency with which they take medication doses so that a given prescription will last longer. In some cases, drugs such as antidepressants are taken on an "as needed" basis in an effort to save money. Each of these decisions made by the patient leads to ineffective drug therapy. A combination of careful monitoring, effective patient counseling and creative effort, on the part of the pharmacist, can often avert noncompliance with chronic medication therapy for mental illness.

INNOVATIVE PACKAGING AND COMPLIANCE

A number of devices have been designed to facilitate patient compliance. These devices target noncompliance in a number of ways. Some function as patient reminders while others offer auxiliary patient information. Still others provide special packaging or offer cost incentive programs. These strategies are not intended to replace direct patient interaction, but rather are meant to augment the pharmacist and/or physician's efforts to insure compliance. While many of these strategies have primarily been used and evaluated in the medically ill (e.g. patients with hypertension, glaucoma, or diabetes), they also have the potential to be useful for the chronically mentally ill.

Increasing complexity of a drug regimen has been associated with higher rates of noncompliance with drug therapy across patient populations. Despite attempts to simplify these regimens, some medications must be given multiple times per day due to their pharmacokinetic or pharmacodynamic profiles. Specific medication container devices as described by Berg et al. (1993), may remind the patient it is time for a dose or simply what doses have been taken that day. However, not all of these devices prompt the patient when it is time for a specific dose. One example is Mediset®, a plastic organizer which has separate compartments for each day of the week and 4 doses per day. This allows patients or family members to prefill medications each week and also keep track of which doses have been taken. A second example is a Counter Cap®. The Counter Cap® is designed to fit a prescription vial or a product bottle and indicates either the day of the week (for single day dosing) or the number of the dose in a given day. Again patients are reminded which doses have been taken as the counter advances each time the vial is opened. Electronic pillboxes are similar to counter caps but signal an alarm when a dosage is due. More complex versions of the pillboxes have a miniature computer screen which can display information or offer visual aides. Each of the above mentioned devices either acts as a prompt for the patient or lessens the confusion when taking multiple doses per day. Patients with mental illness, especially those with schizophrenia or depression, often have memory deficits and may benefit from these interventions.

Innovative methods of medication packaging also have been used to modify compliance behavior. Individual doses are provided in a blister pack which specifies the dosage units and/or days of therapy. Unit dose packaging allows the patient to keep track of doses taken. Also, specific directions are often contained on the package to facilitate compliance with the dosing regimen. This type of packaging has been used mostly with oral contraceptives, antibiotics and corticosteroids which have complex or finite regimens. Recently, Bristol-Meyers Squibb has introduced this type of packaging in marketing the new antidepressant nefazodone. Nefazodone blister packs containing the first two weeks of treatment are provided to physicians for initiation of therapy. A symptom self rating scale is included that alows the patient to monitor improvement. Smith (1989) describes Norwich Eaton's MACPAC® as the most advanced form of compliance packaging. MACPAC® contains blister-pack cards for each daily dose of Macrodantin®. In addition it offers a patient information booklet about urinary tract infections and a reinforcement card placed after the third day of therapy (as this is when most patients are likely to discontinue because of diminished symptoms) which states it is necessary to complete the full course of therapy to fully eliminate the infection. While it has been shown that compliance packaging enhances patient compliance for finite regimens, it has not been proven beneficial or cost effective for long-term maintenance therapy and generally has not been tried with psychiatric medications. However this type of packaging may be beneficial for mentally ill patients who have difficulty remembering how to take their medications or who have trouble with complex regimens.

PSYCHIATRIC PHARMACY SPECIALISTS AS OUTPATIENT CLINICIANS

Pharmacists have made significant strides at reducing noncompliance within a number of non-psychiatric patient groups. There are many examples of pharmacist-run anticoagulation clinics and hypertension clinics that have had a measurable impact on patient outcomes, including reduced hospital readmissions, unscheduled physician visits and ER visits (Gebhart, 1993). Ensuring medication compliance is a significant function of pharmacists in these clinics.

Psychiatry pharmacy specialists are conducting similar medication management clinics in a variety of mental health settings. In some cases, clinics are primarily aimed at management of patients considered psychiatrically stable. In others, pharmacists provide the follow-up needed after psychiatrists have initiated new psychotropic drug therapy. By far, the majority of these clinics are located in Veterans Administration centers and Health Maintenance Organizations.

At a Veteran's Administration hospital in Dallas, Texas, Cynthia Foslien Nash, Pharm.D., has a caseload of over 300 patients she sees routinely in a psychotropic drug maintenance clinic. As a member of a multidisciplinary team, Dr. Foslien Nash plays a key role in both assessing and encouraging compliance with prescribed drug regimens. She interviews patients referred to her clinic to determine their current psychiatric status and any adverse effects they may be experiencing. She interprets serum drug concentrations where appropriate, and integrates this information with her clinical evaluation to assess medication compliance. Dr. Foslien Nash also provides patients with drug information and encourages their continued adherence to prescribed medication regimens.

A recently published report by Ellenor and Dishman (1995) describes an innovative model of pharmaceutical care in psychiatry. At the San Diego Veterans Administration Medical Center in California, psychiatry pharmacy specialists with expanded roles that include prescribing authority, provide medication management for patients in Pharmacy Mental Health Clinics. These clinics were established to address a number of needs, one of which was to improve patients' medication compliance in order to decrease rehospitalization. During clinic visits, pharmacists stress medication compliance with patients. They provide written and oral drug information, calendar schedules, charts, pill boxes or other devices to help improve medication compliance. The pharmacists assure that patients have adequate quantities of medications to last until the next appointment and encourage patients to call the clinic if they experience any illness- or drug-related problems. Utilization of the Pharmacy Mental Health Clinics more than doubled in the first three years that the service was offered, and approximately half of all patient clinic visits for medication management are now scheduled with pharmacists. Intuitively, one would expect that such growth indicates a positive impact of these clinics on the delivery of care to patients within this mental health system. Unfortunately, the report did not include an analysis of patient outcomes or health-systems costs. Assessment of these outcome measures are essential in order to determine the actual value of clinical pharmacy services, and in particular the effect of such services on medication compliance and hospital recidivism rates.

SUMMARY

The focus of pharmacy education is no longer to train highly skilled technicians, but rather to prepare clinicians who will provide valuable services for patients and assume responsibility for the outcomes of their efforts. As members of a therapeutic alliance for the mentally ill, pharmacists are ideally positioned to implement programs that can improve patient adherence to prescribed medication regimens. These programs involve medication education, patient counseling, therapeutic drug monitoring and medication management. Perhaps the biggest challenge facing all of us now is to truly *coordinate* our efforts, and utilize each others' expertise in our common endeavor to overcome the barriers to treatment compliance among patients with chronic mental illness.

REFERENCES

ASHP supplementary standard and learning objectives for residency training in psychiatric pharmacy practice. (1994) *American Journal of Hospital Pharmacists, 51,* 2034–2041.

Berg, J. S., Dischler, J., Wagner, D. J., Raia, J. J., & Palmer-Shevlin, N. (1993). Medication compliance: A healthcare problem. *The Annals of Pharmacotherapy, 27,* S5–S19.

Boczkowski, J. A., Zeichner, A., & DeSanto, N. (1985). Neuroleptic compliance among chronic schizophrenic outpatients: An intervention outcome report. *Journal of Consulting and Clinical Psychology, 53,* 666–671.

Brown, C. S., Wright, R. G., & Christensen, D. B. (1987). Association between type of medication instruction and patients' knowledge, side effects, and compliance. *Hospital and Community Psychiatry, 38,* 55–60.

Canaday, B. R. (1994). *OBRA 90: A Practical Guide to Effecting Pharmaceutical Care* Washington, DC: The American Pharmaceutical Association.

Corrigan, P. W., Liberman, P. L., & Engel, J. D. (1990). From noncompliance to collaboration in the treatment of schizophrenia. *Hospital and Community Psychiatry, 41,* 1203–1211.

Ellenor, G. L., Dishman, & B. R. (1995). Pharmaceutical Care Role Model in Psychiatry — Pharmacist Prescribing. *Hospital Pharmacy, 30*(5), 371–373, 377–378.

Ereshefsky, L. E. (1981) *Patient compliance.* (Continuing Education Vol. 7, No. 3). Texas: College of Pharmacy, The University of Texas at Austin.

Gebhart, F. (1993). Seamless care: Bridging inpatient/outpatient pharmacy. *Hospital Pharmacist Report, 7,* 1, 8.

Hepler, C. D., & Strand, L.M. (1990). Opportunities and responsibilities in pharmaceutical care. *American Journal of Hospital Pharmacy, 47,* 533–543.

Hinkes, R. M., Morales-Llosent, M., & Sadowski, J. E. (1993, December). *Description of a medication teaching group program for mentally ill inpatients.* Poster presented at the American Society of Hospital Pharmacists Mid-Year Meeting, Atlanta, GA.

Kelly, G. R., & Scott, J. E. (1990). Medication compliance and health education among outpatients with chronic mental disorders. *Medical Care, 28,* 1181–1197.

Kelly, E. T., & Trott, J. M. (1979). Effects of mandatory prescription price posting in Connecticut. *Contemporary Pharmacy Practice, 2,* 23–27.

Kleinman, I., Schachter, K., Jeffries, J., & Goldhamer, P. (1993). Effectiveness of two methods for informing schizophrenic patients about neuroleptic medication. *Hospital and Community Psychiatry, 44,* 1189–1191.

Olarte, S. W., & Masnik, R. (1981). Enhancing medication compliance in coffee groups. *Hospital and Community Psychiatry, 32,* 417–419.

Smith, D. L. (1989). Compliance packaging: A patient education tool. *American Pharmacy, NS29,* 126–137.

14

Case Managers and Compliance

MARTHA HODGE

"It means learning how to have power-with rather than power-over those who come to us in distress. It means learning how to work with another person such that neither the clinician nor the client is "in control". Rather both can learn to experience themselves as being heard and responded to as well as being moved and moving the other."
Patricia E. Deegan (1990)

Compliance to case managers means mostly that people are taking their medicines as prescribed or going to the program that was recommended. As a group case managers probably don't think much about their power and influence over and with the people they serve or about the ethics associated with this power. Non-compliance, on the other hand, is discussed on a daily basis because the principle measure of our success is our ability to help people with severe and persistent mental illness live in the community and stay out of hospitals.

Non-compliance is defined by this author as the inability or unwillingness to accept the treatment/service offered; the use of treatment/service in ways other than intended; and/or the full rejection of the service system. A continuing point of confusion for most case managers is the distinction between the terms treatment resistant and non-compliant. For purposes of this chapter, treatment resistant refers to intractable illnesses which are not responsive to treatment rather than the willful rejection of service/treatment.

The following vignettes serve to demonstrate the complex issues that case managers and other staff face on a daily basis and to provide a real life framework for thinking about compliance. (Each of these represent situations faced by this writer in September 1994.)

VIRGINIA

Virginia is a 40+ year old woman who suffers from schizophrenia. She has been in the hospital for the last two years. Yesterday, she had a court hearing where hospital staff requested an extension of her commitment; she was, however, released. The hospital staff feel she is not ready for discharge and urged her to sign in voluntarily. She refused and demanded to be released. Is this non-compliance?

SYLVIA

Sylvia is a young woman diagnosed with both a developmental disability and a serious mental illness. She routinely shares her medicine with her boyfriend so she's always out of medicine before her regularly scheduled appointment. Is this a compliance problem?

BOB

Bob has diagnoses of bipolar disorder and alcohol abuse and has been court ordered to participate in community outpatient treatment. One of the required interventions is partial hospitalization. Bob will attend, but he refuses to participate in group or individual therapy. He doesn't want to "sit around and talk about problems"; he wants to get back to work. The treatment team does not believe that he is ready to return to work. He's about to be "kicked out" of the program for non-compliance.

ALLENE

Allene says she'll take Mellaril, but she absolutely refuses the Moban which has been prescribed. The clinical team, based on prior experience, feels that she is being manipulative and refuses the request. If she persists and doesn't take the Moban, is she non-compliant?

ROBERT

Robert is a 23 year old man with schizophrenia. He is in the county hospital and most recently was homeless. He has repeatedly told staff that he needs a roommate(s) — that he cannot live alone. He also indicated a desire to have someone take care of the cleaning and cooking. He has refused two different efficiency apartments. Staff describe the situation by saying, "he's being difficult, and there are no other placements available". Is refusing a placement that does not meet what he believes are his needs non-compliant?

The remainder of this chapter reviews the historical beginnings of case management and its relationship to deinstitutionalization. Case management is also defined and several models are discussed.

Factors which influence compliance and non-compliance are enumerated with emphasis on developing supportive compliance strategies and establishing helpful relationships. The underlying themes include trying to understand treatment and service from the point of view of the person served, opening the door for two-way exchanges about what might be effective, and offering as many choices and alternatives as possible.

HISTORY

Case management was created in response to the "Great Society" of the late sixties and early seventies which gave rise to much more complicated health and social service systems. It brought optimism that order in a disordered system was possible.

The initial goal of case management was to offer poor and disabled persons a single point of contact with many systems and to reduce inefficiency and duplication of effort. Case management's roots can be traced first, to the social case work model of the thirties (Dill, 1987), and second, to the concept of a Balanced Service System (Miles, 1972) promulgated in the seventies. Its more general acceptance probably resulted from its inclusion in the Joint Commission on Accreditation of Hospitals (JCAH) Standards for Community Mental Health Centers (1976) and NIMH's Community Support Project (Turner & TenHoor, 1978).

It is impossible to date the beginning of deinstitutionalization, but by 1970, people were being released in large numbers from state hospitals. Most had severe mental illnesses, and almost all had spent portions of their lives in institutions of one kind or another and were returning to an increasingly complex world and a non-existent or ineffective community mental health system, designed and funded to serve people with less significant problems. Additionally, medicines and treatment services were not as technologically advanced (the use of decanoate medicines was minimal or non-existent).

The people being released from state hospitals had come to depend on the institution or others for meeting their basic needs. Their community care givers were unprepared, sometimes unwilling, and certainly not paid for the huge task of helping thousands of people manage their mental illness and regain their position in the community.

The absence of positive staff attitudes and the requisite skills to serve former state hospital patients presented a major problem (Bassuk & Gerson, 1978). The social case work model was no longer in vogue; most social workers were being trained as therapists, with case management being relegated to a less important role. There were few staff, with the exception of some state hospital staff who moved to the community, who had even a basic understanding of the problems and burdens associated with severe and persistent mental illness.

Community mental health staff were charged with serving a group of people who had learned to be "good patients" in one setting (the hospital) but who could not sustain the motivation nor, in some cases, perform the tasks associated with meeting their basic needs in the community. It can be argued that many of the people who were labeled as non-compliant after the first wave of deinstitutionalization were, in fact, exhibiting the functional deficits associated with severe mental illness and long term institutional care.

The second group of people to leave state hospitals had more significant impairments, and they found a system even less well prepared to provide assistance. There also was now a large group of people who had never been institutionalized for extended periods of time and who definitely were not socialized to be "good patients" and who objected to many of the treatments or services offered (Savarese et al., 1990). Additionally, substance abuse became more prevalent and has been recognized as a major factor in non-compliance (Drake et al., 1990).

Case managers came to this scene with little training or preparation. The work was ill-defined, and case managers were relegated a low status in organizations. Their role models were well paid staff (or, at least, better paid) who many times openly expressed not only disdain but also despair about the people served by case managers (Lamb, 1988). The functional problems associated with severe mental illness such as vulnerability to stress, poor inter/intrapersonal relationships, inadequate defense mechanisms, and concrete thinking (Stein & Test, 1985) were not being clearly articulated, and these concepts were generally unknown to case managers. (What we have subsequently learned is that many of these functional problems were not related to inabilities, but to lack of experience, stigma, poverty, and life on the fringes of society.)

Paradoxically, the position of case manager was largely created to deal with the very problems associated with non-compliance. Case managers were expected to help people keep their appointments, get their benefits, and attend to the tasks of everyday life. Case management in mental health services grew out of an expectation that people might not be able to meet the demands of community life. Yet, almost immediately, professional staff began worrying that case managers were making people "too dependent" and began an infusion of psychodynamic theory(s) into case management practices and models. The case manager faced a very confusing message, "Get these mentally ill people to do what doctors and therapists say they should do; but don't help them too much in the process". Part of the problem was that professional boundaries for case managers had not been clarified or articulated.

Case managers also faced a community that was in some instances openly hostile; they certainly were trying to obtain services and resources from a limited supply. Rapp (1985) has postulated that success for persons with mental illness is directly related to their access to resources.

The first case managers had "private practice" therapists as their role models and little or no practical direction. They were exposed to a model for compliance that had its roots in coercion and paternalism, taken largely from hospital settings. The use of seclusion and, as needed, medication were standard practices when people objected to or refused treatments, and most staff justified their actions because they were doing what was "best" for the person. There was not a cadre of role models to promote an understanding of the illnesses and the role of the relationship in helping people accept both illness and treatment.

DEFINITION AND MODELS OF CASE MANAGEMENT

Case management is variously defined throughout mental health literature. Even though there is no specific definition or structure of the work, current federal legislation requires states to include the case management function as an important part of their plans for people with severe mental illness (WICHE, 1988). Therefore, the role of the case manager in serving people with psychiatric disabilities has become increasingly significant. The case manager in many systems has as much influence as the physician and can definitely effect treatment and rehabilitation.

"Definitions of case management vary, mostly depending on preferred models and ideological priorities. The definitions generally include the assessment of service problems; provision of access to knowledge, resources, and support; and assurance of continuity of care and quality of care" (Hodge & Draine, 1993, p. 156). For purposes of this discussion, case management is defined as a service that helps people with severe mental illness get and keep the resources and supports that are wanted and needed for community life.

Given this definition and the current state of affairs in managing health care costs, the case manager has two primary functions. First, the mental health case manager has a responsibility for establishing friendly and helpful relationships (referenced as the therapeutic alliance in this book). Friendly and helpful relationships provide a conduit for knowing what is wanted, influencing people and consequently, increasing their compliance with mental health services.

Second, today's case manager has an economic function which involves assisting people in using the right amount of the most efficacious service. The economic function as it relates to compliance is important because many of the people who use the most expensive mental health services (inpatient and crisis) are also frequently labeled non-compliant.

Regardless of the definition or model, most current case management practice is based on some adaptation of the following principles (Hodge, 1994):

Individualization — Services and supports are individualized to meet the specific needs and objectives of the people served.

Outcomes — Case management services are directed towards helping people stay out of the hospital and manage their illness. Helping people find satisfactory homes, jobs and social supports is equally important.

Community based — Much of a case manager's workday is spent out of the office, especially in the environments where the people served live and/or spend their time.

Continuity of service — The system is designed to promote long-term relationships between staff and the people served and to prevent interruptions in service.

Community integration — A consistent theme is connections with people and organizations outside the formal helping system.

Optimism and strengths — The assumptions, "everyone has strengths, and everyone can grow and change," are fundamental.

Choice — The preferences of the person served are considered in so far as possible.

Relationship — The very foundation of the service is a helpful, purposeful, and friendly relationship.

Regulation of service — The system is designed to promote increases and decreases of service/support based on the individual needs of the person at any given time.

Assertive approach — For people who have traditionally refused services or who have been unable to sustain the motivation to seek services, case managers outreach and persist in their efforts to develop a helpful relationship. The assertive approach needs to be used respectfully.

These principles will to some extent undergird most of the models of case management in common practice today.

A summary and adaptation of four models described by Robinson & Bergman (1991) is as follows:

Expanded Broker Model — The principal function of the case manager is linking people to services and organizations. Usually caseloads are fairly high and much of the work is in response to crises. The orientation is maintenance of function and prevention of the use of expensive resources, i.e. hospitalization.

Personal Strengths Model — The principal function of the case manager is helping people recognize or rediscover their potential and their strengths. The premise is that personal strengths can be used to help people reach their goals and that access to resources is of paramount importance in recovery.

Rehabilitation Model — Case managers using this model help people develop "long term views" or "overall goals" and then assist them in a functional assessment to determine the skills, supports and resources necessary for achieving their goal(s). The model has frequently been associated with facility-based services such as psychosocial club houses and other rehabilitation programs. Personal growth, as well as minimizing the negative impact of severe mental illness, are outcomes associated with the rehabilitation model.

Full Support Model — Case managers are a part of an interdisciplinary team that can provide most all of the services and treatments necessary for people who might otherwise be hospitalized or institutionalized. This model has its roots in the famous PACT (Program for Assertive Community Treatment) in Madison, Wisconsin. (Stein [1990] called PACT a system of care rather than a case management model.) This model requires case managers serve small numbers of people and that they have regular access to the physician, nurse, and social worker.

Two vignettes will serve to highlight how a particular model of case management might influence a case manager's response to non-compliance.

ROBERT

Robert is a 43 year old man who suffers from schizophrenia. He has had more than 30 hospitalizations in county and state facilities. He also has been jailed numerous times. He frequently uses marijuana. He refuses all traditional services (even at one point going to a forensic unit rather than complying with an outpatient commitment order).

Expanded Broker — The case manager would continue to call and write form letters requesting Robert to come in and would eventually report problems to the authorities. It is unlikely, however, that Robert would again come to the attention of the authorities unless he broke the law or was so ill that he was committed once again.

Personal Strengths Model — The case manager would look for a success, a preference, an interest, a cultural influence that would foster the beginning of a relationship. If a food like fried chicken turned out to be a preference, the case manager might use fried chicken to help support the developing relationship and encourage taking medicines.

Rehabilitation Model — The model presumes a person who has committed on some level to personal rehabilitation and recovery.

Full Support Model — The professional staff would direct the case manager in those activities most clinically appropriate. In most situations, the professional staff with the principal relationship would outreach and try to obtain compliance through reason (if the person were not acutely psychotic). In other cases, daily medication drops would be paired with small allotments of money or cigarettes, and as a last resort, court orders for forced medications might be obtained.

GLENDA

Glenda is a 33 year old woman who has been diagnosed with both organic and borderline personality disorders. Recently she has been calling the crisis service and 911 several times each evening threatening suicide and/or reporting taking overdoses or cutting on herself. She met with her physician and case manager, and they reached agreement about a crisis plan. She did not follow the plan after the first day. Staff were not surprised since Glenda has always been non-compliant.

Expanded Broker — The case manager would talk with the crisis service and reassure them that these were gestures and that there was little or nothing that could be done. There would probably be lengthy conversations about setting limits.

Personal Strengths Model — The case manager would look for acceptable supports that could be used. Companion services would be considered. Specialized services for women would be offered. Goals would involve smaller steps. For example, going for 12 hours without making a call would be a success. A hierarchy of activities to give support and attention would be developed.

Rehabilitation Model — Peer support and personal responsibility for recovery would be emphasized and most of the initiatives listed above would also be considered. A crisis plan that was explicit in describing staff responses to specific behaviors would be made.

Full Support Model — The professional staff would direct the case manager in those activities most clinically appropriate. There would likely be a thorough psychiatric examination to determine mental status. A crisis plan that was explicit in describing staff responses to specific behaviors would be made. In general there would be close adherence to the existing plan.

These examples are simplified and may be debated clinically, but they do highlight the differences in approach that could be expected depending upon the model of case management that was practiced.

In the ideal world, people are served by the case management model that best meets their immediate needs, i.e. the model will change as needs change. In reality, staffing resources and skills are usually sufficiently limited, making it impossible to be as flexible and responsive as necessary.

FACTORS IN COMPLIANCE

Case managers have been implicitly (explicitly, in some cases) expected to get people to take their medicines. Interestingly this important task has been relegated to the lowest paid and least trained staff.

As principal facilitators of community-based service for people with severe mental illness, case managers have also been expected to find ways to convince people to accept a variety of treatment and rehabilitation approaches. Thoughtful case managers have struggled with urging people to comply with services that seem to be irrelevant and consequently, sometimes find themselves at odds with senior and professional staff. Consider the following example.

JOHN

John is a young Spanish-speaking man who uses almost no mental health services except when he is detained for hospitalization. He'll come to the first appointment after he is released from the hospital, but rarely returns for medication monitoring and individual counseling. Staff describe the situation by saying, "he only comes when he needs something". John's case manager believed that what was offered was not relevant. Her perception of his needs was based on a conversation where he asked for assistance in finding work. The professional staff recommended waiting until John had kept a series of appointments and had demonstrated compliance before assisting him vocationally. Regrettably, case managers report situations similar to this one fairly frequently.

What is the case manager's role in promoting compliance? As an enforcer of compliance with community service/treatment, case managers find themselves in the awkward position of trying to gain a person's trust and at the same time, acting like police. They also know that many mentally ill people who don't comply with services and treatments have had few choices and even less control; and the type and amount of support that has been offered in the past has been so limited.

Is the role clinical? If so, what are the considerations? Are there transference or countertransference issues; or are there cognitive impairments; or is this a case of denial of the illness? Could it be that no partnership between the case manager and person served exists? Is it possible that there is a "bad fit" between the case manager and the person? Is there a therapeutic alliance?

The role of case managers in promoting compliance has largely remained unstated. A few professional journals have referenced compliance in a way useful to case managers. Diamond (1983,1985) wrote two of the first papers that looked at compliance from the point of view of the person served. An optimistic article, "From Noncompliance to Collaboration in the Treatment of Schizophrenia", by Corrigan, Liberman, and Engel (1990), listed potential strategies that could be used by case managers. With these exceptions, the most common message about compliance to case managers has been "get those people to take their medicines". Faced with the absence of much direction, case managers have done remarkably well in trying to influence and assist people in following treatment schedules.

Satisfaction with Services

The acknowledgement of satisfaction as a key factor in compliance is fairly recent, though painfully obvious. It seems unlikely that professionals could have thought that the opinions of the people they serve didn't matter. However, the use of confrontive techniques and professional jargon, and the lack of an educational approach are concrete examples that led to much of the dissatisfaction expressed by the people served and their families.

What exactly does satisfaction with service imply? Does this mean that we should always follow the directions of the person being served? The obvious answer is no. Take for example the person who files harassment charges because the case manager sent a crisis team after a series of suicide threats. Erring on the side of caution with potentially life threatening situations must be the stance of the case manager, even when the wishes and opinions of the person are different. Another example would be a person who requests specialized services when there is no diagnostic or clinical information to support the need.

Some dissatisfaction with service is bound to occur if professionals' perception of support needs are substantially different from those of the people they serve. Money, love, relief from bad feelings, homes, jobs, and friends are at the top of the needs lists of mentally ill people (Estroff, 1987) while staff identify psychiatric treatment and medications, ADL's, case management, and crisis services (Campbell, 1989) as the most important needs.

Satisfaction with treatment and therapists likely grows when person-centered approaches are used; when helping individuals feel better is given the deserved status; and when the therapist promotes a sense of hope that things can be better.

Getting to choose one's helper and/or physician can also increase satisfaction (Andrews et al., 1986). For years, it was assumed to be the problem of the person served when conflicts arose in treatment. More recently, however, it is considered good practice to permit people to change case managers or physicians when good rapport does not exist.

Finally, if some of the burdens of severe mental illness, i.e., stigma, unpleasant side effects of medicines, and poverty are openly acknowledged, people usually feel heard, supported and consequently, satisfied. If people can't be cured, then at least they must experience some positive outcomes in the quality of their lives as a result of the service(s).

Developing Compliance Strategies

Helping people develop the supports for taking medicines, for keeping appointments, for achieving personal goals, and for avoiding substances is recognized as a positive way to influence compliance. Case managers need assistance and direction about who might benefit from these additional supports for compliance. In general, many acute episodes of mental illness are related to stopping prescribed psychotropic medications and/or using/abusing substances. For the person who historically has rejected treatment and becomes acutely ill, questions such as those that follow must be asked.

... What attempts have been made to involve the person in decisions about treatment or service?

... Has outreach to support participation been available?

... How much other support (people, places, things) is available?

... What advantages does community life make possible?

... Have the goals of the person been considered, especially in relation to housing and work?

Most discussions about compliance have been associated with medications. Medication education classes, medication containers, reminders on refrigerators, single daily doses, and decanoate injections are easy, but important strategies. There has been less emphasis on compliance with other forms of treatment (partial care, individual therapy, etc.).

Food is a major compliance support for some people. A man in Ohio managed regularly to get in for his medication injection and a pot of turnip greens and corn bread. For people with organic impairments, arranging transportation and/or taking them for their appointments is probably the best way to improve compliance. The "Friends Connection," a peer companion program for dually diagnosed people (Whitecraft, 1994), is a way to help people avoid substance use.

Compliance strategies must be developed in partnership with the person served. Choice is an important variable. Feelings of control are directly related to the ability to make personal choices. The questions, "What can I do to help you remember to take your medicine," or "which of these supports is most helpful — daily medicine delivery, every other day mediset refills, or daily medicine at the drop-in center?" are far removed from the statement "I'm going to have your medicine delivered every day". This subtle but importance difference in the approach can be a major factor in compliance.

Establishing Friendly, Helpful Relationships

Some of the problems that occur in conjunction with severe and persistent mental illness — loss of power, hope, and a positive sense of self — suggest that an important function of the case manager is developing a meaningful and helpful relationship that is best described as purposeful and friendly. There is always an advocacy component, and the relationship provides the context for the case manager to assist with concrete tasks and to promote compliance with treatment.

Mosher and Burti (1992) defined two of the most important questions that case managers can pose in developing rapport as "What do you want?" and "How can I help you get it?". They also described several relational qualities, including a healing context; a confiding relationship; a mutual understanding of the illness; positive expectations; and successes on which to build, as essential in helpful relationships.

One of the greatest case management challenges faced by this writer came as a result of asking the question "What do you want?" of Abraham who was in his mid-thirties and was described throughout the clinical record as non-compliant, uncooperative, hostile, agitated, and unmotivated. He was also sensitive to neuroleptic medications and experienced akathisia even with small doses. My question provoked the response, "Lady, I want what you got. I want a home, a job, a car, a wife. I don't want to be mentally ill." The challenge was finding something that could give the man enough hope and strength to participate in treatment which might help him realize his dreams. The psychosocial intervention was a supported job for an hour a day for which he was paid minimum wages. The medical intervention was a daily dose of benzodiazepine that he took when he felt his agitation and thinking getting out of control. Sadly the man did not achieve all his goals; to his credit, however, he did increase his time at work to twenty hours a week and he did share a house with some friends.

The advocacy role of case managers involves speaking out in behalf of the people they serve. Helping people get the services and resources to which they are entitled is of paramount importance since people's perception of their needs is often related to the acquisition of goods and services. Advocates push for services that are of an acceptable quality and accessible. They fight stigma and its debilitating effects on people with severe mental illness. They urge people and organizations to develop greater understanding of mental illness.

People who suffer from severe mental illness often count on their case managers to be non-judgemental, but at the same time, to help them see parts of themselves to which they are blind. Case managers may not always help mentally ill people get their way; nor can they support and condone certain actions. However, they must be on the same side of the struggle as the person and must partner with them on many issues. Case managers must express empathy and concern in a way that the person feels respected, supported and strengthened. They must also bring hope and confidence that they will be able to help.

CONCLUSION

Case managers have an important role in influencing people with mental illness to accept efficacious treatment(s) of their choice. Regardless of their academic backgrounds or work experiences, they will need guidance and assistance in dealing with people who are unable to accept or use the services and treatments that will probably benefit them. Emphasis should be on techniques related to helpful relationships and supportive compliance strategies rather than coercion.

Case managers do have an ethical responsibility to weigh the cost and benefit of the service for the person. When case managers and other mental health professionals seek to partner with the people they serve in their efforts to meet their needs as they perceive them, there will probably be fewer people labeled non-compliant.

REFERENCES

Andrews, S., Leavy, A., DeChillo, N., & Frances, A. (1986). Patient/therapist mismatch: We would rather switch than fight. *Hospital and Community Psychiatry, 37,* 918–922.

Bassuk, E., & Gerson, S. (1978). Deinstitutionalization and mental health services. *Scientific American, 232,* 46–53.

Campbell, J. (1989). The well-being project report: Mental health clients speak for themselves. Newhall, CA: The Well-Being Programs.

Corrigan, P. W., Liberman, R. P., & Engel, J. D. (1990). From noncompliance to collaboration in the treatment of schizophrenia. *Hospital and Community Psychiatry, 41,* 1203–1211.

Deegan, P. E. (1990). Spirit breaking: When the helping professions hurt. *The Humanistic Psychologist, 18,* 309.

Diamond, R. J. (1983). Enhancing medication use in schizophrenic patients. *Journal of Clinical Psychiatry, 44,* 7–14.

Diamond, R. J. (1985). Drugs and the quality of life: The patient's point of view. *Journal of Clinical Psychiatry, 46,* 29–35.

Dill, A. (1987). Issues in case management for the chronically mentally ill. In D. Mechanic (Ed.). *Improving mental health services: What the social sciences can tell us.* San Francisco: Jossey-Bass.

Drake, R. E., Osher, F. C., Noordsy, D. L., Hurlbut, S. C., Teague, G. B., & Beaudett, M.S. (1990). Diagnosis of alcohol use disorders in schizophrenia. *Schizophrenia Bulletin, 16,* 57–67.

Estroff, S. (October, 1987). Renewal and Revision: Creating Authentic Communities. Address at the 10th Annual Learning Community. Madison, WI.

Hodge, M. (1994). Framework for the practice of case management at COMCARE. Unpublished document. Phoenix: Regional Behavioral Health Authority.

Hodge, M., & Draine, J. (1993). Development of support through case management services. In R. Flexer & P. Solomon (Eds.), *Psychiatric rehabilitation in practice.* Boston: Andover Medical Publishers.

Joint Commission on Accreditation of Hospitals. (1976). *Accreditation of community mental health service programs.* Chicago.

Lamb, H. R. (1988). One-to-one relationships with the long term mentally ill: Issues in training professionals. *Community Mental Health Journal, 24,* 328–337.

Miles, D. (1972). The balanced service system. Unpublished document. Atlanta: Georgia Division of Mental Health, Mental Retardation, and Substance Abuse.

Mosher, L., & Burti, L. (1992). Relationships in rehabilitation: When technology fails. *Psychosocial Rehabilitation Journal, 15,* 11–17.

Rapp, C. (1985). Research on the chronically mentally ill: Curriculum implications. In Joan Bowker (Ed.), *Education for practice with the chronically mentally ill: What works?* Washington, D.C.: Council on Social Work Education, Inc.

Robinson, G., & Bergman, G. (1991). *Choices in case management: A review of current knowledge and practice for mental health programs.* Washington, D.C.: Mental Health Policy Resource Center.

Savarese, M., Detrano, T., Koproski, J., & Weber, C. (1990). Case management. In P. Brickner, L. Scharer, B. Conanan, M. Savarese, & B. Scanlan (Eds.), *Under the safety net: The health and social welfare of the homeless in the United States.* New York: W.W. Norton.

Stein, L. (1990). Comments by Leonard Stein [special section on the Madison model of community care]. *Hospital and Community Psychiatry, 41,* 649–651.

Stein, L., & Test, M. (Eds.). (1985). *The training in community living model: A decade of experience.* New Directions for Mental Health Services. San Francisco: Jossey-Bass.

Turner, J., & TenHoor, W. (1978). The NIMH community support program: Pilot approach to a needed social reform. *Schizophrenia Bulletin, 4,* 319–348.

WICHE Mental Health Program. (1988). *Guidelines for planning and implementing case management systems: PL99-660, Title V.* Boulder, Colorado: Western Interstate Commission on Higher Education.

Whitecraft, J. (1994). Peer support for consumers with chemical dependency. Presentation at Third National Case Management Conference, Chicago.

NOTE

The assistance of Laurie Curtis, Mary Fleming, and Beth Stoneking, Ph.D, is gratefully acknowledged by the author.

SECTION THREE

People with Special Needs

15

Balancing Compliance with Autonomy: Supporting the Self-Determination Needs of People with Developmental Disabilities

TATIANA DIERWECHTER

INTRODUCTION

Noncompliance is prevalent among people with developmental disabilities and can threaten their ability to function independently (Huguenin, 1993). Compliance, however, can also have negative ramifications. When used to punish, control or suppress choice, it has great potential to thwart growth and skill building. Balancing these conflicting outcomes creates treatment alliances that effectively address the needs of this population. The following incident occurred at a self-advocacy and self-protection training event and illustrates how compliance can be both positive and negative:

> The last of an eight session training event focused on assertiveness. For the warm up exercise participants were asked to share one example of how they had been assertive during the previous week. Many of the participants had difficulty identifying an example. The facilitator assisted them by asking simple questions such as, "Did you choose what you wore today?" and "Did you eat what you wanted for breakfast?" When people answered affirmatively, the group

clapped and praised them. Near the end of the exercise, Laura, a woman with mental retardation who lives in an intermediate care facility exclaimed, "I tried to be assertive, but it didn't work! I told them,' (i.e. the residential staff) that I didn't want to come to this crummy group, but here I am!"

From a professional's perspective, Laura's participation in this group was extremely important. In addition to being a victim of sexual assault and needing assistance in learning basic self-protection skills, the event was one of the few available in the community and was facilitated by an experienced and well respected trainer. Laura clearly resented being forced to participate. Despite the potential benefits of being involved in the group, the skills she was learning ironically were not validated in her living environment.

This chapter will address the tension experienced by members of treatment alliances when identifying service options for people with developmental disabilities. Examples of how compliance has negatively impacted this population throughout history will be highlighted. Using a life cycle perspective, compliance issues in childhood, adolescence, adulthood and old age will be analyzed. Whenever possible, the use of medication as a treatment intervention will be discussed. Because psychotropic medications have potential to produce significant adverse reactions, and are often prescribed for control of maladaptive behaviors without an appropriate psychiatric diagnosis (Zigman, Seltzer & Silverman, 1994), this area warrants special attention. Finally, ways members of treatment alliances can collaborate to effectively meet the needs of people with developmental disabilities will be suggested.

PEOPLE WITH DEVELOPMENTAL DISABILITIES

Like other "special populations," the definition of developmental disabilities has changed. In this chapter, the legal definition of developmental disabilities will be used since it both reflects and shapes the present service delivery system in the United States. Developmental disabilities include:

> Any chronic disability attributable to a mental or physical impairment, or combination thereof, that is manifested before the age of 22, is likely to continue indefinitely and will result in a substantial limitation in function in three or more of the following areas: self care, receptive and expressive language, learning, mobility, self direction, capacity for independent language, economic self sufficiency and necessity for special services that are of extended duration (Longhurst, 1994).

Mental retardation, cerebral palsy, autism, epilepsy and traumatic brain injury are included. Altogether it is estimated that between 1.5 and two percent of the general population have developmental disabilities (Baroff, 1991).

Just like other people, those with developmental disabilities also experience mental health disorders. Although sometimes coinciding, a developmental disability such as mental retardation is very different from mental illness. Mental illness is a psychological disability associated with emotional, social and personality dysfunction. Mental retardation is a cognitive disability caused by the interaction of a person with limited intellectual functioning and their environment. Dually diagnosed, persons with both developmental disabilities and mental illness constitute one of the most underserved populations in the United States (Reiss, 1994). This is true for a number of reasons, including: difficulty diagnosing mental health disorders in individuals with limited or no verbal communication skills, lack of training and experience on the part of professionals in both the mental health and developmental disabilities field, and the erroneous assumption that abnormal behavior is attributable to a developmental disability alone (Crews, Bonaventura & Rowe, 1994). Despite these difficulties, researchers estimate that as many as one-third of persons with developmental disabilities have significant behavioral, mental or personality disorders requiring specialized services, a rate of psychopathology four to six times higher than the general population (Seltzer & Luchterhand, 1994).

HISTORICAL ASPECTS OF COMPLIANCE

People with developmental disabilities have been negatively impacted by complying with treatment throughout modern history. Although patient compliance was often assumed and taken for granted during the 18th and 19th centuries (Blackwell, 1992), this was particularly true for people with developmental disabilities. They were often imprisoned in houses of correction, placed in segregated boarding schools, forced to work and live on farm colonies, and institutionalized in asylums and large public facilities. Laws forbidding marriage and allowing compulsory sterilization also became common (Fishley, 1992). As summarized by Shapiro (1993), people with disabilities represented a hidden, misunderstood minority, often routinely deprived of the basic life choices that even the most disadvantaged members of society take for granted. These individuals could not question or challenge prescribed treatment, resulting in the violation of basic human and civil rights.

Following Word War II, increasing importance was placed on individual autonomy. This was reflected in the civil rights, women's rights and patient's rights movement (Blackwell, 1992). People with developmental disabilities and their families also participated. Previous attitudes that characterized them as "menaces and threats to society, deviant, incapable of learning, and burdens to local communities," (Fishley, 1992) have been replaced with an increasingly common view of them as participating, contributing members of society.

This paradigm shift has dramatically changed the types of services provided. A significantly large number of persons with developmental disabilities have been deinstitutionalized and placed in intermediate care facilities and group homes. The development of supportive living services has allowed them to live in their own apartments and homes. New civil rights protection such as the Americans with Disabilities Act (ADA) and the Individuals with Disabilities Education Act (IDEA) guarantee equal access to education, employment and public accommodations. Better educated students out of integrated classrooms, a new group consciousness and political activism have resulted in more people with disabilities seeking jobs and increasing their daily participation in all aspects of civic and community life. (Shapiro, 1993).

COMPLIANCE OVER THE LIFE CYCLE

While viewing people with developmental disabilities as consumers with choices increasingly dominates the service delivery system (Tower, 1994), the issue of compliance continues to challenge people with developmental disabilities, family members and professionals. In conceptualizing the concept of compliance, Baroff (1991) discussed the basic needs that all humans have, emphasizing self-esteem. Baroff's belief that self esteem is central to good mental health is particularly true for people whose self esteem may be adversely affected by their disability. Baroff also suggests that one of the most important aspects of good self esteem is autonomy. Autonomy, or self efficacy, involves a notion of freedom, the sense that people can exercise choice. Compliance for people with developmental disabilities most often involves the completion of a directive or command within a set time limit (McDonnell, 1993). As previously discussed, their ability to question these requests is often stifled. Dependence rather than independence becomes the adaptive mode (Baroff, 1991).

Given that compliance is most likely to occur when a person has a good relationship with a trusted family member or professional who displays a sustained interest in that person and their well being (Blackwell, 1992), the likelihood that people with developmental disabilities will comply with treatment is generally quite high. Because of the characteristics of developmental disability, people usually require some type of support, informally through family or formally through professionals. Because of the powerful role these people often play in their lives, many individuals comply with treatment that may not reflect their own needs and desires. In the context of a treatment alliance, individual choice making may be overlooked or discouraged.

CHILDHOOD

Because parenting and physical care is critical during childhood, compliance issues most often involve parents and/or primary caregivers. Normally developing children demand self-determination and independence usually by their first year. As parents allow more autonomy, a child reduces its dependence on caregivers and develops new skills (Seligman & Darling, 1989). In contrast, some parents of children with developmental disabilities begin instilling a sense of compliance very early in their child's life. Mental and physical impairments can prolong the period of infancy and associated dependence for a child with a developmental disability and care-givers may struggle to allow more autonomy. The child may then develop an attitude of dependency, expecting others to always provide for her/his needs. Parents sometimes persist in doing for their child what the child could learn to do for themselves, further exasperating the problem (Baroff, 1991).

The following case study shared by a pediatric supervisor at a rehabilitation hospital illustrates this issue:

> Home visitors expended considerable effort establishing contact with Donna and her four year old son, Jeffrey. Donna had allowed therapists to conduct an in-home assessment of Jeffrey's needs and results clearly identified developmental delays. Despite some initial reluctance to bring Jeffrey to the pediatric unit for therapeutic services, Donna's enrolled Jeffrey in the program. Several months later, staff informed their supervisor that Jeffrey was not progressing. It appeared Donna was missing scheduled appointments and did not seem to be repeating "home work" assignments. Assignments included taking Jeffrey for walks in the park and playing on the recreational equipment. When asked, Donna admitted she did not take Jeffrey to the park because she was afraid he would hurt himself on the swings and seesaws. She also believed he would learn these skills on his own without intervention.

Donna's efforts to protect her son from hurting himself resulted in Jeffrey progressing more slowly than anticipated. Jeffrey, like many children with developmental disabilities, may be at risk for exhibiting excessive dependency needs, excessive approval seeking, low self-confidence and an over reliance on others when attempting to solve problems (Reiss, 1994). As summarized by McDonnell (1993), to require complete compliance in children when thoughtful and selective compliance is valued in adults, does not constitute good preparation for future functioning within society.

Just as children with developmental disabilities may more readily comply with adult caregivers, parents of these children often comply with professionals' advice. Prior to the 1960's and 1970's when behavioral psychologists suggested that persons with even severe developmental disabilities were capable of learning, many children were placed in institutions by their parents shortly after birth, usually at the advice of trusted medical professionals (Alper, Schloss & Schloss, 1994). Today, professionals are employed to provide supportive services that allow such children to develop to their fullest potential. Despite this important goal, families can still be negatively impacted when they comply with professional advice. For example:

> An elementary school principal expelled Ellen, a nine year old girl enrolled in a classroom for children diagnosed with cognitive disabilities and emotional disturbance, citing an incident in which Ellen slapped another child during an argument. Representatives from the local educational advocacy organization expressed their concern that

Ellen's response was consistent with her emotional disturbance and she could not be expelled for that reason alone. Several weeks later, the educational advocate contacted the family and was informed that Ellen had been assigned a "home bound placement" as an alternative. The advocate informed Ellen's mother that home bound placements could only be approved with a statement from a physician that a child could not attend school due to medical or physical reasons. Ellen's mother then contacted the principal and insisted that Ellen be allowed to participate in daily classroom activities.

Despite legislation guaranteeing public schooling for all children with disabilities and the increase in educational advocacy efforts by parents, parents are still often excluded from the decision making process and are expected to passively accept the proposed educational program (Alper, Schloss & Schloss, 1994). In this case, Ellen's mother complied with the principal's recommendations for Ellen's educational program only to find later that he had violated the law.

ADOLESCENCE

Perhaps no developmental stage is more challenging for parents. They must begin addressing the issue of sexuality, a usually stressful topic for parents of all children, not just those with special needs, but one that has unique implications for adolescents with developmental disabilities. Compliance becomes a salient issue as many families work diligently to encourage social behaviors that comply with family and societal norms and values around sexuality.

> After discovering that she could not legally sterilize her fifteen year old son, Tim, Judy consulted a psychiatrist who treated Tim with Ritalin, a psychotropic medication often prescribed for children diagnosed with attention deficit disorder. A recent incident at school in which he approached a non-disabled student in the hallway and attempted to hold her hand convinced Judy that the medication was not working. In addition, Tim seemed to be experiencing side effects including loss of appetite and difficulty sleeping. As a result, she contacted a local developmental disability advocacy organization to inquire about sexuality classes. A social worker at the agency reassured Judy that, just like non-disabled young men, Tim seemed to be experiencing the normal thoughts and feelings that accompany puberty. She suggested that additional support and training in friendships, dating and public and private touching might be helpful and she encouraged Judy to enroll Tim in a sexuality training program designed for people with developmental disabilities that her agency sponsored. After 22 group sessions combined with weekly visits with a counselor experienced in serving people with developmental disabilities, Judy reported that Tim's behavior had changed and her concerns had been reduced. Tim was eventually removed from the Ritalin.

Judy's realization that her son was experiencing sexual feelings alarmed her. In addition to the concerns expressed above, Judy worried that his emerging sexuality would lead to escalating inappropriate behavior, perhaps culminating in an unwanted pregnancy or even criminal charges. Judy's initial response was to suppress Tim's emerging sexuality with the use of medication. Given Tim's age, his lack of prior history with any type of socially unacceptable touching, and his lack of access to basic sexuality education, the worker was concerned that Tim was complying with treatment that may not have been appropriate for him. Her greatest concern was that Tim was not diagnosed with attention deficit disorder, the disorder for which Ritalin is primarily intended. In addition, he was experiencing common side effects of the medication while at the same time not benefiting. Like most prescribed medications, it is suggested that Ritalin be given as an integral part of a total treatment program that includes psychological, educational and social measures (Sifteon, 1994). Judy received no other referrals from Tim's psychiatrist upon first contact and only explored other options after she herself decided the medication was ineffective. Fortunately, Judy was open to exploring alternatives and the use of basic sexuality education as an intervention tool met this family's needs.

Perhaps the most disconcerting aspect of compliance as it relates to sexuality is the role it plays in making people with developmental disabilities vulnerable to sexual assault and exploitation. Research suggests that people with developmental disabilities are abused at significantly higher rates than the general population. It is estimated that 86 percent of females and 36 percent of males with developmental disabilities will experience at least one incident of sexual assault in their lifetimes (Patterson, 1991). Children with disabilities are twice as likely to be abused than non-disabled children and the vast majority of offenders are known to the victim (U.S. Department of Health and Human Services, 1993).

Of all the complex factors that contribute to the sexual assault and exploitation of people with developmental disabilities, socialization and training that emphasizes compliance and cooperation with caregivers is perhaps the most concerning (Federer, 1993). As discussed, being unnecessarily dependent on others can negatively influence self image and personal competence. As a result, people with developmental disabilities often feel powerless. In situations involving sexual assault, they may not understand that they could say no much less report an abusive incident (Patterson, 1991).

Given that compliance occurs more frequently when a trusted family member or professional is involved, it is not surprising that the majority of offenders are known to the victim. In addition to family members, a large percent of offenders have contact with victims through specialized developmental disability services (Furey, 1994). The people served often become emotionally attached to professionals and will do whatever is asked to continue receiving attention. Fear of losing one's home or job or being deprived of care also discourages individuals from reporting abuse (Froemming, 1991).

It should be noted that people with developmental disabilities living in large congregate settings are at greater risk for abuse and exploitation than those living in the community. The lack of adequate supervision of residents who are either physically or chemically restrained is of particular concern because of the correlation between sexual abuse and a higher rate of restraint and use of behavior modifying drugs. Although it is not clear if "challenging, disruptive and noncompliant behavior" resulting in physical and chemical restraints is a result of abuse or if people in restraints are simply easier targets for abuse (Furey, 1994), special attention needs to be given to situations where physical and chemical restraints are used to ensure compliance.

ADULTHOOD

Entering adulthood can be particularly problematic. Cultural norms suggest that a person has the capacity to live independently and to function without the support and supervision of others. Common characteristics associated with having developmental disabilities often impede the ability of such people to carry out these goals (Baroff, 1991). As an adolescent with developmental disabilities matures into adulthood, parental anxieties about their son or daughter's general coping skills often intensify. As they did in earlier stages of childhood and adolescence, parents of these adults may react by overprotecting and curbing autonomy.

> Although Richard was almost 33 years old, he had just moved out of his parent's home and into his own apartment. While his self care skills were well developed, Richard's supportive living case manager became exasperated by Richard's mother's efforts to maintain her previous level of involvement. She accepted the placement but questioned the case manager's actions whenever Richard was encouraged to learn new skills. Instead of allowing him to take the bus home for Sunday dinners, she would pick Richard up in her car. When Richard saved money from his job at a local supermarket and used it to buy a jacket, she escorted him to the store and returned it. In addition, she monitored how well he kept his room clean by making regular visits to the apartment. Despite repeated attempts to persuade Richard's mother of the importance of allowing Richard opportunities for independence and choice making, Roger's case manager felt that Richard's eventual return home was inevitable.

Although Richard was his own guardian and legally had the right to continue living in his own apartment and conducting his own affairs, it was very difficult for him to counter the demands his mother placed upon him. Ironically, by complying with parents or other care providers, adults with developmental disabilities often do not have the opportunity to learn those very skills that would ease parental and professional fears (Seligman & Darling, 1989). An additional example highlights compliance issues in adulthood:

> Placed in a state center for the developmentally disabled at the age of five, Susan spent 41 years living in an institution. She described sleeping in a large room with many other children, eating communally and standing naked in line for long periods of time waiting to take showers. As a young adult, she "worked" by taking care of other residents, feeding people, changing their diapers and making beds. Upon

leaving the institution, Susan was placed in a group home where she shortly began exhibiting disruptive behaviors. These included throwing things, screaming and physically assaulting other residents. After running away from the group home, staff referred Susan to a psychiatrist who placed her on Haldol and Mellaril. Susan's aggressive behavior continued, however. She also began "shutting down" verbally, refusing to talk and retreating to her bedroom where she would lay on her bed for hours, missing meals and refusing visitors. At this point, she was diagnosed with bipolar disorder and placed on lithium carbonate. Concerned about the use of multiple medications, Susan's county case manager suggested that an independent consultation be conducted. By charting every behavioral episode, a local specialist helped the staff realize that Susan's outbreaks often occurred at times when she was asked to make choices. As a result, efforts were made to "break down" choices for Susan, starting with simple choices between two different shirts to wear or two different menu items. Within weeks, the number of choices were expanded for Susan and her aggressive behaviors diminished dramatically. Although she continued to benefit from the use of lithium and Haldol, the Mellaril was removed.

Susan struggled with assuming the role of independent adult after years of restricted choice making in an institutional setting. When her behaviors escalated to include threatening and hitting others, she was placed on a series of medications designed to control aggression. This was done without first attempting alternative, less intrusive behavioral or psychological interventions. As discussed by Harper and Wadsworth (1993) this is not unusual. Persons with developmental disabilities residing in group settings are more likely to be administered psychotropic medication than similar persons living in the community, despite the fact that community residents display more severe and frequent behavior problems (Zigman, Seltzer and Silverman, 1994). The number of individuals who receive alternative intervention is quite low, suggesting that psychotropic medication may be an expedient treatment for professionals (Harper and Wadsworth, 1993). Supporting Susan's efforts in choice making allowed her to choose compliance while at the same time gain new skills and reduce her dependence on psychotropic medication.

OLDER ADULTHOOD

For the first time in history, people with developmental disabilities are reaching old age. Improvements in health care and living conditions have dramatically increased the life expectancy of this population. Although persons with more severe disabilities still have shorter life spans, the majority can be expected to live as long as the nondisabled population. As a result, it is now common for a child with a developmental disability to outlive her or his parents (Roberto, 1993).

The majority of older adults with developmental disabilities live with their families. Many have done so since birth (Seltzer and Krauss, 1994). Although the nurturing, support and financial savings to the formal service provider system are invaluable, life long care by one provider can also be detrimental. In addition to having few relationships with people other than family members (Gibson, Rabkin & Munson, 1992) and often experiencing great trauma when forced to relocate after a caregiver either becomes disabled or dies (Roberto, 1993), the lives of older persons with developmental disabilities who live with their parents are often overdetermined. As Edgerton (1994) states, "Not only is their present day organized, arranged and regimented by others, so is tomorrow and the future. Some aging persons with developmental disabilities never escape from the control of others." The following case highlights these concerns:

> Joe is 62 years old. Generally assumed to be mildly mentally retarded, he lived with his mother, Grace, until she recently died from complications associated with a broken hip. Never having learned the kinds of skills that would have allowed him to live alone, Joe's brother and his wife temporarily assumed Grace's caregiving duties. Their lives changed dramatically as they taught Joe how to shave, brush his teeth, and bathe as well as more complex tasks such as washing clothes, cooking simple meals and identifying neighborhood landmarks. When living with Grace, Joe never left the house except to accompany his mother to church. He recently enrolled in the Supplemental Security Income (SSI) program which has allowed him to receive monthly stipends as well as basic health care services. For the first time in 30 years, Joe visited a dentist and received a complete physical examination.

There are many reasons families like Joes' delay the departure of their child. As described by Seltzer and Krauss (1994), continued caregiving may reflect a deep commitment to the idea of the family taking care of its own as well as a realistic assessment of the lack of acceptable residential options and the continued need for support and supervision. Alternatives to home may be judged as unavailable, unsatisfactory, too expensive or having too long a waiting list. Many families had negative experiences with the formal service system and have harbored deep distrust of professionals for years. Finally, there may be great interdependence between a parent and a child that increases with age. A child who provides care and support to frail, elderly parents may play a valuable role in maintaining the independence of the family as a whole. Even when older adults with developmental disabilities express preferences about their present and future living arrangements, they may be disregarded if these are incompatible with parent's attitudes, fears, or anxieties (Roberto, 1993).

Despite these important factors, Joe's complete reliance on his aging mother as the only source of care set the stage for enormous changes as he encountered the consequences of Grace's death. Like Susan, Joe exhibited signs of "learned helplessness," (Nezu, Nezu, & Gill-Weiss, 1992) and was unable to function on his own despite his age and a cognitive level that would suggest enormous potential for independent living. Never having had the opportunity to engage in any aspects of "normal" life, Joe perhaps typifies compliance at its most extreme.

Researchers confirm a tendency towards increasing drug use with advancing age in people with developmental disabilities (Harper and Wadsworth, 1993). Middle aged and older persons in nursing homes and other residential facilities, for example, are more likely to receive psychotropic medication compared to younger persons (Zigman, Seltzer and Silverman, 1994). This contrasts sharply with the generally accepted notion that older people should receive lower dosages of medication to avoid adverse drug reactions. Given that people with a known organic etiology may be more sensitive to medication usage, the potential for inappropriate treatment of older adults who have developmental disabilities with medication may be even greater (Seltzer and Luchterhand, 1994).

Finally, it should be noted that professionals' perceptions are more likely to influence the use of medications than are objective behavior measures or mental health diagnoses (Harper and Wadsworth, 1993). In their study of older adults with developmental disabilities in nursing homes, Zigman, Seltzer & Silverman (1994) conclude that the use of medications is primarily to control behavior problems that staff feel incompetent to handle. Given that medication is often prescribed without determination of an appropriate psychiatric diagnosis, use of medication as a primary source of treatment must always be carefully scrutinized and balanced with other types of behavioral and psychological intervention.

RECOMMENDATIONS FOR IMPROVING THE TREATMENT ALLIANCE

This chapter has reviewed how compliance positively and negatively impacts the lives of people with developmental disabilities. Historical factors as well as examples throughout the life span suggest that compliance, despite its many benefits, has enormous potential to suppress autonomy and choice making, qualities that are recognized in the general population as positive and necessary for independent living. The role of medication in this process has also been highlighted because of the great potential for misuse in this population.

The advent of the disability rights movement has brought new attention to the critical issue of compliance, challenging the way it has been used in the past to control people and creating new opportunities for people with developmental disabilities to learn assertiveness and self advocacy skills. Consumers, family members and professionals have participated in this movement and are called upon to continue addressing the issue of compliance within the context of treatment alliances.

There are many ways members of treatment alliances can further this goal. For example, training opportunities for professionals must be expanded, particularly for direct care providers who work the closest with people but usually have the least access to continuing professional education. Historical information about this population, a review of legislation and service models that have changed the way people with developmental disabilities are viewed, and the use of nonaversive treatment approaches can provide professionals with a strong theoretical foundation, helping them to balance both the positive and negative aspects of compliance.

Professionals also need support and assistance in delivering family centered services. As described throughout this chapter, families, particularly older ones, bring very different values, beliefs and traditions to the caregiving process, particularly where autonomy is concerned. These often contrast with the expectations of professionals and can be a cause of great tension and conflict. Because a family centered approach emphasizes respect for diversity and focuses on strengths and priorities, it facilitates the development of trust between families and professionals and can be very helpful in bridging these differences (Rounds, Weil and Bishop, 1994). Interestingly, consumers, family members and professionals interviewed for this chapter validated the important role trust plays in enhancing treatment alliances. A basic tenet of most helping professions, establishing trust involves listening to concerns, providing complete information regarding options, recognizing the difficulty of changing and/or utilizing unfamiliar supports and accepting decisions that families make (Seligman and Darling, 1989). Tower (1994) encourages human service agencies to formalize this family centered approach by establishing ombudsman or advocacy assistance programs to resolve conflicts. Insuring consumer interests are represented on advisory committees and boards of directors is also critical. By promoting consumer involvement, agency and consumer goals become more congruent (Roberto, 1993).

In addition to training professionals, people with developmental disabilities and their family members need access to self-advocacy training. Defined as "teaching people how to make decisions and choices that affect their lives so they can become more independent," self advocacy training can begin counteracting years of socialization that has encouraged dependency (Longhurst, 1994). Because of the role compliance plays in making people with developmental disabilities vulnerable to sexual assault, self-advocacy training in this area is especially important. Family members can also benefit from training that encourages them to challenge the image of professionals as "experts" and to take on a more entrepreneurial role when securing services. This includes seeking information, identifying service options, weighing outcomes and ultimately making decisions that reflect the family's needs and priorities (Seligman & Darling, 1989). Direct care providers can also model good self advocacy skills, teaching strategies for affective communication, and coaching them through the maze of policies and procedures that people with developmental disabilities and their families often encounter (Tower, 1994).

Finally, consumers, family members and professional service providers must engage in political and systems advocacy. In addition to raising awareness about the needs of people with developmental disabilities and their families, implementation of recent legislative achievements such as the American with Disabilities Act (ADA) and the Individuals with Disabilities Education Act (IDEA) must be continued and expanded. Treatment alliance members must also advocate for the development and funding of adequate community supports at the local, county, state and national levels. Parents of adolescents, for example, may feel more comfortable addressing sexuality issues if they are aware of comprehensive sexuality education opportunities. Older families may be more likely to plan for the future if high quality, alternative residential services are available. Unfortunately, limited and diminishing resources make it difficult to meet the present needs of this population and increasing political pressure to make further cuts in these programs means even the continuation of existing levels of service cannot be assumed. Services such as these are integral to the ability of people with developmental disabilities to participate successfully in integrated, everyday life. People with developmental disabilities, family members and professional service providers must become effective public advocates. Instead of achieving higher degrees of conformity or control in what are often unappealing and unchallenging segregated environments (McDonnell, 1993), the task of treatment alliance members is to change the environment of people with developmental disabilities so that self-determination and choice making become as important as compliance.

REFERENCE

Alper, S., Schloss, P. J., & Schloss, C. N. (1994). *Families of students with disabilities: Consultation and advocacy*. Boston: Allyn and Bacon.

Baroff, G. S. (1991). *Developmental disabilities: Psychosocial aspects*. Austin: Pro-ed.

Blackwell, B. (1992). Compliance. *Psychotherapy & Psychosomatics, 58,* 161–169.

Crews, W. D., Bonaventura, S., & Rowe, F. (1994). Dual diagnosis: Prevalence of psychiatric disorders in a large state residential facility for individuals with mental retardation. *American Journal on Mental Retardation, 98* (6), 688–731.

Edgerton, R. B. (1994). Quality of life issues: Some people know how to be old. In Seltzer, M. S., Krauss, M. W., & Janicki, M. P. (Eds.). *Life course perspectives on adulthood and old age* (pp. 3–18). Washington, DC: American Association on Mental Retardation.

Federer, D. (1993). The dangers of learned compliance. *Connections, July*, 5.

Fishley, P. (1992). I am john. *Health and Social Work, 17* (2), 151–157.

Froemming, R. (1991). *Sexual abuse of adults with developmental disabilities: Legal issues and proposals for change*. Madison: Wisconsin Council on Developmental Disabilities.

Furey, E. M. (1994). Sexual abuse of adults with mental retardation: Who and where. *Mental Retardation, 32* (3), 173–180.

Gibson, J. W., Rabkin, J., & Munson, R. (1992). Critical issues in serving the developmentally disabled elderly. *Journal of Gerontological Social Work, 19* (1), 35–49.

Harper, D. C. & Wadsworth, J. S. (1993). Behavioral problems and medication utilization. *Mental Retardation, 31* (2), 97–103.

Huguenin, Nancy, H. (1993). Reducing chronic non-compliance in an individual with severe mental retardation to facilitate community integration. *Mental Retardation, 31* (5), 332–339.

Longhurst, A. (1994). *The self advocacy movement by people with developmental disabilities: A demographic study and directory of self advocacy groups in the United States.* Annapolis Junction, MD: American Association on Mental Retardation Publication Center.

McDonnell, A. P. (1993). Ethical considerations in teaching compliance to individuals with mental retardation. *Education & Training in Mental Retardation, March,* 3–13.

Nezu, C. M., Nezu, A. M., & Gill-Weiss, M. J. (1992). *Psychopathology in persons with mental retardation: Clinical guidelines for assessment and treatment.* Champaign, IL: Research Press Company.

Patterson, P. M. (1991). *Doubly Silenced: Sexuality, sexual abuse and people with developmental disabilities.* Madison: Wisconsin Council on Developmental Disabilities.

Reiss, S. (1994). *Handbook of challenging behavior: Mental health aspects of mental retardation.* Worthington, OH: IDS Publishing Corporation.

Roberto, K. A. (Ed.). (1993). *The elderly caregiver: Caring for adults with developmental disabilities.* Newbury Park, CA: Sage Publications.

Rounds, K. A., Weil, M., & Bishop, K. K. (1994). Practice with culturally diverse families of young children with disabilities. *Families in Society: The Journal of Contemporary Human Services, January:* 3–14.

Seligman, M., & Darling, R. B. (1989). *Ordinary families, special children: A systems approach to childhood disability.* New York: Guilford Press.

Seltzer, G. B., & Luchterhand, C. (1994). Health and well-being of older persons with developmental disabilities: A clinical review. In Seltzer, M. S., Krauss, M. W., & Janicki, M. P. (Eds.). *Life course perspectives on adulthood and old age* (pp. 3–18). Washington, DC: American Association on Mental Retardation.

Seltzer, M. S., & Krauss, M. W. (1994). Aging parents with coresident adult children: The impact of lifelong caregiving. In Seltzer, M. S., Krauss, M. W., & Janicki, M. P. (Eds.). *Life course perspectives on adulthood and old age* (pp. 3–18). Washington, DC: American Association on Mental Retardation.

Shapiro, J. (1993). *People with disabilities – forging a new civil rights movement.* New York: Times Books.

Sifteon, D. W. (1994). *The PDR family guide to prescription drugs.* Montavale, NJ: Medical Economics Data Production Company.

Tower, K. D. (1994). Consumer-centered social work practice: Restoring client self-determination. *Social Work, 39* (2), 191–196.

U.S. Department of Health and Human Services. (1993). *A report on the maltreatment of children with disabilities.* (Contract No. 105-89-1630). Washington, DC: National Clearinghouse on Child Abuse and Neglect Information.

Zigman, W. B., Seltzer, G. B., & Silverman, W. P. (1994). Behavioral and mental health changes associated with aging in adults with mental retardation. In Seltzer, M. S., Krauss, M. W., & Janicki, M. P. (Eds.). *Life course perspectives on adulthood and old age* (pp. 67–91). Washington, DC: American Association on Mental Retardation.

16

Treatment Compliance in Schizophrenia: Issues for the Therapeutic Alliance and Public Mental Health

NEAL COHEN

The proven efficacy of the neuroleptics in treating patients with psychosis and preventing relapse makes the problem of treatment compliance among the population who have schizophrenia a significant public mental health issue. Patient compliance with a prescribed treatment regimen is a complex phenomenon that implies a sense of trust and commitment to work collaboratively with a psychiatrist and other caregivers. Given the nature of the illness, people with schizophrenia experience problems in the development of trust associated with a limited and cautious attachment to others. Therefore, the ability of the patient with schizophrenia to engage with an individual clinician or treatment team is often fraught with difficulties that may require intervention strategies to facilitate ongoing involvement with treatment (Stoudemire & Thompson, 1983).

Chen (1991) has described the multiple manifestations of noncompliance among people with severe mental illness in community treatment settings. These include the failure to accept the aftercare discharge plan derived from a psychiatric hospitalization, both in "no show" or missed appointments with clinic referrals from inpatient services (26–50% of scheduled appointments at outpatient clinics result in no-shows; Allan, 1988; Burgoyne, Acosta, & Yamamoto, 1983; Kluger & Karras, 1983) and from emergency services (32–75% no-show rate; Axelrod & Wetzler, 1989; Jellinek, 1978). Another significant component of noncompliance is the frequency of dropout from treatment settings. Studies demonstrate that between 9 and 40 percent of patients never return following one clinic appointment (Atwood & Beck, 1985; Craig & Huffine, 1976) and between 30–60%

239

drop out of treatment within the first year (Atwood & Beck, 1985; Larsen, Ngayen, & Green, 1983; Swett & Noones, 1989) with the majority occurring within the first four visits (Baekeland & Lundwall, 1975; Swett & Noones, 1989).

The literature has consistently demonstrated the importance of outpatient treatment for people with persistent mental illness in the prevention of relapse and rehospitalization (Caton, 1982; Fink & Heckerman, 1981). There is, however, a paucity of studies that systematically examine the components of treatment in order to identify the benefit of drug treatment in combination with specific, well-defined psychosocial interventions (Hogarty, Anderson, & Reiss, 1986). Most outcome studies do not distinguish psychosocial interventions from pharmacotherapeutic interventions, and noncompliance with treatment and with medication are usually viewed as synonymous.

Barofsky and Bulson (1980) report no difference in the compliance with treatment of patients with psychiatric illness in comparison to other patients with chronic medical conditions. Despite the equivalency among patients with chronic illness in their noncompliance with treatment efforts, there appears to be a distinctly strong aversion to neuroleptic medication among patients who have schizophrenia that has a major bearing upon vulnerability to relapse and rehospitalization. Soskis (1978) reported upon a cohort of patients with schizophrenia who were much better informed than inpatients with medical disorders about the drugs they were receiving; however, only 56% of the patients with schizophrenia stated that they would take the medication if they had the choice, as compared with 93% of the inpatients with medical disorders. While psychoeducational efforts regarding medications are thought to be essential to secure compliance from patients with schizophrenia, there remains a very large percentage of patients whose objections are rooted in subjective complaints of not feeling like themselves, and believing themselves to be limited in their functioning as a consequence of compliance with standard medication (Hogan, Awad, & Eastwood, 1983).

The problem of medication noncompliance among patients with schizophrenia has not widely been addressed in the training of psychiatric residents, which has largely emphasized hospital treatment. Patients who refuse antipsychotic drug therapy in the hospital are usually treated over their objection by following legal procedures that override their right of treatment refusal (Zito, Routt, Mitchell, & Roerig, 1985). The national trend toward shorter lengths of stay for inpatient services places even greater emphasis upon getting the patient treated with suitable pharmacotherapy to control psychotic symptoms. As Awad (1993), Strauss (1989), Van Putten, May and Marder (1984) report, patient complaints of drug-induced dysphoria are generally given short shrift. The reasons for drug refusal among hospitalized patients remain controversial. In an earlier report, Van Putten (1978) identified the emergence of extrapyramidal symptoms as significantly contributing to medication noncompliance in the patient with schizophrenia. However, in a study comparing patients who refuse with those who consent to neuroleptic treatment, Marder et al. (1983) found that drug refusers did not have a history of severe medication side effects but were more hostile, more mistrustful of the treatment team, and less likely to believe that they were ill. Appelbaum (1982) has pointed out that there is no single reason for drug refusal, which comprises a group of behaviors that depend on a patient's experiences, clinical state, and other variables. Van Putten, May and Marder (1984) reported that for patients who have schizophrenia, a dysphoric response to the first dose was found to be a powerful predictor of future noncompliance. Furthermore, a persistent dysphoric response was associated with a poor clinical outcome. There was consistency in the patients' subjective responses throughout therapy, suggesting that these responses to antipsychotic medication be acknowledged and attempts made to attenuate them through use of anti-parkinsonian medications or dosage adjustments. A recent review by Awad (1993) supports a correlation between altered subjective state on neuroleptics, medication compliance, and therapeutic outcome.

The rejection of medications and treatment by patients with schizophrenia has often been linked to a lack of awareness of illness, often described as "lack of insight." As a consequence of this denial, patients with schizophrenia may refuse to enter the hospital when ill, refuse to accept medications or discontinue medications immediately upon discharge. Insight has been associated with greater expressed willingness to take medication (McEvoy, Aland, & Wilson, 1981), greater compliance with medication regimens (Lin, Spiga, & Fortsch, 1979) and less need for hospitalization if symptoms of relapse emerge (Heinrichs, Cohen, & Carpenter, 1985). These findings suggest a readiness for schizophrenic patients with insight to accept and collaborate with treatment. In a study by McEvoy, Apperson et al. (1989) insight in a group of acutely psychotic schizophrenic patients remained consistent over time even as these patients recovered. This finding suggests that psychotic symptoms per se did not interfere with these patients' ability to recognize their illness and need for treatment. In a follow-up study on these patients' clinical course after discharge from the hospital (McEvoy, Fretner et al., 1989), good insight was associated with greater treatment compliance with treatment after 30 days in the community and less frequent rehospitalization.

The etiology of the awareness of illness deficit in schizophrenia is poorly understood. In a recent review article, Amador et al. (1991) describe a number of neuropsychological deficits that bear a striking resemblance to poor insight in schizophrenia. When differentiated from a psychological coping mechanism, insight and unawareness of illness may be recognized as a cognitive marker for subtyping patients with schizophrenia and for developing strategies for clinical intervention that will teach better recognition of the illness and early signs of relapse.

Weiden, Shaw, and Mann (1986) conceptualized neuroleptic noncompliance as occurring in "active", "passive", or "rational" patients. The noncompliant patient with schizophrenia who experiences dysphoric neuroleptic-induced side effects is seen as a "rational" patient whose decision is derived from an intact judgment. The "active" refuser expresses opposition to neuroleptic treatment early in treatment. This rejection of treatment with neuroleptics may derive from a lack of insight or awareness of illness for which pharmacotherapy is indicated. Seen in persons with acutely psychotic and/or residual psychotic symptoms, "active" refusal may be expressing a family or cultural attitude that rejects treatment as stigmatizing by labeling the individual as mentally ill. The "passive" patient accepts medications during hospital treatment but over time stops taking neuroleptics as a consequence of dropping out of treatment. Chronic psychotic symptomatology with a predominance of negative symptoms (avolitional, anhedonic, and amotivational states) is most characteristic of the passive response.

The subtyping of neuroleptic noncompliance has implications for treatment and intervention strategies. Weiden, Shaw, and Mann, (1986) recommend an assessment of noncompliance that makes inquiry into the patient's subjective responses to neuroleptics, history of treatment emergent extrapyramidal symptoms, longitudinal course of psychotic symptomatology, and the patient's personal, cultural, and family attitudes toward mental illness and treatment. With a comprehensive assessment of noncompliance history available, the clinician has an opportunity to anticipate the issues that may well compromise the therapeutic relationship and lead to termination of treatment. Kane (1986) describes the resistance of many clinicians to discussing issues of medication noncompliance with their patients as reflecting a belief that "making too much of the (neuroleptic) adverse effects will encourage the patient to discontinue medication." (p. 578). An open communication of attitudes toward medication allows for some relevant psychoeducational effort that can strengthen the therapeutic alliance and allow the treatment to continue in an honest and more informed manner.

TREATMENT FIT AND BARRIERS TO TREATMENT COLLABORATION

As a public mental health issue, noncompliance with treatment and medication among patients with schizophrenia and severe mental illness must be addressed in terms of the availability of and access to relevant services in the community. After decades of deinstitutionalization, a new generation of patients has emerged for whom the revolving door of readmission to inpatient settings has become a persistent pattern of service utilization. Repeated admission becomes an inevitable outcome when patients are unable to participate in treatments that are poorly conceived and a clear mismatch with the needs of people with serious mental illness, especially those living in poverty and without meaningful social supports.

Patients repeatedly admitted and labeled as noncompliant are stigmatized by mental health professionals who view them as resistant or lacking motivation to accept the treatment that clinicians offer. When assessed in psychiatric emergency rooms, these patients are often stereotyped as untreatable, and admission is avoided. Instead, they receive a prescription and an appointment at a community mental health clinic, usually several weeks in the future. In a fragile state and with a tenuous hold on reality, these patients do not keep their appointments but return to the emergency room within days or weeks. They are now admitted to the hospital, but a chart note documents their noncompliance with treatment (Cohen, 1993).

This all-too-familiar scenario derives from the failure to offer an appropriate intervention that might allow a better outcome. More appropriate interventions might involve crisis intervention in a holding unit of the emergency room, an assertive outreach team to engage the patient after release from the emergency room, or a crisis residence to maintain the closest level of supervision and supportive structure outside the hospital. With only medication and psychotherapy, the traditional tools of treatment, clinical staff often regard these patients as unable to be helped. Considering their noncompliance with such treatments, they may even be viewed as being responsible for their plight.

The stigma imposed on such patients is related to the futility that clinicians feel when their interventions fail. The iatrogenic orgin of this clinical and systems mismatch needs to be recognized if we are going to stop blaming the victim for noncompliance with dysfunctional or limited service systems. The promulgation of new treatment models can serve as an antidote to the futility felt by clinical staff and also can give these patients access to more relevant services (Cohen, 1993).

Talbott, Bachrach and Ross (1986) also discussed the consequences of patient interactions with mental health systems as vital to the creation of the "fit" necessary to influence compliance. The balance or equilibrium among the elements of the treatment situation (i.e. patient, clinician, and mental health systems) requires flexibility or resiliency in systems as much as in patients. This interactive model of compliance/noncompliance has been echoed in more recently reported multidimensional models which are concerned with strategies to overcome barriers to treatment collaboration (Blackwell, 1992; Corrigan, Liberman, & Engel, 1990).

Despite the promulgation of interactive models of compliance, the pejorative or stigmatizing view of noncompliance still often prevails among clinicians who regard the patient as responsible for their plight. Many clinicians continue to experience the treatment of people with severe mental illness as frustrating, hopeless and unrewarding (Corrigan, Liberman, & Engel, 1990; Talbott, 1987). Mirabi, Weinman, and Magnetti, (1978) reported that in a survey of 436 mental health professionals, 85 percent preferred not to treat patients with "chronic" illness. This frequently held negative attitude is especially troubling because it can easily lead to a paternalistic or adversarial relationship with the patient (Friedman, 1985). Since positive therapeutic alliances are found to lead to greater acceptance by patients of the treatment regimen (Frank & Gunderson, 1990), the larger public mental health aspect of patient noncompliance requires greater educational efforts with mental health professionals to overcome clinician resistances and to promote greater collaborative practice styles with the severely mentally ill (Corrigan, Liberman and Engel, 1990).

THE TRAINING EXPERIENCE

Psychiatric residents especially need to be able to work therapeutically with patients who have persistent illness, many of whom have histories of being refractory to treatment. Pressures abound to turn such patients away from emergency rooms because of anticipated complicated and lengthy stays in the hospital, or to transfer them to long-term care settings such as state psychiatric hospitals. While individual patient histories may provide a rationale for such actions, the message to our psychiatric residents is unmistakable: treat only those patients who have strong social supports, high levels of functioning, and good prognosis (Cohen, 1990). As the field moves further in this direction, the treatment challenges posed by patients with severe mental illness who have histories of noncompliance and recidivism are in danger of receiving increasingly less attention.

A recent glimmer in this therapeutic darkness is the finding that the drug Clozapine has significant therapeutic action for patients who were previously resistant to treatment (Kane, et al., 1988). In response to this advance, staffs are examining their caseloads to select candidates for therapeutic trials of novel medications. Furthermore, advances in psychosocial rehabilitation technology offer new hope for the reintegration of patients into stable community life.

Besides the potential therapeutic benefit to be derived from these new approaches, a collective gain for patients lies in the discovery of an antidote to the therapeutic nihilism that has made "chronic" an adjective synonymous with "hopeless." Residents can learn a great deal about treatment responses (successes and failures) through a broad clinical exposure to patients with long term or recurrent illness. The commitment of clinicians to work collaboratively with people who have severe mental illness is critical to lifting the stigma and negative reactions that interfere with treatment partnerships which can produce treatment regimens acceptable and relevant to the goals of clinicians and patients alike.

THE HOMELESS MENTALLY ILL

Cohen (1992) discussed the significant advances that modern medicine has made through the struggle against major epidemics. The plagues of cholera, tuberculosis, and polio all resulted in new treatments and preventive measures, while AIDS awaits a therapeutic breakthrough. By unlocking the mechanisms of its viral pathogenesis, AIDS researchers may very well have an impact on the future of cancer therapeutics. The potential for a major advance in the therapeutics of severely mentally ill persons is now at hand as a consequence of another epidemic. A dramatic increase in the number and visibility of homeless people wandering the streets of both urban and rural areas was noted in the 1980s (Cohen & Marcos, 1992). Numerous studies of subpopulations of the homeless consistently find a substantial degree of mental impairment although rates range widely. Fischer, Drake and Breakey (1992) reported that severe mental illness was 20 times more prevelant among homeless populations than among those living in impoverished households. It is clear that this epidemic-like growth in the number of homeless mentally ill persons includes many with severe psychiatric impairments who are the most visible victims of failed deinstitutionalization policies.

As a result of greater than one decade of significant experience with the homeless mentally ill, psychiatry is now beginning to develop a new therapeutic armamentarium for persons with severe mental illness. For example, our understanding of the role of the outreach team in linking disaffiliated persons to needed community-based resources has been advanced by model programs concerned with the care of the homeless mentally ill. Similarly, the necessity of housing the homeless is now influencing psychiatry to accept an integral role in developing models of supportive housing in the maintenance of severely impaired persons with mental illness in the community. In the past few years the National Institute of Mental Health has established priority funding for research that will advance a new technology of psychosocial rehabilitation for homeless mentally ill persons. These efforts to address the suffering of the homeless mentally ill should eventually pay dividends in psychiatry's aim to treat and ultimately prevent serious and persistent mental illness. Psychiatry, like medicine, must learn all that it can from its own epidemic in order to help the even more numerous but less visible victims of mental illness.

The homeless mentally ill are a diverse group of people who differ in as many characteristics as they share. Diagnosis, chronicity, social networks, work history and skills, level of functioning, and current symptomatology all vary widely. The resistance of many to treatment services is partially derived from a fear and mistrust of institutions and the professionals associated with them. As a result, gaining the trust of homeless mentally ill persons is basic to the work of all treatment models. Without any cooperation from the homeless person in making a clinical assessment, the mental health professional will be able to judge only the most obvious aspects of the person's level of functioning and relationship to the immediate environment.

The noncompliance of the homeless mentally ill with traditional community mental health services highlights the importance of outreach intervention teams to fill gaps in mental health services by providing the services that no one else provides. The work is extremely labor intensive, often involving two or more staff members spending entire days with one individual. The teams must be flexibly designed to provide those services that a particular group or individual is missing.

The outreach team aims to build a relationship in which even the most fragile and disaffiliated homeless person may feel trust and respect. The approach should be non-threatening and respectful of the individual's place in the community, even though he or she is homeless. The initial encounter sets the tone for what the individual may continue to expect from the outreach team. Giving a homeless person a warm cup of coffee, a sandwich or piece of fruit, or an item of clothing makes the offer of assistance seem relevant and understandable. Often, the outreach team using this approach may spend months dropping off items of food or clothing for a homeless person who may say little, if anything, to them.

Although the task may appear simple and repetitive, clinicians who do this work must possess a variety of skills and have the capacity to be flexible about their roles in the team. Clinical staff may sometimes question whether food preparation or delivery is an appropriate component of their job description. Viewing the team's work at a surface level, however, means missing the complexity and dynamics of the relationship to the homeless individual (Cohen & Marcos, 1992).

Having a specific expertise derived from a limited, discipline-oriented training and perspective is inadequate to perform the many tasks facing the outreach team. The most successful approach blends diverse perspectives into a holistic systems view directed at the total person and the set of problems in need of a solution.

The powerful influence of the social ecology and institutional context within which homeless persons survive has an impact on clinical work with these populations. Gounis and Susser (1990), and Grunberg and Eagle (1990) describe the pervasiveness of demoralization among long-term shelter residents who have developed patterns of behavioral passivity and dependency like the ones so prevalent among patients of long-term stay hospitals. This phenomenon, known as "shelterization", acts as a barrier preventing mental health workers from engaging homeless persons.

Many homeless persons report that they believe the streets are safer than the predatory environment of large public shelters. A psychopathology featuring social withdrawal, apathy, and psychomotor retardation was found to be commonplace among many people who are homeless and mentally ill and who preferred life on the streets to institutional alternatives, such as shelters, group homes, long-term care facilities, and so on (Cohen et al., 1986). The presence of severe deficit symptoms and deterioration in functioning highlights the difficulty in engaging and treating this population of homeless mentally ill (Cohen & Sullivan, 1990). Even when neuroleptic medications can be given, severe isolation and withdrawal often persist, blocking the patient's engagement in therapeutic services.

CONCLUSIONS

The strategies that are employed to engage even the most difficult-to-treat homeless mentally ill persons are representative of the therapeutic flexibility necessary to extend to people with schizophrenia and severe mental illness. For those in an acute psychological crisis, going to a clinic, hospital, or emergency room may be too difficult a step. Other mentally ill persons may be chronically disaffiliated from or difficult to reach through traditional community-based services. Life in a community is far more complex and less easily controlled than life in an institution. People are free to stay away from clinic appointments, reject medications, and refuse engagement in mental health services. An engagement strategy must always be devised from the knowledge of specific aspects of a person's life in that community. Services must be flexible, "living", and responsive to the needs of high-risk patients — where they are, and when they are needed. In the vast majority of individuals with schizophrenia for whom neuroleptic medication and psychosocial interventions can significantly ameliorate symptomatology and enhance quality of life, addressing the issue of compliance with treatment is critical to the necessary task of tailoring treatment to each individual. The therapeutic alliance is strengthened by this intervention and becomes the vehicle for maintaining the treatment as a collaboration of individuals willing to overcome barriers and resistances that will arise and recur.

REFERENCES

Allan, A. T. (1988). No-shows at a community mental health clinic: A pilot study. *International Journal of Social Psychiatry, 34*, 40–46.

Amador, X. F., Strauss, D. H., Yale, S. A., & Gorman, J. M. (1991). Awareness of illness in schizophrenia. *Schizophrenia Bulletin, 17*(1), 113–132.

Appelbaum, P. S. (1982). Clinical aspects of treatment refusal [abstract]. *Proceedings of the 135th Annual Meeting of the American Psychiatric Association*. Washington, D.C., APA Press.

Atwood, N., & Beck, J. D. (1985). Service and patient predictors of continuation in clinic-based treatment. *Hospital and Community Psychiatry, 36*, 865–869.

Awad, A. G. (1993). Subjective response to neuroleptics in schizophrenia. *Schizophrenia Bulletin, 19* (3), 609–617.

Axelrod, S., & Wetzler, S. (1989). Factors associated with better compliance with psychiatric aftercare. *Hospital and Community Psychiatry, 40*(4), 397–401.

Baekeland, F., & Lundwall, L. (1975), Dropping out of treatment: A critical review. *Psychological Bulletin, 82*, 738–783.

Barofsky, I., & Bulson, R. D. (1980). *The Chronic Psychiatric Patient in the Community: Principles of Treatment*. New York: Spectrum.

Blackwell, B. (1992). Compliance. *Psychotherapy and Psychosomatic, 58*, 161–169.

Burgoyne, R. W., Acosta, F. X., & Yamamoto, J. (1983). Telephone prompting to increase attendance at a psychiatric outpatient clinic. *American Journal of Psychiatry, 140*, 345–347.

Caton, C. L. (1982). Effect of length of inpatient treatment for chronic shizophrenia. *American Journal of Psychiatry, 139*, 856–861.

Chen, A. (1991). Noncompliance in community psychiatry: A review of clinical interventions. *Hospital and Community Psychiatry, 42*(3), 282–287.

Cohen, N. L., Hardesty, A., Putnam, J., & Sullivan, A. (1986). Homeless mentally ill: Issues of clinical measurement. Paper presented at the annual meeting of the American Psychiatric Association, Washington, D.C.

Cohen, N. L., & Marcos, L. R. (1986). Psychiatric care of the homeless mentally ill. *Psychiatric Annals, 16*(12), 729–732.

Cohen, N. L. (1990). Taking psychiatric training back to the future. *Hospital and Community Psychiatry, 41*(12), 1289.

Cohen, N. L., & Sullivan, A. M. (1990). Strategies of intervention and service coordination by mobile outreach teams. In N.L. Cohen (Ed.), *Psychiatry Takes to the Streets*. New York: Guilford, pp. 63–79.

Cohen, N. L. (1992). What we must learn from the homeless mentally ill. *Hospital and Community Psychiatry, 43*(2), 101.

Cohen, N. L., & Marcos, L. R. (1992). Outreach intervention models for the homeless mentally ill. In H. R. Lamb, L. L., Bachrach, & F. I. Kass (Eds.), *Treating the Homeless Mentally Ill* (pp. 141–157). Washington, D.C.: APA.

Cohen, N. L. (1993). Stigmatization and the "noncompliant" recidivist. *Hospital and Community Psychiatry, 44*(11), 1029.

Corrigan, P. W., Lieberman, R. P., & Engel, J. D. (1990). From noncompliance to collaboration in the treatment of schizophrenia. *Hospital and Community Psychiatry, 41*(11), 1203–1211.

Craig, T. J., & Huffine, C. L. (1976). Correlates of patient attendance in an inner-city mental health clinic. *American Journal of Psychiatry, 133*, 61–65.

Draine, J., & Solomon, P. (1994). Explaining attitudes toward medication compliance among a seriously mentally ill population. *Journal of Nervous and Mental Disease, 182*(1), 50–54.

Fink, E. B., & Heckerman, C. (1981). Treatment adherence after brief hospitalization. *Comprehensive Psychiatry, 22*, 379–386.

Fischer, P. J., Drake, R. E., & Breakey, W. R. (1992). Mental health problems among homeless persons: A review of epidemiological research from 1980 to 1990. In H. R. Lamb, L. L. Bachrach, & F. I. Kass (Eds.), *Treating the Homeless Mentally Ill* (pp. 75–93). Washington, D.C.: APA.

Frank, A. F., & Gunderson, J. G. (1990). The role of the therapeutic alliance in the treatment of schizophrenia: Relationship to course and outcome. *Archives of General Psychiatry, 47*, 228–238.

Friedman, R. S. (1985). Resistance to alternatives to hospitalization. *Psychiatric Clinics of North America, 8*, 471–481.

Gounis, K., & Susser, E. (1990). Shelterization and its implications for mental health services. In N. L. Cohen (Ed.), *Psychiatry Takes to the Streets*. New York: Guilford, pp. 231–255.

Grunberg, J., & Eagle, P. F. (1990). Shelterization: How the homeless adapt to shelter living. *Hospital and Community Psychiatry, 41*, 521–525.

Heinrichs, D. W., Cohen, B. P., & Carpenter, W. T., Jr. (1985). Early insight and the management of schizophrenic decompensation. *Journal of Nervous and Mental Disease, 173*, 133–138.

Hogan, T. P., Awad, A. G., & Eastwood, R. (1983). A self-report scale predictive of drug compliance in schizophrenics: Reliability and discriminative ability. *Psychological Medicine, 13*, 177–183.

Hogarty, G. E., Anderson, C. M., & Reiss, D. J. (1986). Family psychoeducation, social skills training, and maintenance chemotherapy in the afterecare treatment of schizophrenia: One-year effects of a controlled study on relapse and expressed emotion. *Archives of General Psychiatry*, 43, 633–642.

Jellineck, M. (1978). Referrals from a psychiatric emergency room: Relationship of compliance to demographic and interview variables. *American Journal of Psychiatry*, 133, 61–65.

Kane, J. M. (1986). Prevention and treatment of neuroleptic noncompliance. *Psychiatric Annals*, 16(10), 576–579.

Kane, J., Henigfeld, G., Singer, J., & Meltzer, H. (1988). Clozapine for the treatment-resistant schizophrenic: A double-blind comparison with chlorpromazine. *Archives of General Psychiatry*, 45, 789–796.

Kluger, M. D., & Karras, A. (1983). Strategies for reducing missed appointments in a community mental health center. *Community Mental Health Journal*, 19, 137–143.

Larsen, D. L., Ngayen, T. D., & Green, R. S., (1983). Enhancing the utilization of outpatient mental health services. *Community Mental Health Journal*, 19, 305–320.

Lin, I. F., Spiga, R., & Fortsch, W. (1979). Insight and adherence to medication in chronic schizophrenics. *Journal of Clinical Psychiatry*, 40, 430–432.

Marder, S. R., Mebane, A., Chien, C., Winslade, W. J., Swann, E., & Van Putten, T. (1983). A comparison of patients who refuse and consent to neuroleptic treatment. *American Journal of Psychiatry*, 140(4), 470–472,

McEvoy, J. P., Aland, J., & Wilson, W. H. (1981). Measuring chronics schizophrenic patients' attitudes toward their illness and treatment. *Hospital and Community Psychiatry*, 32, 856–858.

McEvoy, J. P., Apperson, L. J., Appelbaum, P. S., Ortlip, P., Brecofsky, J., Hammill, K., Geller, J. L., & Roth, L. (1989). Insight in schizophrenia: Its relationship to acute psychopathology. *Journal of Nervous and Mental Disease*, 177(1), 43–47.

McEvoy, J. P., Fretner, S., Everett, G., Geller, J. L., Appelbaum, P. S., Apperson, L. J., & Roth, L. (1989). Insight and the clinical outcome of schizophrenic patients. *Journal of Nervous and Mental Disease*, 177, 48–51.

Mirabi, M., Weinman, M. D., & Magnetti, S. M. (1978). Professiosnal attitudes toward the chronic mentally ill. *Hospital and Community Psychiatry*, 36, 404–405.

Soskis, D. A. (1978). Schizophrenia and medical inpatients as informed drug consumers. *Archives of General Psychiatry*, 35, 645–649.

Strauss, J. S. (1989). Subjective experiences of schizophrenia: Toward a new dynamic psychiatry. *Schizophrenia Bulletin*, 15, 178–179.

Stoudemire, A., & Thompson, T. L. (1983). Medication noncompliance: Systemic approaches to evaluation and intervention. *General Hospital Psychiatry*, 5, 233–239.

Swett, J., & Noones, J. (1989). Factors associated with premature termination from out-patient treatment. *Hospital and Community Psychiatry*, 40, 947–951.

Talbott, J. A., Bachrach, L. L., & Ross, L. (1986). Noncompliance and mental health systems. *Psychiatric Annals*, 16(10), 596–599.

Talbott, J. A. (1987). The chronic mentally ill: What do we know and why aren't we implementing what we know? In W. W. Menninger, & G. T. Hannah (Eds), *The Chronic Mental Patient*. Washington, D.C.: APA.

Van Putten, T. (1978). Drug refusal in schizophrenia: Causes and prescribing hints. *Hospital and Community Psychiatry, 29*, 110–112.

Van Putten, T., May, P. R., & Marder, S. R. (1984). Response to antipsychotic medication: The doctor's and the consumer's view. *American Journal of Psychiatry, 141*(1), 16–19.

Weiden, P. J., Shaw, E., & Mann, J. J. (1986). Causes of neuroleptic noncompliance. *Psychiatric Annals, 16*(10), 571–575.

Zito, J. M., Routt, W. W., Mitchell, J. E., & Roerig, J. L. (1985). Clinical characteristics of hospitalized psychotic patients who require antipsychotic drug therapy. *American Journal of Psychiatry, 142*(7), 822–826.

17

Lithium Compliance in Manic-Depressive Illness[1]

KAY REDFIELD JAMISON

Many patients with affective illness seem to have little or no difficulty in taking potent daily medications for an indeterminate period. They do not appear to be unduly concerned about potential or actual side effects, nor do they seem to struggle with the existential issues that might reasonably be raised when a person is required to take powerful mind- and mood-altering drugs. Because of temperament or past experience, they do not protest or ignore their physicians' recommendations but often are grateful for the medications and thank the doctors who prescribe them. Often such patients state that lithium or antidepressants have rescued them from chaos, despair, debilitating hospitalization, or suicide. Compliant patients are an interesting, although inadequately studied, group. Certainly they are a source of gratification to their physicians. For every patient who follows the treatment course, however, there is at least one who does not — one who resists, protests, objects, takes too little, takes too much, or takes none at all. Clearly, this behavior negates the therapeutic efficacy of lithium.

We focus on lithium for several reasons: (1) The consequences of lithium noncompliance[1] are profound and can be life-threatening. (2) Lithium often is prescribed on an exceptionally long-term or lifelong basis. (3) Lithium noncompliance is a frustrating, common, and perplexing clinical problem. (4) Poor lithium compliance is almost certainly the single most important factor in poor treatment response. (5) Essentially no compliance research has been carried out on carbamazepine (Lenzi et al., 1989) or sodium valproate.

The consequences of noncompliance are clinically equivalent to those of untreated or inadequately treated manic-depressive illness: recurrence and intensification of affective episodes that are often accompanied by interpersonal chaos, alcohol and drug abuse, personal anguish and family disruption, financial crises, conjugal failure, psychiatric hospitalization, suicide, and violence. This point may be obvious, but it is frequently ignored. Unlike unresponsiveness, however, noncompliance is reversible and can usually be changed through experience, education, learning, and psychotherapy.

In addition to the costs in human suffering brought about by noncompliance, the potential economic costs to society are staggering. Reifman and Wyatt (1980) estimated that the use of lithium in the decade between 1969 and 1979 saved the United States $4 billion through reductions in medical costs and restoration of productivity. A recent updating of these figures, in 1989 dollars, suggests a saving of more than $40 billion from 1969 to 1989 (Wyatt, personal communication). Noncompliance substantially undermines potential economic gains. From a practical point of view, the development of effective techniques to deal with lithium non-compliance has major implications for insurance companies and health maintenance organizations.

Another consequence of lithium noncompliance is the probable bias of research findings in clinical studies related to lithium. Frank and colleagues (1985) stressed that investigators "have an obligation to account for nonadherent patients in their analyses" (p. 42) by specifying how many and which patients fail to comply (patient, history of illness, and therapist variables). Data should be analyzed with and without end-point analysis techniques.

In this chapter, we approach the discussion from the perspective of the clinician, by first detailing strategies for dealing with lithium noncompliance. In the second section, we review research findings from anecdotal and systematic observations (rates, correlates, and results of interventions).

CLINICAL MANAGEMENT

Patient Factors

Risk factors for lithium noncompliance, summarized from studies reviewed later, are presented in Table 17.1. Generally, compliance appears to increase with age, which coincides with a period of increasing risk of episodes recurring. The first year after the initiation of lithium treatment is a particularly high-risk period of stopping lithium against medical advice. A constellation of related mood variables seem to predict noncompliance: missing the highs, elevated mood in its own right, and a history of grandiose delusions. There is some evidence that patients experiencing proportionately more manic than depressive episodes are more likely to be noncompliant.

Table 17.1. Risk Factors for Lithium Noncompliance[a]

- First year of lithium treatment
- History of noncompliance
- Younger
- Male
- Fewer episodes
- History of grandiose, euphoric manias
- Elevated mood
- Complaints of "missing highs"

[a]Summary based on studies of both bipolar and unipolar patients.

Medication Factors

Patients report that weight gain, cognitive impairment, tremor, increased thirst, and lethargy are their major reasons for stopping lithium. They mention gastric irritation, nausea, vomiting, and diarrhea less often. The frequency of these side effects and their importance in noncompliance are reviewed later in the chapter. The effects of lithium on personality are also relevant to compliance, since some patients become less sociable, outgoing, active, and elated while taking the drug.

Conceivably, some of the lethargy and memory difficulties attributed to lithium actually may be symptoms of the unrecognized, atypical, retarded depressive relapses that lithium sometimes fails to prevent. Along with cognitive problems and hopelessness secondary to the depression, lethargy and cognitive difficulties caused by lithium can increase the likelihood of medication noncompliance. Concomitant chronic use of antidepressants sometimes increases episode frequency. Discouraged by the episodes, patients may stop taking lithium, or they may fail to recognize these mini-episodes and ascribe the accompanying emotional blunting to lithium.

The similarity of lithium-induced changes in cognitive functioning and energy levels to the symptoms of affective illness may cause the opposite problem as well. Some complaints from patients are mistakenly attributed entirely to breakthrough depressions or other manifestations of illness. Although difficult to differentiate clinically, in research settings cognitive side effects of lithium have been observed in normal subjects, as well as in patients with affective disorders.

Misunderstandings about lithium can arise between patients and physicians because psychiatrists tend to stress the medical side effects of lithium (e.g., thyroid and renal effects, polyuria, tremor). This emphasis may stem from early studies when clinical investigators were very concerned about the long-term somatic effects of lithium but paid relatively little attention to side effects that many patients find more distressing, such as weight gain, decreased energy, slowing of cognition, decreased memory and concentration, and diminished enthusiasm.

Even though some cognitive effects may be unavoidable and untreatable, they must be taken seriously and corrected to the extent possible. In some instances, lithium-induced hypothyroidism may be responsible for decreased energy and slowed intellectual functioning. This condition can be treated easily. In other cases, when too little lithium leads to breakthrough depressions or too much lithium leads to mild neurotoxicity, subtle titration of the dosage or adjunctive treatment with anticonvulsant medications can improve the problem substantially.

Special reinforcement schedules intrinsic to lithium treatment force clinicians to contend with a singularly difficult set of problems:

- Lithium (unlike analgesics, neuroleptics, or benzodiazepines) has delayed therapeutic actions: 5 to 7 days for an antimanic effect, usually 3 to 5 weeks for an antidepressant effect.

- Lithium has no known intrinsic reinforcing qualities, either immediate or delayed.

- Patients are expected to stay on the drug for an indeterminate time, much of it in a more or less normal state, with no immediate felt need for the drug.

- If a patient stops the medication, the negative consequences of noncompliance (recurrences of the affective illness) are often long-delayed (there is no immediate negative reinforcer).

- The onset of lithium treatment often is paired with unpleasant events (psychosis, hospitalization, family problems).

- If lithium is first prescribed for a manic episode, the natural history of the illness predicts that the patient is at significant risk for a postmanic depression, which further pairs the onset of lithium treatment with unpleasant psychological and physical experiences.

- The cessation of lithium is often accompanied by relatively immediate positive experiences, either because of the disappearance of side effects or because of breakthrough hypomania (often a contributing factor in lithium non-compliance in the first place).

Treatment Issues

Guidelines for maximizing lithium compliance are summarized in Table 17.2. Sackett and associates (1985) emphasize the "uniformly dismal performance of clinicians" in predicting and assessing compliance in their patients. They found that detecting which patients are noncompliant could be done more quickly, less expensively, and

Table 17.2. Guidelines for Maximizing Lithium Compliance

Monitor compliance
   Regular lithium levels
   Inquire frequently
   Encourage queries and concerns from patients and families

Side effects
   Forewarn
   Treat aggressively (especially hypothyroidism and tremor)
   Minimize lithium level

Education
   Early symptoms of mania and depression
   Unremitting and worsening course of (untreated)
      manic-depressive illness

Medication
   Minimize number of daily doses
   Pillboxes (7 day), especially if on two or more medications
   Involve family members in administering, if appropriate
   Written information about lithium and side effects
   (Limited) patient-titration of lithium level

Adjunctive psychotherapy

Self-help groups

about as well simply by asking patients about taking their medications as by using drug levels. To increase the reliability of patients' responses, they suggest an interview format that makes the admission of noncompliance socially acceptable; for example, "Most people have trouble taking all of their pills. Do you have any trouble taking all of yours?" The physician should order lithium level determinations regularly and inquire frequently about possible problems with compliance and concerns about the medication.

Also critical are the attitudes toward lithium of all physicians and psychotherapists involved in patient care. In general, clinicians who are ambivalent about the role of biological factors in the causation and treatment of affective disorders tend to convey their ambivalence to their patients and possibly contribute to unsatisfactory compliance. Findings from a study by Cochran and Gitlin (1988) underscore the importance of the role of the patient's psychiatrist in ensuring compliance. The results of their study suggest that the more strongly the psychiatrist believes in the treatment regimen, the more likely the patient is to comply. The problem is further compounded by the antagonism toward lithium and other psychoactive medications on the part of some mental health workers, who may subtly or overtly sabotage drug compliance. In contrast, clinicians with an extreme biological bias may oversell lithium and thereby pave the way to patient disillusionment when minor relapses occur, or they may underestimate the role of psychological factors in the illness and its treatment and overlook subjective symptoms, like emotional dulling or memory disturbance, that many patients find extremely troublesome. The evidence from studies in general medical settings and lithium clinics suggests that physicians may inadvertently contribute to lithium noncompliance by failing to educate the patient and family. A clear understanding of manic-depressive disease, its course without treatment, and the role of lithium in attenuating this course (Frank et al., 1985) can enhance compliance.

Psychotherapy is important in the treatment of patients with illness, specifically in encouraging lithium compliance. Patients taking lithium tend to place a far greater value on adjunctive psychotherapy than do clinicians, and noncompliant patients have been shown to regard psychotherapy as highly useful in helping them adhere to a regimen of lithium treatment (Jamison et al., 1979). Consistent with these observations are findings that show that patients treated with cognitive therapy more often took their lithium as prescribed than did patients who did not receive psychotherapy (Cochran, 1982). Because of their compliance, the psychotherapy patients also had fewer affective episodes and fewer hospitalizations. Self-help groups, such as those organized by the National Depressive and Manic-Depressive Association, are beneficial to many patients and their families.

REVIEW OF THE LITERATURE

Rates of Lithium Noncompliance

Of the more than 10,000 articles written about lithium, fewer than 50 deal in a substantive way with noncompliance. This lack of research is extraordinary, given the extent of the problem. There is little information about how many patients stop taking lithium against medical advice, for what reasons they stop, for how long, at what point in their therapeutic regimen or mood cycles, and whether there are sex and age differences in reasons for noncompliance or incomplete compliance. Little systematic research has been done on patients' perceptions of the positive and negative consequences of taking the drug, regularly, and the effect of these perceptions on actual patterns of lithium use.

Rates of lithium noncompliance, summarized in Table 17.3, range from 18 to 53 percent. These rates, although high and of concern, are lower than those cited for patients given tricyclic antidepressants alone, 32 to 76 percent, although tricyclic noncompliance rates are considerably lower, ranging from 10 to 47 percent, when the medications are used in combination with psychotherapy (Park and Lipman, 1964; Pugh, 1963; Jacob et al., 1984; Frank et al., 1985; Overall et al., 1987). Drop-out rates for carbamazepine range from 31 to 50 percent (Fawcett and Kravitz, 1985; Placidi et al., 1986; Luznat et al., 1988).

Table 17.3. Rates of Lithium Noncompliance

Study	%
Angst et al., 1970	18[a]
Van Putten, 1975	20–30
Bech et al., 1976	24
Jamison et al., 1979	47[b]
Connelly et al., 1982	25
Cochran, 1982	52
Vestergaard & Amdisen, 1983	23[a]
Jamison et al., unpublished	28[b]
Frank et al., 1985	
Danion et al., 1987	53
Maarbjerg et al., 1988	23[a]
Lenzi et al., 1989	51[c]

[a]Within the first 6 months of treatment
[b]Differences in the socioeconomic status (SES) of the patients probably account for the differences in the two Jamison et al. studies (more noncompliance among lower SES patients)
[c]Compared with 38% of those patients taking carbamazepine

Clinical Reports of lithium Noncompliance

The first reported instance of lithium noncompliance in a manic-depressive patient was the first patient treated with the drug. After recounting the initial dramatic success of lithium, Cade, years later, described the subsequent course:

> It was with a sense of the most abject disappointment that I readmitted him to hospital 6 months later as manic as ever but took some consolation from his brother who informed me that Bill had become over confident about having been well for so many months, had become lackadaisical about taking his medication and finally ceased taking it about 6 weeks before. (1978, p. 13)

Several anecdotal reports of lithium noncompliance have been published, along with proposed explanations. Polatin and Fieve (1971) emphasized that a patient often attributes decreases in creativity and productivity to lithium. They also stressed the role of denial in chronic, serious illnesses. Fitzgerald (1972) speculated that refusal to take lithium stemmed from intolerance of reality-based depressions, preference for a hypomanic way of life, or provocation from a spouse or other family member who also missed the patient's hypomanic episodes. Van Putten (1975), in addition to stressing the preference for hypomania, saw the importance of side effects and lithium-induced dysphoria, characterized by a driveless, anhedonic condition. Like Schou and colleagues (1970), he suggested that depressive relapses, as well as a tendency to feel well and to see no further need for medication, were significant variables in lithium refusal. Grof and associates (1970) found that the majority of their patients who stopped lithium had been free of relapse and felt no need to continue. Schou and Baastrup (1973) cited several reasons for lithium noncompliance: decreased energy, enthusiasm, or sexuality, increased marital difficulties, and a common perception that life was flatter and less colorful than before lithium treatment. Some of these complaints no doubt result from direct effects of lithium on the illness, and some are due to side effects. Kerry (1978) suggested that the social stigma associated with manic-depressive psychosis may lead to rejection of lithium, the most concrete symbol of the illness.

Cochran (1982) found that patient concerns clustered around the following issues:

• Personal control: frustrations with the "medical model," which they perceived as more focused on symptoms than personal gains, and insufficient emphasis on the establishment of alternative means of control, such as changes in diet or reduction in stress

• Changes in life brought about by successful lithium treatment: missing of highs, impact of stabilization on relationships

• Lack of predictability in the course of the illness, possible breakthrough episodes, and length of time on lithium and discomfort about having to be passive in light of possible impending episodes

• Issues concerning lithium, such as safety, mechanism of action, side effects, and efficacy

Cochran noted that, during treatment of noncompliance, patients often followed a pattern in their ability and willingness to articulate their attitudes toward lithium. Initially, they discussed their appreciation of lithium and expressed little ambivalence. By the third session, however, patients frequently spoke of massive ambivalence about lithium and considerable concern about future compliance. Miklowitz and colleagues (1986) found that:

> Medication compliance was not by itself significantly associated with illness course in this sample, but did tend to mediate the relations between family factors and 9-month clinical outcome. Specifically, when the family environment to which the patient returned following hospitalization was negative, patients were at high risk for a poor clinical outcome regardless of whether they were medically compliant. However, a neutral or benign family environment was associated with a good clinical outcome only when the patient consistently adhered to his/her medication regimen. (p. 631)

Data-Based Studies of lithium Noncompliance

UCLA STUDIES

In a more systematic exploration of the clinical reports described previously, Jamison and colleagues (1979) pursued two obvious sources of information and experience: the attitudes of patients themselves (47 lithium patients from the Affective Disorders Clinic at the University of California, Los Angeles) and, independently, the attitudes of clinicians experienced in the use of lithium (50 physicians, each of whom had treated at least 50 patients with lithium). Nearly one half of the patients reported having stopped taking lithium at some time against medical advice, and 34 percent of those said that they stopped more than once. Of those who reported that they had not stopped, more than 90 percent stated that they had never considered doing so. These findings raised the possibility that patient practices in medication compliance tend to divide into two distinct subgroups. (The pattern of full compliance may be fundamentally different from the three other patterns of late compliance, intermittent compliance, and complete noncompliance.)

Demographic Findings. In the UCLA study, no significant differences were found in sex, age, education, or income between the 22 patients who reported that they discontinued lithium treatment against medical advice and the 25 who continued. Patients with a history of mania (bipolar I) tended to be less compliant than those with a history of hypomania (bipolar II). The number of months on lithium was the only variable that differentiated significantly between the groups. More patients reported discontinuing lithium during long-term treatment. This finding may simply reflect the effect of increasing the period at risk for noncompliance.

Perceived Effectiveness of Lithium. Both groups of patients reported lithium to be highly effective in preventing recurrences of mania and effective, although somewhat less so, in preventing recurrent depressions. Ninety-six percent of the clinicians and 73 percent of the patients found lithium an extremely or very effective treatment for mania. More patients (40 percent) than clinicians (24 percent), however, regarded lithium as an effective treatment for depression. No significant relationship existed between perceived effectiveness and reported compliance.

Motivation for Continuing Lithium Treatment. Both the compliant and noncompliant patient groups indicated that fear of depression was a stronger reason for staying on lithium than fear of mania. The clinicians concurred in this perception.

Perceived Importance of Psychotherapy. Fifty percent of the patients considered psychotherapy to be "very important" in lithium compliance, but only 27 percent of the clinicians, most of whom were practicing psychotherapists. This finding may suggest a tendency among clinicians to value the potency of an effective medication so highly that they underestimate the psychological aspects of the illness and their impact on medication compliance. Nevertheless, over half the clinicians indicated that they almost always encouraged patients to seek adjunctive psychotherapy.

Side Effects of Lithium. Clinicians rated side effects as more important in noncompliance than did patients who reported discontinuing lithium therapy. Both patients and clinicians viewed lethargy, impairment in coordination, and lithium-induced tremor as important in noncompliance. Patients regarded dulling of senses as equally important, whereas clinicians emphasized weight gain. Three of the four side effects most important to clinicians (tremor, weight gain, and nauseas and vomiting) are all relatively somatic in nature, perhaps reflecting a tendency for patients to mention physical rather than cognitive changes. Conversely, clinicians may be reluctant to acknowledge substantial cognitive changes, or perhaps they view such changes as manifestations of affective episodes (as indeed they can be) rather than of medication. Female patients regarded lethargy and dulling of senses as significantly more problematic, which may reflect the often unrecognized lithium-induced hypothyroidism more often present in women than in men.

Psychodynamic Issues. Nearly two thirds of physicians thought that lithium noncompliance was "somewhat" or "very" related to patients acting out their denial of a serious lifelong illness. Other physicians believed that noncomplying patients were acting out psychodynamic factors in therapy. A few thought that anger at the therapist or at a significant other was also an important reason for a patient stopping lithium against medical advice.

General Reasons for Noncompliance. Table 17.4 lists in order of importance the reasons for noncompliance cited by the entire patient

Table 17.4. Rank Orders of General Reasons for
Noncompliance: UCLA Study

Rank Order	Total Patient Sample (N = 47)	Patients Who Reported Discontinuing Lithium Treatment (N = 22)	Independent Clinician Sample (N = 50)
1	Bothered by idea that moods are controlled by medication	Bothered by idea that moods are controlled medication	Felt well, saw no need for lithium
2	Felt depressed	Missed highs[a]	Missed highs
3	Bothered by idea of chronic illness	Felt depressed	Bothered by idea of chronic illness
4	Felt less attractive to spouse	Bothered by idea of chronic illness	Felt less creative
5	Felt well, saw no need for lithium	Felt well, saw no need for lithium	Felt less productive
6	Hassle to take medications[a]	Hassle to take medications[a]	Bothered by idea that moods are controlled medication
7	Missed highs	Felt less attractive to friends	Hassle to take medication
8	Felt less creative	Felt less creative	Felt less attractive to friends
9	Felt less productive	Felt less productive	Felt depressed
10	Felt less attractive to friends	Felt less attractive to spouse	Felt less attractive to spouse

[a]$P < 0.05$. Patients who actually discontinued lithium rated these reasons significantly more important than did patients who did not stop lithium.

From Jamison et al., 1979

sample, by the group that had reported noncompliance, and by the clinicians. (When patients reported that they had always complied, they were asked to give reasons that might cause them not to comply). From the patients' perspective, the four most important reasons for noncompliance were:

- A dislike of medication controlling their moods
- A dislike of the idea of having a chronic illness, symbolized by the necessity for lithium therapy
- Feeling depressed
- Side effects, particularly lethargy, decreased coordination, and dulling of senses

Patient and clinician perceptions seldom disagreed, but when they did, they were significant. Patients were much more bothered than clinicians believed them to be by their moods being controlled by medication. Those patients who reported discontinuing lithium were more likely to report missing highs and the hassle of taking medications. On the other hand, patients generally perceived that a decrease in productivity, creativity, and attractiveness to spouse or friends was not that important. This finding contrasts with prevailing notions about reasons for noncompliance, and it suggests that many patients do not necessarily equate highs with creativity or productivity. From the clinicians' point of view, the three most important reasons for lithium noncompliance were:

- The patient felt well and saw no need to continue the medication
- The patient missed the highs of hypomania
- The patient was bothered by the idea of having a chronic illness

Although men and women in this sample showed no overall significant differences in reasons for noncompliance, the women were more likely to stress "missing highs" and "bothered by the idea of moods being controlled by medication". It may be that women perceive more desirable benefits from their highs because they show more extensive changes from baseline experience in such areas as sexuality, energy, and productivity. Some corroborating evidence for this hypothesis has been presented (Jamison et al., 1980). Furthermore, women may be accustomed to accepting extremes of moods and emotions as within the bounds of normal feminine and culturally sanctioned experience; consequently, they may be upset by the idea of external control. As a result of the natural history of bipolar illness, women may also experience more frequent mini-episodes, leading to further accommodation of mood swings, if not actual acceptance and learned modulation.

Men, on the other hand, may regard fluctuating moods as aberrant and, therefore, legitimately subject to external or medical control. Although not systematically studied, the legal and financial sequelae of affective episodes may be more extensive for men than for women. Differences in cultural expectations and the phenomenology of the illness may partially account for this attitude among men, as may their higher ratio of mania/depressive episodes, more aggressive and destructive behavior when manic, and greater physical strength.

UCLA-COLUMBIA STUDY

Jamison and colleagues, in an unpublished study, extensively examined 71 manic-depressive patients from two very different geographic, social, and economic settings. One group of 31 patients came from an affluent private practice, and the other group of 40 came from a public university clinic.

Despite significant geographic and socioeconomic differences in the results, overall the two groups were impressively similar. In the discussion that follows, data from patients in both samples were combined.

Overview of Findings. Two patient variables were significantly related to lithium compliance. Older patients were more compliant ($p < 0.05$), and women were far more compliant than men ($p < 0.007$). There was no significant relationship between compliance and IQ, ethnicity, marital status, income, or religious background.

The 1979 UCLA study did not examine the relationship between illness variables and lithium compliance. The UCLA-Columbia study found that the number of both depressive ($p < 0.05$) and manic ($p < 0.05$) episodes was significantly related to compliance. The more affective episodes a patient had, the more likely he or she was to report compliance, even though more episodes also meant more time had passed in which the patient could have been noncompliant. Almost certainly, this finding reflects an early high-risk period for noncompliance and a tendency to have to experience one or more recurrences of illness before the initial denial alters appreciably. The study showed no relationship between compliance and polarity of the first episode, type of mania or hypomania (euphoric, dysphoric, mixed), or the extent of perceived positive aspects of hypomania. Unlike the earlier study, there were no differences in the rates of compliance between patients with bipolar-I and bipolar-II disorders.

Attitudes toward treatment also differed. Compared with compliant patients, those who were not more often reported feeling that psychotherapy was important in complying with a lithium treatment schedule ($p < 0.02$). Noncompliant patients were more likely to say they stopped lithium because they felt well ($p < 0.01$). Far more than compliant patients, they perceived taking lithium as a hassle ($p < 0.02$). On a semantic differential test of attitudes toward lithium, antidepressants, and psychotherapy, there were no significant differences. There also were no differences in the experience of lithium side effects.

The following psychological measures revealed no significant differences between the compliant and noncompliant groups: Beck Depression Inventory, Manic-Depressive Scale, Eysenck Personality Inventory, Breskin Rigidity Test, Aesthetic Preference Scale,

Sensation-Seeking Scale, Internal-External Locus of Control, and the Jenkins Activity Survey, a measure of Type A or potentially cardiac-prone behavior.

Side Effects. The earlier UCLA study neglected to include memory problems in the listing of lithium side effects, reflecting the fact that cognitive effects were seldom mentioned in the lithium literature at that time. Because patients complained of memory problems, however, the UCLA-Columbia study included them. Patients said these problems were the most important reason for stopping lithium against medical advice. Fully one third found memory problems very important in noncompliance, compared with only 18 percent who believed polyuria to be a significant contributor. Ironically, polyuria is probably the most studied of the lithium side effects and changes in cognitive functioning one of the least. Weight gain and problems with coordination and tremor were also cited as very important in noncompliance.

General Reasons for Noncompliance. Table 17.5 outlines several reasons for lithium noncompliance in the UCLA-Columbia study. Patients who had stopped taking lithium were asked why, and those who had not stopped were asked what might make them do so. The results vary somewhat from the earlier UCLA study, which did not frame questions about side effects in the same way as did the UCLA-Columbia study (where they were given as the most important reason for stopping lithium against medical advice). The perception of decreased creativity ranked as a more important side effect in the

Table 17.5. Rank Orders of Reasons for Lithium Noncompliance: UCLA-Columbia Study[a]

Rank Order	Reasons for Noncompliance (N-71)
1	Side effects[a]
2	Indefinite intake/chronicity of illness
3	Less creative
4[b,c]	Felt well, saw no need to take lithium
5	Less productive
6	Missed highs
7	Less interesting to spouse
8	Disliked idea of moods being controlled by medication
9[d]	Hassle to remember to take medication
10	Felt depressed, thought mood would improve

[a]See Table 17.8 for rank ordering of the importance of individual side effects in noncompliance
[b]Males > females, $p < .05$
[c]Those who stopped lithium > those who did not, $p < .01$
[d]Those who stopped lithium > those who did not, $p < .02$

From Jamison et al., unpublished

UCLA-Columbia study, perhaps reflecting a greater proportion of professional and creative individuals in the New York private practice group. Dislike of being on medication ranked as less important than in the earlier investigation, again perhaps because of the different nature of the patient populations. Differences in social attitudes toward mood disorders over the past several years also may have had an effect.

OTHER STUDIES

Several other studies that have examined correlates of lithium compliance are summarized in Table 17.6.

Demographic Variables. A variety of compliance measures has been used across a range of clinical settings and predictive variables. Few demographic variables (age, sex, income, education) predict lithium compliance consistently, an observation in line with results of medication compliance studies in general. Among the exceptions to this rule are the findings that being married was associated with better compliance (Connelly et al., 1982), that women were much more likely than men to be compliant (Jamison et al., unpublished data), and that compliance increases with age (Frank et al., 1985; Jamison et al., unpublished data). The last factor coincides with a greater risk period of affective recurrences. The UCLA-Columbia study also found that better compliance was associated with a larger number of affective episodes requiring treatment. Thus, increasing compliance may be secondary to decreasing denial as the illness continues to recur. A related possibility is that it reflects the fact that the severity of consequences ultimately leads to better compliance.

Relative Proportion of Manic to Depressive Episodes and Other Illness Factors. A pattern evolves for the one consistent illness predictor, a constellation of elevated mood variables. Jamison and colleagues (1979) found that "missing of highs" was one of the few factors significantly differentiating compliant from noncompliant patients. Connelly and colleagues (1982) reported that noncompliance was associated with elevated mood, although the direction of causality was not specified, and Lenzi and associates (1989) found that grandiosity was significantly associated with noncompliance. Rosen and Mukherjee (unpublished data) found that noncompliance was associated with a history of grandiose delusions. Although grandiosity predicts a good acute response to lithium, they hypothesized that:

> The presence of grandiose delusions increases the probability of both an acute response to lithium carbonate in the manic phase and rapid drop-out from lithium prophylaxis thereafter ... personality factors (denial of dependency, etc.) which are expressed as grandiosity in the acute manic phase of the illness also operate to promote discontinuance of medication in the prophylactic period of treatment.

This condition is borne out by a study in bipolar-I disorder that showed lithium compliance to be less likely in those who experienced recurrent manic episodes (without evidence for clinical depression)

Table 17.6. Correlates of Lithium Compliance: Data-Based Studies

Study	Patient N	Measures of Compliance	Correlates of Lithium Compliance	Factors Unrelated to Compliance
Jamison et. al., 1979	47 (38 BP)	Patient self-report	Noncompliant patients significantly more likely to miss "highs" ($p < .05$) or regard medication as a "hassle" ($p < .05$)	Age, sex, education, income, BPI vs BPII[a], side effects
Cochran, 1982	26 BP	Blind judge examining self-report data, physician ratings, reports from significant others, lab values, chart notations	None	Age, sex, education. Found compliance was a better predictor of attitudes than attitudes were of compliance
Connelly et al., 1982	48 (40 BP)	Lithium level 0.5–1.5 mEq/1; Attendance at 75% or more clinic appointment for 9 months	Noncompliance associated with elevated mood ($p < 01$). Compliance associated with men ($p < .01$) and a perception of the continuity of care ($p < .05$)	Education, age, diagnostic sub-categories, side effects, Health Belief Model Score
Frank et al., 1985	216 BP	Not specified	Compliance associated with increasing age ($p < .05$), being married ($p < .05$), higher education ($p < .05$), history of good compliance ($p < .002$)	Previous interepisode functioning, duration of previous episodes, age at first onset, number of previous episodes

Table 17.6. Correlates of Lithium Compliance: Data-Based Studies

Study	Patient N	Measures of Compliance	Correlates of Lithium Compliance	Factors Unrelated to Compliance
Danion et al., 1987	73 (36 BP)	Lithium level below 0.5 and above 1.0; psychiatrist estimate of compliance	Noncompliance associated with low intellectual level, cognitive deficit, affective relapses, personality disorders	Age, sex, polarity, severity, duration, side effects
Maarbjerg et al., 1988	133 (61 BP)	Patient considered non-compliant if not taking lithium six months after start of treatment	Noncompliance associated with early onset of illness, large number of previous hospital admissions, personality disorder, substance abuse	Diagnostic subgroup
Lenzi et al., 1989	67[b] (53 BP)	Lithium and carbamazepine plasma levels	Compliance associated with social support, unpleasant psychotic experiences, treatment for depressive episode. Noncompliance associated with treatment for mania, grandiosity and hypochondriacal concerns	Diagnostic subgroup, nature of medication side-effects

Table 17.6. Correlates of Lithium Compliance: Data-Based Studies

Study	Patient N	Measures of Compliance	Correlates of Lithium Compliance	Factors Unrelated to Compliance
Rosen & Mukherjee, unpublished	56	Number of months on lithium	Noncompliance associated with history of grandiose delusions ($p < .001$). Compliance associated with increasing age ($p < .05$), history of ECT ($p < .001$), history of state hospitalization ($p < .05$), symptomatic decreased need for sleep ($p < .05$)	Family history, diagnosis, frequency of previous episodes
Jamison et al., unpublished	71 BP	Patient self-reports, physician ratings	Compliance associated with increasing age ($p < .05$), females ($p < .01$), number of depressive episodes requiring treatment ($p < .05$), number of manic episodes ($p < .05$), higher occupational status ($p < .02$) Noncompliance associated with more positive experiences when manic (for women, $p < .05$)	Ethnicity, marital status, income, religious back-ground, polarity of first episode, type of mania or hypomania, degree of positive experience associated with hypomania, BPI vs BPII, side effects, attitudes toward treatments, Beck Depression Inventory, Eysenck Personality Inventory, BRT, Aesthetic Preferences, Sensation Seeking, Internal-External Locus of Control, Jenkins Activity Survey

[a]Although there was a tendency for BPI patients to be less compliant.
[b]35 patients on lithium, 32 patients on carbamazepine, all female.

than in those who experienced both disabling depressive and manic episodes (Lenzi et al., 1989). Other illness factors, such as polarity of episodes, severity, family history, diagnostic subtype, and frequency of affective episodes are not clearly related to compliance.

Subjective Complaints and Lithium Compliance

> The subjective experience was primarily one of indifference and slight general malaise. This led to a certain passivity. The subjects often had a feeling of being at a distance from their environment, as if separated from it by a glass wall. The subjective feeling of having been altered by the treatment was disproportionately strong in relation to objective behavioral changes. The subjects could engage in discussions and social activities but found it difficult to comprehend and integrate more than a few elements of a situation. Intellectual initiative was diminished and there was a feeling of lowered ability to concentrate and memorize; but thought processes were unaffected, and the subjects could think logically and produce ideas. —Mogens Schou[2]

In this section, data on frequently reported subjective complaints associated with lithium treatment are presented. Conceptual and methodological problems are common in the literature of lithium side effects, where important variables are often unspecified, unclear, or uncontrolled, for example, serum lithium level, duration of lithium treatment, use of other medications or nonprescription drugs, diagnosis, age, and gender. The degree and type of inquiry into side effects (spontaneous report, checklists, scaled measures of frequency and severity) vary enormously from study to study, and control subjects rarely are included in the design. Prelithium profiles of side effects (a baseline before lithium) are seldom obtained, making the subsequent interpretations of lithium side effects difficult. Differentiating the simple presence or absence of a side effect from its severity or relationship to noncompliance is even less common.

Several authors stress the worrisome problem of distinguishing lithium side effects from the symptoms of the underlying affective disorder.[3] Abou-Saleh and Coppen (1983) found, for example, that drug-free depressed patients reported more side effects than both control subjects and lithium-treated patients and that subjective side effects reported by lithium-treated patients were related to their affective symptoms and personality variables. Lyskowski and colleagues (1982), on the other hand, found that the presence of noneuthymic mood was not associated with changes in the incidence of side effects.

The rates of the most frequently reported lithium side effects are presented in Table 17.7. In the 12 reviewed studies, 35 to 93 percent of the lithium-treated patients reported subjective complaints from their medication. The pooled percentage, based on a total of 1,035 patients, is 74 percent. Lyskowski and coworkers (1982), in a longitudinal study of 67 patients, found that 7 percent were free from all side effects, 63 percent had only mild complaints, and 30 percent reported persistent moderate or severe side effects (especially polyuria and thirst). The persistent side effects were not related to age, age at onset of illness, severity of illness, or duration of lithium treatment.

SOMATIC EFFECTS OF LITHIUM

In our review, slightly more than a third of patients (36 percent) complained of excessive thirst, the most commonly reported lithium side effect. Polyuria (30 percent) and tremor (27 percent) were the next most frequent somatic complaints, followed by weight gain (19 percent), drowsiness/lethargy (12 percent), and diarrhea (9 percent). When asked the importance of a given side effect in stopping lithium, patients showed a different pattern (Table 17.8). Of the somatic side effects, they perceived weight gain and problems with coordination and tremor as the most likely to lead to noncompliance, followed by polyuria, tiredness/lethargy, dulling of senses, blurred vision, and nausea and vomiting.

The difference between acknowledging the presence of a side effect and perceiving it as troubling and likely to lead to noncompliance is further underscored by the findings of Gitlin, Cochran, and Jamison (1989). They asked 49 patients with bipolar disorder to indicate whether they had experienced various side effects while on lithium. The five most frequently cited side effects were thirst, excessive urination, weight gain, dry mouth, and fatigue. When asked which side effects were actually most bothersome a significantly different list emerged: weight gain, mental confusion, poor concentration, mental slowness, and memory problems. Four of the five most bothersome lithium side effects were cognitive.

COGNITIVE EFFECTS OF LITHIUM

Disturbance of memory was the most important "late" side effect observed in our patients, not on account of its frequency but because it was very troublesome. Contrary to the other side-effects of lithium which were usually not reported by the patients unless the therapists asked specifically about them, memory dysfunction was an inconvenience patients did complain about. This symptom was not associated with a mild depressive phase, as one might hypothesize, since all patients who complained of memory reduction were clearly normothymic and were only receiving lithium prophylactically. (p. 263) —Christodoulou et al., 1977

In the review of studies summarized in Table 17.7, memory problems were the third most frequently cited side effect (28 percent of patients). In one study, fully one third of patients reported that memory problems were very important in their decisions to stop lithium against medical advice (Jamison et al., unpublished data). Memory problems were more important than any other side effects in noncompliance (Table 17.8).

Table 17.7. Lithium Side Effects: Percentage of Patients with Subjective Complaints

Study	Patients N	Excessive Thirst	Polyuria	Memory Problems	Tremor	Weight Gain	Drowsiness	Diarrhea	None
Schou et al., 1970[a]									
Initial treatment									
(<1wk)	30	18[a]	18[a]		16	0			4
Extended (1–2 yr)	100	23[a]	23[a]		4	11			65
Bech et. al., 1976	39	62	38	38	51				
Ghose, 1977	50	42		52	34	18	24	8	
Bech et al., 1979[b]	26	62		46	65				
Johnston et al, 1979	49	45[a]	45[a]		31				37
Bone et al., 1980	69	23	38		25		13	10	18
Vestergaard et al., 1980[c]	237	70			45	20		20	10
Lyskowski et al., 1982									
Cross-sectional analysis	142[d]	32	25	3[e]	7	7	6	3	10
Longitudinal analysis	67[f]	13	15	0	10	3	1	0	7
Abou-Saleh & Coppen, 1983									
Males	30	36		57	39		36		
Females	64	49		44	51	34			

Table 17.7. Lithium Side Effects: Percentage of Patients with Subjective Complaints

Study	Patients N	Excessive Thirst	Polyuria	Memory Problems	Tremor	Weight Gain	Drowsiness	Diarrhea	None
Duncavage et al., 1983	21	48	57		14	43		10	19
McCreadie & Morrison, 1985	40	38	30	45	28	43	23	30	35
Page et al., 1987	59	36[a]	36[a]	39	39	36		17	
Jamison et al., unpublished	71		18[g]	33[g]	32[g]	30	24[g]		
Total N	1,094								
Pooled Percentages[h]		35.9	30.4	28.2	26.6	18.9	12.4	8.7	26.2

[a] Polyuria and excessive thirst combined as a single symptom
[b] Patients with Meniere's disease; no history of psychiatric illness
[c] Two-thirds of patients on other medications in addition to lithium
[d] One rating only
[e] Mental confusion
[f] ≥3 ratings
[g] Percent rated as "very important" in lithium noncompliance
[h] Pooled percentages based on patients taking lithium only

Table 17.8. Importance of Side Effects in Lithium Noncompliance

Rank Order[a]	Side Effect	Very Important %	Unimportant %
1	Memory problems	33	22
2	Weight gain	30	28
3	Coordination/tremor	32	31
4	Polyuria	18	17
5	Tiredness/lethargy	24	25
6	Dulling of senses	29	32
7	Blurred vision	26	40
8	Nausea/vomiting	23	40

On the mean scores, there were no significant differences by sex or intelligence

[a]For means of scale scores, ranging from 1 (unimportant) to 5 (very important)

Data from Jamison et al., unpublished

SUMMARY

Noncompliance to lithium among patients with manic-depressive disorder is costly to themselves, those who know them, and society as a whole. Patients who fail to comply are usually young, early in their illness, reluctant to give up their highs, or prone to frequent elevated moods and grandiose delusions. Patients themselves cite medication side effects (e.g., weight gain, cognitive impairment) and several psychological factors as their major reasons for stopping lithium.

Clinicians wishing to increase lithium compliance can take several steps: minimize, whenever possible, the lithium level, minimize and treat aggressively the drug's side effects, track the patient's compliance, examine their own ambivalence about lithium maintenance, educate patients and their families about manic-depressive illness and the role of lithium in attenuating its course, use alternative medication, and encourage adjunctive psychotherapy.

NOTES

1. Parts of this chapter were published originally in Jamison and Goodwin (1983a,b) and Jamison and Akiskal (1983).

2. From Schou's description of lithium's effects on himself and other researchers during an early experimental trial (Schou, 1968, p. 78).

3. Bech et al., 1979; Abou-Saleh and Coppen, 1983; Vestergaard, 1983; Jefferson and Greist, 1987.

REFERENCES

Abou-Saleh, M. T., & Coppen, A. (1983). Subjective side-effects of amitriptyline and lithium in affective disorders. *British Journal of Psychiatry, 142*, 391–397.

Angst, J., Weis, P., Grof, P., Baastrup, P. C., & Schou, M. (1970). Lithium prophylaxis in recurrent affective disorders. *British Journal of Psychiatry, 116*, 604–614.

Bech, P., Thomsen, J., Prytz, S., Vendsborg, P. B., Zilstorff, K., & Rafaelsen, O. J. (1979). The profile and severity of lithium-induced side effects in mentally healthy subjects. *Neuropsychobiology, 5*, 160–166.

Bech, P., Vendsborg, P. B., & Rafaelsen, O. J. (1976). Lithium maintenance treatment of manic-melancholic patients: Its role in the daily routine. *Acta Psychiatrica Scandinavica, 53*, 70–81.

Bone, S., Roose, S. P., Dunner, D. L., & Fieve, R. R. (1980). Incidence of side effects in patients on long-term lithium therapy. *American Journal of Psychiatry, 137*, 103–104.

Cade, J. F. J. (1978). Lithium-Past, present and future. In F. N. Johnson & S. Johnson, eds. *Lithium in Medical Practice*. Baltimore: University Park Press, pp. 5–16.

Christodoulou, G. N., Siafakas, A., & Rinieris, P. M. (1977). Side-effects of lithium. *Acta Psychiatrica Belg, 77*, 260–266.

Cochran, S. D. (1982). Strategies for preventing lithium noncompliance in bipolar affective illness. Doctoral dissertation, University of California, Los Angeles.

Cochran, S. D., & Gitlin, M. J. (1988). Attitudinal correlates of lithium compliance in bipolar affective disorders. *Journal of Nervous and Mental Disease, 176*, 457–464.

Connelly, C. E., Davenport, Y. B., & Nurnberger, J. I. Jr. (1982). Adherence to treatment regimen in a lithium carbonate clinic. *Archives of General Psychiatry, 39*, 585–588.

Danion, J. M., Neunreuther, C., Krieger-Finance, F., Imbs, J. L., & Singer, L. (1987). Compliance with long-term lithium treatment in major affective disorders. *Pharmacopsychiatry, 20*, 230–231.

Duncavage, M. B., Nasr, S. J., & Altman, E. G. (1983). Subjective side effects of lithium carbonate: A longitudinal study. *Journal of Clinical Psychopharmacology, 3*, 100–102.

Fawcett, J., & Kravitz, H. M. (1985). The long-term management of bipolar disorders with lithium, Carbamazepine, and antidepressants. *Journal of Technology Assessment Health Care, 6*, 31–35.

Fitzgerald, R. G. (1972). Mania as a message: Treatment with family therapy and lithium carbonate. *American Journal of Psychotherapy 26*, 547–553.

Frank, E., Prien, R. F., Kupfer, D. J., & Alberts, L. (1985). Implications of noncompliance on research in affective disorders. *Psychopharmacology Bulletin, 21*, 37–42.

Ghose, K. (1977). Lithium salts: Therapeutic and unwanted effects. *British Journal of Hospital Medicine, 18*, 578–583.

Gitlin, M. J., Cochran, S. D., & Jamison, K. R. (1989). Maintenance lithium treatment: Side-effects and compliance. *Journal of Clinical Psychiatry, 50*, 127–131.

Goodwin, F. K., & Jamison, K. R. (1990). *Manic-Depressive Illness*. New York: Oxford University Press.

Grof, P., Cakulis, P., & Dostal, T. (1970). Lithium dropouts: A follow-up study of patients who discontinued prophylactic treatment. *International Pharmacopsychiatry, 5,* 162–169.

Haynes, R. B., Taylor, D. W., & Sackett, D. L., eds. (1979). *Compliance in Health Care.* Baltimore: The Johns Hopkins University Press.

Jacob, M., Turner, L., Kupfer, D. J., et al. (1984). Attrition in maintenance therapy for recurrent depression. *Journal of Affective Disorders, 6,* 181–189.

Jamison, K. R., & Akiskal, H. S. (1983). Medication compliance in patients with bipolar disorders. *Psychiatric Clinics of North America, 6,* 175–192.

Jamison, K. R., & Goodwin, F. I. (1983a). Psychotherapeutic treatment of manic-depressive patients on lithium. In: M. Greenhill & A. Gralnick eds., *The Interrelationship of Psychopharmacology and Psychotherapy.* New York: Macmillan, pp. 53–74.

Jamison, K. R., & Goodwin, F. K. (1983b). Psychotherapeutic issues in bipolar illness. In: L. Grinspoon, ed.: *Psychiatric Association Annual Review.* Volume II. Washington, D.C.: American Psychiatric Press, pp. 319–345.

Jamison, K. R., Gerner, R. H., & Goodwin, F. K. (1979). Patient and physician attitudes toward lithium: Relationship to compliance. *Archives of General Psychiatry, 36,* 866–869.

Jamison, K. R., Gerner, R. H., Hammen, C., & Padesky, C. (1980). Clouds and silver linings: Positive experiences associated with primary affective disorders. *American Journal of Psychiatry, 137,* 198–202.

Jefferson, J. W., Greist, J. H., Ackerman, D. L., & Carroll, J. A. (1987). *Lithium Encyclopedia for Clinical Practice.* Second edition. Washington, D.C.: American Psychiatric Press.

Johnston, B. B., Dick, E. G., Naylor, G. J., & Dick, D. A. T. (1979). Lithium side-effects in a routine lithium clinic. *British Journal of Psychiatry, 134,* 482–487.

Kerry, R. J. (1978) Recent developments in patient management. In: F. N. Johnson & S. Johnson, eds. *Lithium in Medical Practice.* Baltimore: University Park Press, pp. 337–353.

Lenzi, A., Lazzerini, F., Placidi, G. F., Cassano, G. B., & Akiskal, H. S. (1989). Predictors of compliance with lithium and carbamazepine regimens in the long-term treatment of recurrent mood and related psychotic disorders. *Pharmacopsychiatry, 22,* 34–37.

Luznat, R. M., Murphy, D. P., & Nunn, C. M. H. (1988). Carbamazepine vs lithium in the treatment and prophylaxis of mania. *British Journal of Psychiatry, 153,* 198–204.

Lyskowski, J., Nasrallah, H. A., Dunner, F. J., & Bucher, K. (1982). A longitudinal survey of side effects in a lithium clinic. *Journal of Clinical Psychiatry, 43,* 284–286.

Maarbjerg, I. C., Aagaard, J., & Vestergaard, P. (1988). Adherence to lithium prophylaxis: I. Clinical predictors and patients reasons for nonadherence. *Pharmacopsychiatry, 21,* 121–125.

McCreadie, R. G., & Morrison, D. P. (1985). The impact of lithium in South-West Scotland: I. Demographic and clinical findings. *British Journal of Psychiatry, 146,* 70–74.

Miklowitz, D. J., Goldstein, M. J., Nuechterlein, K. H., Snyder, K. S., & Doane, J. A. (1986). Expressed emotion, affective style, lithium compliance, and relapse in recent onset mania. *Psychopharmacology Bulletin, 22,* 628–632.

Overall, J. E., Donachie, N. D., & Faillace, L. A. (1987). Implications of re-strictive diagnosis for compliance to antidepressant drug therapy: Alprazolam versus imipramine. *Journal of Clinical Psychiatry, 48*, 51–54.

Page, C., Benaim, S., & Lappin, F. (1987). A long-term retrospective follow-up study of patients treated with prophylactic lithium carbonate. *British Journal of Psychiatry, 150*, 175–179.

Park, L. C., & Lipman, R. S. (1964). A comparison of patient dosage devia-tion reports with pill counts. *Psychopharmacology, 6*, 299–302.

Placidi, G. F., Lenzi, A., Lazzerini, F., et al. (1986). The comparative efficacy and safety of carbamazepine versus lithium: A randomized, double-blind trial of 83 patients. *Journal of Clinical Psychiatry, 47*, 490–494.

Polatin, P., & Fieve, R. R. (1971). Patient rejection of lithium carbonate prophylaxis. *Journal of the American Medical Association, 218*, 864–866.

Pugh, R. (1983). An association between hostility and poor adherence to treatment in patients suffering from depression. *British Journal of Medical Psychology, 56*, 205–208.

Reifman, A., & Wyatt, R. J. (1980). Lithium: A brake in the rising cost of mental illness. *Archives of General Psychiatry, 37*, 385–388.

Sackett, D. L., Haynes, R. B., & Tugwell, P. (1985). *Clinical Epidemiology: A Basic Science for Clinical Medicine.* Boston: Little, Brown & Company.

Schou, M. (1968). Lithium in psychiatric therapy and prophylaxis. *Journal of Psychiatric Research, 6*, 67–95.

Schou, M., & Baastrup, P. C. (1973). Personal and social implications of lithium maintenance treatment. In: T. A. Ban, J. R. Boissier, G. J. Gessa, H. Heimann, L. Hollister, H. E. Lehmann, I. Munkvad, H. Steinberg, F. Sulser, A. Sundwall, & O. Vinar, eds. *Psychopharmacology, Sexual Disorder and Drug Abuse.* Amsterdam and London: North Holland Publishing Co., pp. 65–68.

Schou, M., Baastrup, P. C., Grof, P., Weis, P., & Angst, J. (1970). Pharmaco-logical and clinical problems of lithium prophylaxis. *British Journal of Psychiatry, 116*, 615–619.

Van Putten, T. (1975). Why do patients with manic-depressive illness stop their lithium? *Comprehensive Psychiatry, 16*, 179–183.

Van, Putten, T., Crumpton, E., & Yale, C. (1976). Drug refusal in schizo-phrenia and the wish to be crazy. *Archives of General Psychiatry, 33*, 1443–1446.

Vestergaard, P., & Amdisen, A. (1983). Patient attitudes toward lithium. *Acta Psychiatrica Scandinavica, 67*, 8–12.

Vestergaard, P., Amdisen, A., & Schou, M. (1980). Clinically significant side effects of lithium treatment: A survey of 237 patients in long-term treat-ment. *Acta Psychiatrica Scandinavica, 62*, 193–200.

18

Facilitating Compliance in Alcoholism Treatment

ALLEN ZWEBEN and DAVID BARRETT

Our joint interest in compliance stems from involvement in establishing and implementing an innovative treatment program for alcohol abusing clients in a community-based health care facility that serves a large managed health care population. Individuals are typically referred to this program after it has become apparent that alcohol use may be interfering with the resolution of other problems afflicting them such as marital, employment, and medical difficulties. Many of these clients are initially unaware of the seriousness of their alcohol problems as well as the need for formal help. They often appear to be ambivalent about participating in a specialized treatment program. Given the perceptions of these individuals about their alcohol use it is often difficult to sustain them in treatment. Consequently, it has been necessary to design specific procedures and strategies in order to help these clients. The issues and content dealt with in this chapter represent an outgrowth of our clinical and research experiences in this treatment program. Case material is derived from the clients seen in this program.

BACKGROUND AND RELEVANT RESEARCH ON THE COMPLIANCE MODEL IN ALCOHOLISM TREATMENT

Changing Alcohol Client Populations

Within the past two decades, there has been an expansion of the boundaries of alcohol treatment services. Health maintenance organizations and insurance carriers are now required by law in many states to provide alcoholism treatment services along with other medical services. Companies have added alcoholism counseling in their benefits package. Courts are currently requiring that first-time drinking and driving offenders undergo an alcohol assessment, education, and treatment. Veterans Administration hospitals have included alcohol and other drug treatment services in the repertoire of services (Parry, 1992).

These outreach efforts have contributed to changing the kinds of client populations currently seen in alcoholism treatment (Sobell & Sobell, 1993; Weisner & Room, 1984; Heather & Robertson, 1983). Clients now treated in alcohol treatment programs are much more diverse in terms of demographics, problem dimensions, and severity (Sobell & Sobell, 1987; Sobell & Sobell, 1993; Heather & Robertson, 1983). Rather than the chronic, severely debilitated person with alcohol problems, the vast majority of clients presenting for treatment are individuals experiencing what has been termed "alcohol-related difficulties" (Sobell & Sobell, 1987; Sobell & Sobell, 1993). These individuals are afflicted with differing levels of severity of problems stemming from the drinking behavior. They may be experiencing mild, moderate, or severe consequences without symptoms of physical dependence (e.g., withdrawal and tolerance) (Holt et al., 1980). Such consequences may pertain to interpersonal (e.g., family conflict), intrapersonal (e.g., guilt about drinking), legal (e.g., drinking and driving), and employment (e.g., missing days of work) difficulties. Unlike people with chronic alcohol problems, a sizeable number of these clients have a stable pattern of employment and living situation (Heather & Robertson, 1983; Heather, 1989), factors which help to promote the rehabilitation process.

A substantial number of individuals with alcohol problems are initially seen for ancillary difficulties that may be related to or accompanying the drinking. Such clients may have been treated for a variety of issues such as marital and family conflict, interpersonal problems, and job stress before their alcohol problems are detected. This is not uncommon in managed health care settings that deal with a variety of emotional or mental health difficulties along with alcohol problems.

Because their concerns are centered on issues which initially brought them to the facility, many of these clients do not perceive their drinking as problematic or requiring formal help. Consequently, conventional approaches are usually ineffective (Miller, Benefield, & Tonigan, 1993). Tactics commonly used such as confrontation or "breaking down denial," and "labeling" are met with resistance. These less impaired individuals do not readily identify with or accept the "alcoholic" label and its corresponding notions of "powerlessness," lifelong abstinence, and ongoing attendance at AA (Miller, 1985). Such ideas represent a radical departure of their perceptions about drinking behavior. Thus, it is not surprising that a sizeable proportion of these clients are reluctant to enter or remain in alcoholism treatment.

Client Retention Rates

Only a small proportion of subjects remain in treatment past the third treatment session. Rates of early drop-out from alcohol treatment (e.g., less than four sessions) range from 44 to 75% in treatment programs in North America and the United Kingdom (cf., Thom et al., 1992; Rees, Beech, & Hore, 1984). Rates of successful referrals range from 10% to less than 30%. For example, Goldberg et al. (1991) discovered that counselors in a general medical setting were able to set up a referral appointment for only 11% of the identified clients with alcohol problems. In this study, potential clients were merely asked whether or not they would be willing to meet with an alcoholism counselor. Soderstrom and Crowley (1987) attempted to enroll victims of alcohol-related trauma in an alcohol abuse treatment program. Despite the damage caused by their drinking, only 30% of these individuals were successfully enrolled. Finally, one study focusing on alcohol treatment referrals among general practitioners in Great Britain showed that only 12–18% of the individuals referred attended at least one time (Thom et al., 1992). Together, these studies indicate that innovative and creative methods are needed to recruit and retain clients in alcoholism treatment.

DEFINITION OF COMPLIANCE

In the alcoholism treatment literature a positive relationship between drinking improvement and compliance has been established; those clients who remain in treatment usually fare better than those who terminate prematurely. However, in our model, compliance is viewed as a facilitative or incremental goal rather than a final goal of treatment. A facilitative goal is defined as "necessary but not sufficient" to produce change (Nelsen, 1984). Within this context compliance is defined in terms of *having clients receive adequate exposure* to treatment in order to derive maximum benefits. Thus, the compliance strategies presented are aimed at facilitating client engagement, participation in, and completion of treatment.

PERSPECTIVES ON COMPLIANCE IN ALCOHOLISM TREATMENT LITERATURE

From a standpoint of a "disease" model of alcoholism, compliance problems in treatment may stem from "personality traits." Individuals are viewed as having an underlying "character structure" that is counterproductive to engaging and sustaining a therapeutic relationship (Miller, 1985). These clients have been described as "counterdependent," meaning that they are fearful and distrustful of intimate relationships (Baekeland, Lundwall, & Shanahan 1973). Mechanisms of denial, rationalization, and projection are commonly employed by people with alcohol problems to refute concerns expressed about drinking and to prevent them from forming a therapeutic alliance. A commonly-held belief among traditional counselors is that alcohol clients need to "hit bottom" (i.e., experience severe consequences stemming from the drinking) before engaging productively in treatment.

Our own views of compliance problems differ a great deal from the "trait" perspective. We recognize that compliance problems stem

from a combination of social, contextual, and interactional issues.
Concerning social matters, clients whose lives are severely dis-
rupted by financial, legal, employment matters may be too overwhelmed to attend sessions regularly (Zweben, Pearlman, & Li,
1982; Zweben & Li, 1981). Others may lack family, friends, and other
supports necessary to sustain a commitment to treatment. In regard
to contextual matters, clients may encounter obstacles in the setting
that may interfere with help-seeking behavior. Individuals may be
confronted with inconvenient office hours, a long and complicated
intake process, indifferent staff members, long waiting lists, and
poor transportation facilities. Such conditions may result in client
inaction with respect to addressing the alcohol problems (Beckman
& Kocel, 1982). With respect to interactional matters, the high degree of discrepancy between practitioner and client may exist concerning such matters as the level of harm associated with drinking,
the etiology of the problem, and methods for changing the alcohol
consumption pattern (Zweben et al., 1988). Failure to resolve these
differences may result in a client terminating treatment prematurely.
Clients are more likely to remain in treatment when these differences are mutually resolved (Zweben & Li, 1981).

COMPLIANCE MODEL

The present chapter is focused on interactional strategies effective
in enhancing client commitment and participation in treatment
using the principles of motivational psychology and techniques of
brief intervention (cf., Heather, 1989; Bien, Miller, & Tonigan, 1993;
Miller, 1985; Miller & Rollnick, 1991). Discrepancies between client
and therapist are resolved by allowing the client the opportunity to
reevaluate existing beliefs in light of objective data concerning the
severity of the alcohol problem. Clients are asked to comment on a
variety of issues related to the drinking behavior such as family conflict, employment problems, and unhealthy lifestyle in order to trig-
ger an internal conflict between the individuals' own views and the
day-to-day activities regarding the drinking (Cooney, Zweben, &
Fleming, 1995). Individuals are forced to struggle with the fact that
their drinking behavior is interfering with their fundamental goals
and values (e.g., causing harm to his/her family). A resolution of
this conflict usually occurs once the client makes a commitment to
change as evidenced by entering and remaining in treatment. Such a
decision helps to reduce the dissonance in the client and restore his/
her emotional equilibrium (e.g., self-respect, "peace of mind," etc.)
(Becker, 1985; Orford, 1985).

An essential ingredient of the compliance model involves enhancing the client's self-efficacy. Self-efficacy is defined as the client's belief that there are available alternatives to the alcohol abusing life
style and more importantly, alternatives *that she or he can reasonably implement* (Bandura, 1977). A client who has a sufficient degree of self-efficacy will more likely recognize the risks associated

with *not* changing the behavior and consequently be ready to take the necessary steps to reduce the risk. Without an adequate degree of self-efficacy, clients may continue to deny or avoid the alcohol problem and remain resistant to help. This is often interpreted as lack of motivation, but more accurately reflects personal doubts about his/her ability to change in the face of obstacles and stressful situations (Rollnick, Heather, & Bell, 1982).

Another component of the compliance model is the emphasis on client choice. Commitment to treatment is enhanced by encouraging client's thinking about the suitability of drinking goals and the steps necessary to meet these goals. The client is asked what is he/she is willing to do in order to reduce the problems resulting from alcohol abuse. What alternative behaviors is he or she willing to adopt? The aim is to reach an agreement about the sequence of action steps that need to be taken in order to stabilize the drinking behavior and eliminate the problems that prompted them to seek treatment. Successful negotiation of a treatment contract means that the client actually believes that his or her own interests and not the practitioner's interests are being served (Sobell & Sobell, 1987).

OVERVIEW OF THE COMPLIANCE STRATEGIES

Regardless of the amount of time spent in treatment, the therapist might expect compliance problems. The therapist needs to continually identify and address current or potential problems that may interfere with a client's commitment. The compliance strategies outlined in Table 18.1 are employed differentially. Particular techniques are related to compliance issues arising in treatment. In this way, clients are helped to remain in treatment.

Table 18.1.

A. Outline of Compliance Strategies
   1. Discovering the Client's Beliefs
   2. Addressing Discrepancies
      a. Assessing the client's beliefs
      b. Feedback on objective tests
      c. Reflective listening
      d. Affirming and normalizing
   3. Forging a Consensus about Treatment Goals and Plans
      a. Role induction
      b. Identifying proximal goals
      c. Delaying decision-making
   4. Supporting the Client's Coping and Social Resources
   5. Addressing Potential Barriers to Compliance
      a. Immunizing the client against negative reactions to treatment

COMPLIANCE STRATEGIES

Discovering the Client's Beliefs

Clients enter treatment with certain beliefs about their problem and expectations of what will and should take place (Rees, 1985). Failure to comply is often related to a lack of agreement between the therapist and client about the cause and severity of the alcohol problems and the amount and type of treatment that may be necessary (Zweben et al., 1988). Health care practitioners are encouraged to conduct an initial assessment of the client's belief's about the alcohol problem, the chain of events that brought them to the treatment setting, and their prior experiences with the available treatments (Meichenbaum & Turk, 1987). The therapist might ask the client to consider how particular treatments could be useful in dealing with the identified problems and how family members would react if they became engaged in such treatments. In this way, the therapist can gauge the individual's and family's receptivity to the type and amount of treatment offered.

Information about the client's beliefs can be incorporated into a standard health habits questionnaire in which drinking is one of several health care domains explored. Measures of consumption levels and related consequences can be incorporated into the heath care assessment in order to identify differing levels of severity of alcohol-related problems. Other measures to include pertain to social support, high risk drinking situations, and self-efficacy. These measures are used to identify the client's individual coping and social resources that can support his/her commitment in undertaking the requisite action steps. The interested reader is referred to Cooney, et al. (1995) and Miller, et al. (1995) for up-to-date information on screening and assessment tools for alcohol problems.

The therapist is advised to maintain a neutral posture in the interview in order to allow the client maximum opportunity to explore their own views and perceptions. The therapist is cautioned not to introduce his or her own values and beliefs for this may negatively impact on the intervention.

Case Example: Mary is a 32 year old divorced mother of two. She lives with her boyfriend John and daughters age 8 and 6. She was referred by her primary care physician who asked for a consult before he prescribes medication for stress and anxiety.

THERAPIST: You were referred by Dr. Jones, is that right?

MARY: Yes, he is afraid I might abuse my tranquilizers.

T: What does he see that worries him?

M: I had a script before. It never lasted a month. I just wasn't careful about them.

T: What happened that got you started on them at first?

M: I was going through my divorce, and I just kept losing it. I used them to get to sleep; but after awhile, I started using them to relax, or just to feel good.

T: You started using them for reasons beyond the reason that the doctor prescribed them. What did you think about that?

M: I got worried! My mother was a pill popper. I didn't want to end up like she did. Besides, I used to smoke a lot of dope. So I know how hard it is to kick a habit.

T: So you have had some personal experience with addictive behavior; is that right? What happened?

M: Yeah! My mother finally went to treatment. She quit about 10 years ago. For me, I just figured it was time to quit. I was 19 years old and had a kid on the way.

T: I think you're saying that you were no longer a kid and that you had responsibilities that required you to give up that lifestyle. It seems like just deciding was enough. Right?

M: That's exactly right! I had lots of friends who had kids, but they kept right on partying. I didn't want my kids to grow up in the same kind of home that I was raised in. It was easy.

T: You wanted to be a good parent. That meant you had to straighten up. What happened? How did you do it?

M: I just stopped. It's just a matter of will-power. Besides, I was getting married. It was no big deal.

Comment: The therapist asks open-ended questions reflecting and clarifying the client's response. Teaching or leading is avoided as rapport is established. The goal here is to discover facts and the client's beliefs. Interpretation, if offered, is done in a tentative fashion checking the client's reaction.

Addressing Discrepancies

Discrepancies often exist between the client and therapist concerning the presence and seriousness of the problem as well as the solutions for resolving them. These differences may be due to a lack of readiness on the part of the client to address the alcohol problems (Prochaska & DiClemente, 1984). This may stem from: (1) low awareness of the alcohol problems; (2) low self-efficacy about changing the drinking behavior; (3) lack of relevant skills for dealing with issues related to the drinking behavior (e.g., coping with an abusive spouse); and/or (4) appropriate or realistic concerns about the suitability of the proposed action plan for overcoming the abusive behavior (e.g., referral to a Twelve-Step treatment program). The therapist needs to give considerable attention to these individual factors in formulating hypotheses about how to deal with compliance problems.

Assessing the client's beliefs. The therapist reviews information obtained on the client's beliefs about the severity of the alcohol problems and related events. The therapist explores how the client interprets various events that may be contributing to the abusive behavior. At the same time, he or she examines the client's willingness to change the circumstances associated with drinking. This enables the therapist to gauge the individual's receptivity to the type of treatments currently offered. It permits the therapist to devise a working hypothesis about what kinds of goals and action plan may be feasible or acceptable (Beckman & Kocel, 1982; Jordan & Oei, 1989; Pfeiffer, Feuerlein, & Brenk-Schulte, 1991).

T: What happened that you began to feel anxious?

M: You can't do that forever (drinking and partying) you know. I started to burn out. My mom was on my back for leaving my girls with her on the weekends. And it cost me a lot of money.

T: Your mom saw that it was interfering in your life; and she began to complain. What do you think about that?

M: I didn't see it then, but I can admit it now. I was abusing it; I had a problem.

T: What happened? How did you get out of it?

M: I didn't really. I met John, my boyfriend. He moved in with me about 8 months ago. My problems started soon after that.

T: Things didn't get better when John moved in.

M: Not really. I didn't go out as much, but he likes to drink so we just drank at home. I never drank at home before he came.

T: I think you are saying that was a big change for you and not a good change. Is that right?

M: I'll say! Before I would go out to enjoy myself; to get away from the stress of being a single mother. Now it's stressful all of the time. I never get away from it.

Comment: This is the beginning of a problem statement; one that can be objectified and addressed in treatment. The therapist can explore potential obstacles (social support, confidence, other resources).

Feedback on objective tests. Feedback on objective tests can have a powerful impact on client beliefs. This is usually done prior to decision-making about treatment goals. Information is presented on the risks associated with the drinking practices along with various life events that may contribute to the continuation or cessation of the behavior. Comparisons are made between what the client perceives and what the data indicate. This process helps to rectify a client's erroneous beliefs about the drinking behavior. It helps the client to recognize his or her own ambivalence about making the necessary changes in order to modify the drinking practices. This is an important step in helping to establish realistic goals with the client.

In our case example, the therapist offers feedback on an alcohol screening questionnaire:

T: Let me tell you about the tests you took. First, the amount you drink in a typical week exceeds what is generally considered safe. In a typical week you usually drink about 24 standard drinks. That means you routinely drink more than 97% of women in the U.S. The nights that you have 2–3 beers your blood alcohol level is about .08. This is enough to affect judgement, mood, and coordination. So it isn't surprising that you report problems even with your more moderate nights. On the weekends you routinely drink above the limit of legal intoxication. These two factors together — the weekly totals and your peak blood alcohol level — put you at risk for more serious problems in the future especially if you drink when you are taking prescription medication. You look surprised.

M: Wow, I can't believe it; 97%! Is that right?

T: You're surprised. We're confident these numbers are accurate; it is based on a nation-wide household survey.

M: What does that mean? I mean, what should I do?

T: That's a good question; but not an easy one. What this says is your drinking puts you at risk for more serious alcohol-related problems. Let's consider what happens if you continue drinking as you are?

M: I just see trouble. I don't have the same will power that I used to. It gets harder to stop at two beers.

Comment: The therapist avoids giving specific advice by anticipating that Mary will need time to absorb the limited feedback that has been given.

Reflective listening. As clients are interviewed, they will reveal information that is inconsistent with their values or beliefs which can lead to a sense of personal discomfort. For example, a client may desire to maintain current drinking habits despite concerns expressed about its negative impact on the family. The use of reflective listening can be useful; the therapist identifies and accepts the ambivalence the client may be experiencing. In demonstrating a receptivity to client views, the therapist fosters a "working alliance."

Affirming and normalizing. With clients who are not receptive, strategies such as affirming and normalizing can be effective. For example, a client who expresses disbelief about the feedback is met with reflection and a request to "say more." Such elaboration may reveal a lack of confidence in his or her own ability to change the negative drinking pattern. The therapist needs to affirm and normalize this uncertainty. For example, a therapist might comment that it is not unusual for some clients to feel uncomfortable or unprepared to take the recommended action steps given the fact their initial views of the drinking differ a great deal from the feedback

data. Techniques such as reflective listening, affirming, and normalizing are helpful in establishing a working alliance, an important
ingredient in facilitating a client's commitment.

T: I can see this is a dilemma for you. I have a lot of respect for the
     way you have cooperated with this assessment and with your
     ability to be honest with yourself. This is a complicated issue; if
     there were an easy answer, I think you would have come up
     with it on your own. At the same time, you have overcome
     problems in the past. I think you have a lot of determination
     and personal strength when you do something.

M: You are right. I can do it if I decide to. I just wasn't expecting to
     spend so much time talking about alcohol. I'm kind of in shock.

T: That's to be expected. I know you are still concerned about your
     anxiety. And I understand what you mean about being in a state
     of shock. You came to talk about anxiety and depression, not
     alcohol.

M: Yes. Stress may be what brought me here, but I know that my
     drinking is contributing to the problem.

Comment: Openly and respectfully acknowledging that the focus
has shifted from Mary's original concern keeps the treatment process somewhat related to the client's initial concerns. Affirming client strengths (e.g., honesty) enhances client self-efficacy even in
situations where there may be potential disagreement about treatment goals. Cooperating with Mary's goals will increase the likelihood that she will stay in treatment and gain awareness about her
problem drinking.

FORGING A CONSENSUS ABOUT TREATMENT
GOALS AND PLANS

Role induction. The technique of role induction can be used to
reduce discrepancies between therapists and clients and to forge a
consensus about treatment goals (cf., Zweben & Li, 1981; Zweben
et al., 1988). It can be effective where the client lacks a clear understanding of how the alcohol problems are to be addressed in treatment (Zweben & Li, 1981). Role induction involves giving the client
information about the goals and strategies of the intervention. The
therapist provides the client with a rationale about how the treatment
offered is relevant to his or her particular needs, capabilities, and resources. Client's perceptions about what is being offered is checked
against information presented on the treatment regimen (e.g., length
of stay, client-therapist roles and responsibilities, and kinds of issues
to be examined). In this way, client misperceptions of treatment are
reduced and a treatment contract can be formulated.

Identifying proximal goals. Clients often feel overwhelmed by the
magnitude of the tasks involved in attaining the drinking goals. This
stress may stem from a lack of confidence on the part of the clients in

their abilities to implement the proposed action plan. Many clients lack both experience and skill in sequencing and prioritizing specific actions necessary to achieve treatment goals. It is often difficult for clients to develop an incremental action plan that is consistent with the ultimate aims of abstinence or nonproblem drinking.

The therapist can assist the client by breaking down a long-term goal into manageable tasks. This allows treatment components to be added in a step-wise fashion (Meichenbaum & Turk, 1987). This is achieved by asking the client what he or she wants to do. Clients often identify an action that is relevant to their immediate circumstances and likely to lead to an outcome which (in terms of their own perceptions) is immediately rewarding. For example, if both therapist and client agree that abstinence is the safest goal, the therapist should examine intermediate steps that will lead to achieving this. The therapist examines the pros and cons of each of these short-term goals to reaffirm the client's own role in decision-making. It is important to ask about the expected consequences of change because the client's "outcome expectation" is a critical determinant of whether the action is initiated (Bandura, 1977).

T: Are you saying that you want to stop drinking at home, but still drink when you are in social situations?

M: Yes, but I know I can't go out and get hammered on the weekends like I have at times in the past.

T: So you want to abstain at home, but you also want to change how you drink when you are out with John or your friends. How will this help?

M: If I stop drinking at home, John and I will have to start dealing with each other. We've been living together, but we don't ever really talk about things; and we have a lot to talk about!

T: What do you see as your next step?

M: I have to go home and talk to John. I have to tell him that I really need to make some changes before I lose it.

T: What will you say to him?

M: I have to stop drinking; and I need your help.

T: What do you think he will say?

M: He'll say "fine." He'll go along with whatever I decide.

Comment: The client is helped to break down the treatment into incremental steps. She believes that abstaining from alcohol in the home will enable her to improve communication with John. She also believes that improving communication is an important step in changing the negative drinking pattern. The goal of stabilizing the drinking pattern becomes less overwhelming or more manageable.

Delaying decision-making. When clients are reluctant to agree on recommended treatment goals, it is important not to pressure them. There is a danger that the client will make a commitment to the proposed plan before he or she feels confident about implementing it. As a result, the client may have difficulty in returning for future sessions.

Rather than continuing to negotiate, the therapist supports the client's inaction while reinforcing his or her willingness to express these misgivings. The therapist stresses that such behavior is consistent with having the client play an active role in decision-making. The therapist may "compliment" the client for openly expressing his/her differences about the proposed treatment plan. This prevents the client from agreeing prematurely with the plan in order to appease the therapist, and it allows the client greater opportunity to weigh the costs and benefits. An individual confronted with an aversive task such as changing an alcohol abusing lifestyle may be better prepared to react positively over time (Zweben et al., 1988).

SUPPORTING THE CLIENT'S COPING AND SOCIAL RESOURCES

The health care practitioner facilitates compliance by eliciting client participation in decision-making activities related to the carrying out of negotiated goals (Meichenbaum & Turk, 1987). Such involvement is essential in enhancing a client's commitment to change. Focus is placed on identifying the range of possible change options and exploring the feasibility of these alternatives. Data derived from the assessment battery is used in identifying and choosing alternatives for dealing with "high risk" situations. Such events include those situations in which the client has demonstrated control over drinking behavior such as spending leisure-time with his or her children. Throughout the session, the client is continually reinforced for his or her involvement in the interview for the purpose of increasing his or her participation and commitment to the treatment program (Chang, 1994).

At the same time, the client is given an opportunity to identify relationships such as family members, relatives, and friends that can be utilized to encourage and sustain a client's commitment. The therapist should provide direction for obtaining the support of significant others such as informing family members about the drinking problem, inviting family members to the treatment sessions, and participating in family events that are incompatible with drinking (e.g., attending church). In cases where a social support network is lacking, the therapist can provide specific referrals to augment the client's support network. Linking the client with such resources as AA Fellowship programs can be important in helping to forestall early drop-out from treatment. The client should be requested to schedule an appointment with the referral source before he or she leaves the treatment session. Such concrete action helps to reinforce the client's commitment. At subsequent appointments, the therapist should inquire about progress and satisfaction with the referral recommendation to firm up the commitment.

T: I think you are hoping John will support your decision. I'm wondering who else can help you?

M: I have a lot of help. My mom and sister. Even my ex-husband Gary. They have all expressed some concern about what I was doing, and would all like to see me get back on track.

T: So even though you didn't come here because of your drinking, you know other people have been concerned and will support you. How can they help if this is harder than you think?

M: I have to let them help. I've kind of shut them out, especially when it comes to talking about John. I didn't want them interfering.

T: So if things stay rough with John, you will have to become more independent from him and rely more on your family for support. I think you also have to remember to rely on your own strengths. You've done this at least once before, when you were 19 and stopped smoking marijuana. Both of these factors together can be a help to you, regardless of what John does.

Comment: Mary reveals a social resource she has neglected. The therapist affirms her coping skills by reminding her of her experience resisting social pressure.

ADDRESSING POTENTIAL BARRIERS TO COMPLIANCE

Immunizing the client against negative reactions to treatment. The therapist needs to be sensitive to compliance problems stemming from "second thoughts" or negative reactions occurring outside the treatment session. Clients often experience anxieties and fears after leaving the session as a result of unresolved matters being addressed. Such problems may stem from a lack of confidence about ability to handle events associated with the abusive drinking pattern (e.g., low self-efficacy). These delayed responses may be related to a lingering concern about the suitability of the action plan for resolving the alcohol problem. For example, a client may agree with the therapist about the need to spend more time with his family instead of his "drinking buddies." However, after leaving the session he may have "second thoughts" about following through. He may decide that he is not ready to handle ridicule from his so-called "buddies" by refusing to stop at a bar and drink with them after work. Thus, he may decide to drop-out of treatment rather than discuss this potentially "embarrassing" matter.

Clients with a prior history of noncompliance would be appropriate candidates for employing immunization. Such clients often commit themselves to a treatment regimen without resolving an underlying ambivalence about how the alcohol problems are to be addressed in the treatment sessions. Many of these clients withdraw from treatment prematurely in part, to avoid dealing with these concerns. In these cases, the therapist "normalizes" these potential difficulties and helps prepare the client to deal with them. Various options can be offered for handling these delayed responses such as maintaining a log of reactions, discussing them in subsequent sessions, and sharing these negative thoughts with family members. To reinforce the client's role in decision-making, the therapist indicates that "not returning to treatment" is one of the alternatives to consider when encountering negative thoughts. However, the latter should be coupled with a reminder about the potential consequences of this decision. When linked with real or potential consequences, the "leaving treatment" option usually loses its appeal and clients often find other alternatives more acceptable to them.

T: Let's talk about where you go from here. You've identified both anxiety and drinking as problems you want to change. My main concern now is that you may leave here and have second thoughts about what we discussed today. Sometimes people prematurely commit themselves to certain goals and later decide they really don't want to do it. While they are here, they feel okay but once they leave something happens to change their mind. What do you think?

M: That sounds like me. I've changed my mind before. I'm afraid if I try to do too much I'll fall on my face. Then I feel like giving up.

T: Yes. This is quite common. When things get tough, people often do not want to return to therapy. They feel they let people down. Do you see this happening to you?

M: No, I think since we talked about it, I can't see this happening. But you never can tell.

T: If it does happen, if you feel like not returning, what can you do?

M: I guess I can talk to John or my family, or I can talk to you about it at the next session.

Comment: The therapist immunizes the client against delayed negative reactions to therapy. The intent is to normalize the reaction and to prepare the client to deal with it in a more productive way than leaving treatment prematurely.

SPECIAL CONSIDERATIONS

It should be noted that many of the issues encountered with clients in our own setting are similar to those experienced with dually diagnosed clients in other programs (described by Drake and his colleagues in their work with dually diagnosed clients) (Drake et al., 1990; Drake et al., 1993; Drake & Noordsy, 1994). As is the case in our own program, dually diagnosed clients typically lack an awareness of the seriousness of the drinking problems and consequently, experience a sense of discrepancy between their own and the therapists' perceptions about the alcohol involvement. Despite the severity of their alcohol problems, these clients often reveal a reluctance to address these problems. Thus, confrontation tactics widely utilized in alcoholism treatment programs are typically avoided with dually diagnosed clients in favor of indirect, empathic, collaborative approaches for purposes of maximizing their participation in treatment. Such tactics are consistent with the motivational strategies employed in our own program and have been shown to be effective with dually diagnosed clients (Drake et al., 1993). In sum, although our present motivational model has been implemented primarily with individuals having alcohol abuse as a primary disorder, we believe that its basic components are also applicable to individuals who have severe psychiatric as well as substance abuse disorders.

SUMMARY

In this chapter, we have described practical strategies that can be employed systematically to facilitate a client's engagement in alcoholism treatment. These strategies are aimed at discovering the client's beliefs about causes and severity of the alcohol-related problems, assessing those beliefs in light of objective information, and formulating hypotheses about what techniques might be beneficial in engaging the client in treatment. Motivational counseling techniques such as reflective listening, affirming, and normalizing are utilized to establish a treatment alliance. With clients who remain uncooperative or hesitant about accepting or following a proposed action plan, tactics such as delaying decision-making, immunization, and developing proximal goals can be useful. Plans are made to utilize the clients' social support network to buttress their coping or decision-making capacities. The therapist encourages a sense of autonomy and well-being on the part of the client throughout treatment. We hope that a major benefit of these compliance strategies will be to relieve the therapist of some of the day-to-day frustrations in dealing with these "resistant" clients, help prevent "burn-out," and lead to an increased sense of optimism toward treating these difficult clients.

REFERENCES

Baekeland, F., Lundwall, L., & Shanahan, T. J. (1973). Correlates of patient attrition in the outpatient treatment of alcoholism. *Journal of Nervous and Mental Disease, 157,* 99–107.

Bandura, A. (1977). Self-efficacy: Toward a unifying theory of behavioral change. *Psychological Review, 84,* 191–215.

Becker, M. G. (1985). Patient adherence to prescribed therapies. *Medical Care, 23*(5), 539–555.

Beckman, L. J., & Kocel, K. M. (1982). The treatment-delivery system and alcohol abuse in women: Social policy implications. *Journal of Social Issues, 38*(2), 139–151.

Bien, T. H., Miller, W. R., & Tonigan, J. S. (1993). Brief interventions for alcohol problems: A review. *Addiction, 88*, 315–336.

Chang, P. (1994). Effects of interviewer type on compliance: An analogue study. *Journal of Counseling Psychology, 41*, 74–82.

Cooney, N. L., Zweben, A., & Fleming, M. F. (1995). Screening for alcohol problems and at-risk drinking in healthcare settings. In R. K. Hester, & W. R. Miller (Eds.), *Handbook of alcoholism treatment approaches* (2nd edition, pp. 45–60). Boston: Allyn and Bacon.

Drake, R. E., Bartels, S. J., Teague, G. B., Noordsy, D. L., & Clark, R. E. (1993). Treatment of substance abuse in severely mentally ill patients. *The Journal of Nervous and Mental Disease, 181*(10), 606–611.

Drake, R. E., McHugo, G. J., & Noordsy, D. L. (1993). Treatment of alcoholism among schizophrenic outpatients: 4-year outcomes. *American Journal of Psychiatry, 150*(2), 328–329.

Drake, R. E., & Noordsy, D. L. (1994). Case management for people with coexisting severe mental disorder and substance use disorder. *Psychiatric Annals, 24*(8), 427–431.

Drake, R. E., Teague, G. B., & Warren, S. G., III. (1990, June). Dual diagnosis: The New Hampshire Program. *Addiction and Recovery*, 35–39.

Goldberg, H. I., Mullen, M., Richard, K. R., Psaty, B. M., & Ruch, B. P. (1991). Alcohol counseling in a general medicine clinic. *Medicine Care, 7*, JS49–JS56.

Heather, N. (1989). Psychology and brief interventions. *British Journal of Addiction, 84*, 357–370.

Heather, N., & Robertson, I. (1983). *Controlled drinking*. London: Methuen.

Holt, S., Steward, I. C., Dixon, J. M. J., Elton, R. A., Taylor, T. V., & Little, K. (1980). Alcohol and the emergency service. *British Medical Journal, 281*, 638–640.

Jordan, C. M., & Oei, T. P. S. (1989). Help-seeking behaviour in problems drinkers: A review. *British Journal of Addiction, 84*, 979–988.

Meichenbaum, D., & Turk, D. (1987). *Facilitating treatment adherence: A practitioners handbook*. New York: Plenum.

Miller, W. R. (1985). Motivation for treatment: A review with special emphasis on alcoholism. *Psychological Bulletin, 98*, 84–107.

Miller, W. R., Benefield, R. G., & Tonigan, J. S. (1993). Enhancing motivation for change: A controlled comparison of two therapist styles. *Journal of Consulting and Clinical Psychology, 61*, 455–461.

Miller, W. R., & Hester, R. K. (1995). Treatment for alcohol problems: Toward an informed eclecticism. In R. K. Hester, & W. R. Miller (Eds.), *Handbook of alcoholism treatment approaches* (2nd edition, pp. 1–11). Boston: Allyn and Bacon.

Miller, W. R., & Hester, R. K. (1989). Inpatient alcoholism treatment: Rules of evidence and burden of proof. *American Psychologist, 44*, 1245–1246.

Miller, W. R., & Rollnick, S. (1991). *Motivational interviewing: Preparing people to change addictive behavior*. New York: Guilford Press.

Miller, W. R., Westerberg, V., & Waldron, N. (1995). Evaluating alcohol problems in adults and adolescents. In R. K. Hester, & W. R. Miller (Eds.), *Handbook of alcoholism treatment approaches* (2nd edition, pp. 61–88). Boston: Allyn and Bacon.

Nelsen, J. (1984). Intermediate treatment goals as variables in single-case research. *Social Work Research and Abstracts, 20*(3), 3–10.

Orford, J. (1985). *Excessive appetites: A psychological view of addictions.* New York: John Wiley & Sons.

Parry, R. E. (Ed.). (1992). *Screening for alcoholism in the Department of Veterans Affairs* (technical report). Department of Veteran's Affairs, Veterans Health Administration, Health Services Research and Development Service.

Pearlman, S., Zweben, A., & Li, S. (1989). The comparability of solicited versus non-solicited clients in alcoholism treatment research. *British Journal of Addiction, 84*, 523–532.

Pfeiffer, W., Feuerlein, W., & Brenk-Schulte, E. (1991). The motivation of alcohol dependents to undergo treatment. *Drug and Alcohol Dependence, 29*, 87–95.

Prochaska, J. O., & DiClemente, C. C. (1984). *The transtheoretical approach: Crossing traditional boundaries of therapy.* Homewood: IL: Dow Jones-Irwin.

Rees, D. W. (1985). Health beliefs and compliance with alcoholism treatment. *Journal of Studies on Alcohol, 46*(6), 517–524.

Rees, D. W., Beech, H. R., & Hore, B. D. (1984). Some factors associated with compliance in treatment of alcoholism. *Alcohol and Alcoholism, 19*, 303–307.

Rollnick, S., Heather, N., & Bell, A. (1982). Negotiating behavior change in medical settings: The development of brief motivational interviewing. *Journal of Mental Health, 1*, 24–37.

Sobell, M. B, & Sobell, L. C. (1993). *Problem drinkers: Guided self-change treatment.* New York: Guilford Press.

Sobell, M. B., & Sobell, L. C. (1987). Conceptual issues regarding goals in the treatment of alcohol problems. *Drugs and Society, 1*(2/3), 1–38.

Soderstrom, C. A., & Crowley, R. A. (1987). A national alcohol and trauma center survey. *Archives of Surgery, 122*, 1067–1071.

Thom, B., Brown, C., Drummond, C., Edwards, G., & Mullan, M. (1992). The use of services for alcohol problems: General practitioner and specialist alcohol clinic. *British Journal of Addiction, 87*, 613–624.

Weisner, C., & Room, R. (1984/1985). Financing and ideology in alcohol treatment. *Social Problems, 32*(2), 167–184.

Zweben, A., & Barrett, D. (1993). Assessment and brief advice as a treatment for alcoholic and spouse. In T. J. O'Farrell (Ed.), *Marital and family therapy in alcoholism treatment* (pp. 421–455). New York: Guilford Publications.

Zweben, A., Bonner, M., Chaim, G., & Santon, P. (1988). Facilitative strategies for retaining alcohol-dependent clients in outpatient treatment. *Alcoholism Treatment Quarterly, 5*(½), 3–24.

Zweben, A., & Li, S. (1981). The efficacy of role induction in preventing early dropout from outpatient treatment of drug dependency. *American Journal of Drug and Alcohol Abuse, 8*(2), 171–183.

Zweben, A., Pearlman, S., & Li, S. (1982). Reducing attrition from conjoint therapy with alcoholic couples. *Drug and Alcohol Dependence, 11*, 321–331.

19

Compliance and the Treatment Alliance in the Elderly Patient with Severe Mental Illness

DONALD P. HAY, LINDA K. HAY, JULIE RENNER,
KARL FRANSON, RAKHSHANDA HASSAN and
PEGGY SZWABO

INTRODUCTION

This chapter is the result of the combined efforts of six faculty members working within the same Division of Geriatric Psychiatry. Each contributor has a different role to play in the care of geriatric psychiatry patients and we frequently request each other's assistance to create the best outcome. This chapter is a true interdisciplinary product!

The chapter focuses on the extensive and far ranging issues for elderly patients with serious mental illness regarding the effectiveness of a treatment alliance to result in adherence or compliance for treatment recommendations.

In the outpatient section we learn that stigma or the perception of myths strongly influences the acceptance of psychiatry and its treatments. There are also practical issues, including transportation, weather, or limitations of chronic illness that affect adherence to treatment recommendations.

The section on medications also describes the significant effect of the stigma of the illnesses and of the "mood altering drugs." Other problems specific to the elderly include increased forgetfulness and poor vision. Of concern for the elderly patient are the real and imagined side effects which may lead to both under- and/or over compliance. Recommendations include family support systems and the need for improved instruction. Also of significant concern is the need for maintenance medication with continued use of the medication in its proper dosage form.

The section on inpatient issues also refers to stigma as a primary concern, along with the need for information to flow to and from the family and/or nursing home. Some recommendations to improve diagnosis and treatment include post-admission conferences, pre-discharge conferences and continued evaluation of the affect, behavior, and cognition of the elderly patient such that appropriate treatment recommendations can be made.

Stigma also heads the list of the section on ECT, and the recommendations called for include the need for significant education before, during and after ECT, as well as the focus on appropriate utilization of, and follow-through for continuation and maintenance ECT.

The section on day hospital treatment highlights the need for effective transition from inpatient to outpatient treatment, which is extremely complicated and has a high potential for breakdown and noncompliance. Recommendations for the prevention of relapse include education regarding the use of medication and a focus on continuation of care for post-hospitalization.

The section on consultation and liaison treatment reports that hospitalization is extremely stressful for the elderly patient, considering frequent multiple system disease, decreased nutrition, decreased strength and mental function, as well as problems with polypharmacy. The primary concerns continue to be the diagnosis and treatment of anxiety, delirium, dementia and depression. Specific concerns include the request for competency evaluations, as well as addressing the issue of elderly individuals refusing further medical treatment.

All of the above issues, as reflected in these sections, continue to be of significant concern for the providers of mental health care to this very special population.

OUTPATIENT

The compliance of the elderly population in outpatient treatment programs is related to several factors. First are effects having to do with knowledge of and acceptance of psychiatry, psychiatric medications, and psychotherapy. Since awareness and study of the special psychiatric issues of the older adult have been late to develop relative to those of younger adults, this population may be unaware of its own psychiatric needs and may be less motivated to seek and maintain treatment.

There is also the perpetuation of myths related to the elderly including the impression that depression, difficulties with thinking, sleeping, and anxiety are to be expected, and for this reason treatment is not needed. This may serve to diminish the elderly persons cooperation in seeking and complying with treatment as well as to prejudice practitioners who do not diagnose and treat these disorders as frequently as others. Sadly, it has been reported that more than 80% of elderly individuals who completed a suicide had visited their primary care physician within a month of their death, and 20% had done so within 24 hours (AARP, 1989).

There are a variety of practical concerns which make it difficult for elderly patients to comply with treatment. These include transportation limitations, weather concerns, and the effects of chronic illness. Many older individuals and their spouses are unable or reluctant to drive. Relying on family members or public transportation may be an additional burden for the patient who, by virtue of psychiatric illness, is already experiencing a sense of helplessness. The outpatient treatment team may increase the burden of transportation issues by recommending limitation of driving by the patient for safety reasons.

Elderly outpatients cancel appointments more often than younger patients as a result of inclement weather. Cold, ice, and rain in the winter as well as heat in the summer may provide barriers to travel especially for those with physical disabilities, and for those requiring walkers, canes, and wheelchairs. The elderly outpatient is also more reluctant to travel during increased traffic and may prefer morning or early afternoon visits secondary to easy fatiguability.

The elderly experience more *chronic* physical illness than younger populations. Outpatient appointments are frequently canceled as a result of medication side effects, as well as hospitalizations for concomitant medical illness.

There is only limited reporting with regard to outpatient compliance specific to the elderly. One study in older male problem drinkers found that subjects who had late-onset alcohol related problems and whose spouses also participated in counseling were more likely to comply than those whose spouses did not participate (Atkinson, Tolson & Turner, 1993). Secondly, patients who experienced an extremely serious problem such as having been arrested but who received support from spouses were more likely to be compliant.

Psychotherapy for the elderly requires extreme flexibility by the therapist. One report describes the reluctance of an older man to engage in psychotherapy. A 78 year old depressed man would not come to the outpatient office for psychotherapy but agreed to meet for breakfast with the psychologist. This meeting allowed for assessment and continued with successful cognitive therapy (Shute, 1986).

MEDICATIONS

The elderly population uses a disproportionate amount of medication due to a greater incidence of chronic diseases. Twenty-five percent of all prescription medications are taken by patients 65 years or older. It is particularly important for the elderly psychiatric population to take their medicine correctly for reasons of individual as well as family or community safety and reduction of unnecessary hospitalizations. It is often more difficult for an elderly individual to follow medication regimens due to the sheer number of medications prescribed as well as the increased probability of side effects including short term memory loss.

Although the elderly patient population is deemed to be more physician reliant, this does not appear to correlate with an improvement in medication compliance. Issues such as increased forgetfulness, poor vision, increased number of chronic illnesses, are typically cited as causes of noncompliance in the elderly population. Geriatric mental health patients may be at an increased risk due to self-neglect from an underlying psychiatric condition such as depression, psychosis or dementia. For example, it was reported by Peterson (1986) that anger and depression were possible factors underlying uncooperativeness in this population.

McMullin Ross & Rees (1991) reviewed compliance during long-term therapy in community patients who knowingly stopped psychotropic medications. The reasons for discontinuance among patients who lived alone included "felt medication disagreed with him/her or suffered physical side effects; medication was not making him/her feel better; felt better so thought medication was no longer needed; thought he/she was taking too much medication." The study also evaluated medication utilization among elderly patients with psychiatric disorders who had caregivers. The reasons for noncompliance in this group included "poor cognitive function; medication not making him/her feel better; felt better, so thought medication no longer needed". The investigator concluded that proper counseling and continued counseling of both those living alone and those with caregivers may have been of benefit in increasing compliance.

Wood (1986) suggested that the key to compliance is to remove both the stigma about taking mood-altering drugs and guilt about the disorder. She recommended educating the patient about the appropriateness of the medications and positive side effects, as well as securing the family's support.

Medication side effects and intolerance to adverse drug reactions is a leading cause of medication noncompliance. Thus, the selection of medication is often based on the side effect profile of these medications. However, despite the clinicians best efforts, these adverse effects may cause problems, even when the clinician "starts low and goes slow." Many times the psychotropic drugs elicit complaints of sedation, dizziness and headache as well as gastrointestinal distress. This is because the elderly have a seemingly lower tolerance level to anticholinergic effects. (Wantanabe & Davis 1990). These adverse effects typically have a temporal relationship to taking the dose and therefore are easily identifiable to the patient as a side effect. Some of these effects are self-limiting and if so clinicians can encourage the patient to remain compliant until the effect subsides. Because the clinician is typically aware of the increased sensitivity of the elderly, noncompliance and low dosages may lead to false treatment failures. Therapeutic drug monitoring (Tonkin & Bochner 1994, Orsulak & Kolodner 1989) may provide useful information to the clinician when the patient has failed therapy. The elderly are known to require lower doses to achieve therapeutic concentrations and are also more likely to become toxic at conventional dosages.

Fortunately, the pharmacokinetics of psychotherapeutic agents often allow for once daily dosing. Yet, some patients do mistakenly take too much medication. A recent review of compliance during long-term therapy demonstrates that noncompliance takes many different forms (Urquhart, 1994). For example, over compliance among elderly psychiatric patients may increase the likelihood of adverse drug reactions and toxicity.

INPATIENT

Working with patients on a geriatric psychiatry unit is complicated by some issues specific to the elderly. The higher incidence of dementia in the elderly alone or in combination with depression results in cognitive impairment such that patients are not able to provide adequate information about their situation. For this reason, geriatric psychiatry shares some elements with child psychiatry in that the family members are always invited to participate in the information gathering as long as the patient consents. This factor plays a critical role in compliance. Many older adults today still view psychiatry with skepticism and fear due to stigmatization. Whereas younger adults are more familiar with biochemical theories of neurotransmitter deficiency in the brain, such as, "depression is an illness," many older individuals fear psychiatric involvement as a sign of inadequacy at the least, or as a signal of impending incompetency, at the worst. The greater fear is that if seen by a psychiatrist, they will be found incompetent and sent to an institution. For this reason, a significant number of older adults will not come to a psychiatric inpatient setting by choice. This is a situation in which the family can play a significant role. Work on compliance begins prior to admission and is a function of a team effort with the patient, family, psychiatrist, and other team members working together for a smooth transition to the inpatient setting.

Since most admissions of geriatric patients include numerous questions from family members, the admission process can be overwhelming, not only for patient and family, but also for the inpatient team. For this reason, we have adopted a technique called the "Post Admission Conference or P.A.C." At the time of admission, we tell the family that within five working days we will hold a "PAC," with opportunity for any or all family members to come in for a time-limited session (usually one-half hour). The family members are given two alternative dates and times in an attempt to meet their needs. This conference is more in-depth than initial phone calls, and includes our accumulated knowledge of the history, the diagnostic impression, the treatment plan, and the prognosis. At the conference we ask the family for input so that we can work collaboratively. Prior to the PAC we request that questions regarding these items be held until the meeting so that we can answer them with adequate information including results of basic laboratory and other studies, work-up, or consultations. This technique reduces apprehension, fear, and at times mistrust or anger from the family due to unanswered or perfunctorily-answered early phone calls and visits.

Similarly, prior to the end of hospitalization a "Predischarge Conference" — "PDC" is held, again with invitation to the family. At the PDC we recap the course of the hospitalization, what our findings were, what treatments were initiated, and renew our prognosis and post-discharge treatment recommendations. This is again offered as a half-hour session and is set up one or more days prior to discharge. By virtue of the "PAC" and the "PDC" we have been able to diminish and usually eliminate most of the fears, anger, and misgivings on the part of the family. It also reduces the complaint "I never get to see my relative's doctor." The Postadmission and Predischarge Conferences also include an invitation to the nursing home staff and we work with them collaboratively. As a result of this technique we receive fewer angry phone calls from either the family or the nursing home staff (usually 24 to 48 hours after discharge from the hospital) stating concern that "my mother" or "the patient" is "no better and perhaps worse than when we sent her to you." Both the PAC and the PDC help to maintain continuity of care and thereby a treatment alliance that promotes compliance.

During the hospitalization, we frequently reassess the Affect, Behavior, and Cognition of the patient. These "ABC's" are the elements of continuing change for the geriatric psychiatry patient. We use standardized scales such as the Geriatric Depression Scale (Yesavage & Brink, 1983) or the DSM-IV symptoms of major depression, which have been summarized in an acronymic mnemonic "CEASE SAAD" for the affective assessment (see Table 19.1). For

Table 19.1.

CEASE SAAD

Using the Scale

C   Concentration difficulties (8)*

E   Energy low (6)*

A   Anxiety high (5)*

S   Spontaneous crying (1)*

E   Early morning awakening (4)*

S   Suicidal (9)*

A   Appetite disturbed (3)*

A   Anhedonia (2)*

D   Derogatory feelings and guilt feelings (7)*

---

*Number in parenthesis corresponds to the DSM-IV.

Each of the above categories must be assessed by questioning the patient as to their subjective awareness of these symptoms or as reported by family members or friends when the patient is unable to answer the questions. If the patient is unable to verbalize their symptoms it is helpful to supply them with choices for their answers. An example for "Concentration" is to ask the patient if they can read the newspaper or watch their favorite television show.

Table 19.2.

WISDOM

Using the Scale

W world spelled backwards

I   items (3) of memory

S serial sevens

D date of birth

O orientation

M memory of presidents

Each of the above categories must be assessed by questioning the patient:

W spell the word "world" backwards

I   repeat 3 items and ask again in a few minutes

S subtract 7 from 100, subtract 7 from 93, subtract 7 from 86

D what is your date of birth

O today's date, full name, location

M current president, previous two presidents

---

behavior we look to nursing reporting as well as the "Cohen-Mansfield Agitation Inventory (Cohen-Mansfield, 1988)" or the "Behave AD" (Reisberg, et al., 1987), and for assessment of cognition we recommend the Folstein Mini Mental State Examination (Folstein, Folstein & McHugh., 1975), the Blessed Dementia Scale, or any other easily utilizable scale. We use a short mental status form called "Wisdom" which assesses areas of orientation and disorientation as a easily utilizable tool to assess these areas on a regular basis (see Table 19.2). By virtue of reassessing the "ABC's" frequently, we are able to keep track of the patient's functioning, and by so doing can increase compliance, since we are not ignoring any one area during the hospitalization or at the time of discharge.

ECT

Electroconvulsive therapy (ECT) presents multiple challenges to compliance in the elderly. The first obstacle to surmount is resistance to the ECT treatment itself due to fears about the nature and effects of the treatment intensified by public stigma. Studies reveal that up to

75% of patients express negative feelings about ECT. Specific fears include permanent memory loss, brain damage, or death (Fox, 1993).

Interestingly, two distinct types of fear have been noted. The understandable pre-treatment fear is differentiated from a pathologic fear in patients previously treated with ECT, even if they had a good response. Some of the most vehement refusals of ECT are characterized by this type of fear. Disorientation experienced by patients upon awakening from the ECT treatment has been postulated as an initiator of fear. Clinical observations suggest that patients rarely speak about this and require direct questioning. Clinical characteristics of the patients who experience fear of ECT, such as anxiety or personality disorder, have not been distinguished, but such information might enhance compliance by alerting clinicians to patients who may be especially reluctant to accept ECT. Fears about ECT, although common, do not affect outcome (Fox, 1993).

Fears may be ameliorated by education. The patient and the family must first be instructed in a manner consistent with the standards of informed consent: the patient or patient's guardian and the patient's family (with the patient's permission) must understand the following:

(1) the nature of the psychiatric condition for which the ECT is being prescribed,

(2) the nature, process, and anticipated results of ECT,

(3) the medically significant risks of ECT including and risk of death (1/10,000 patients) or serious harm, and alternative treatments or procedures, and

(4) the chances of success or failure of the proposed and alternative treatments and procedures.

These disclosures should be made by the attending psychiatrist and should be documented (Campion, 1993).

Despite implementation of this educational model attitudinal factors may interfere such that patients and families often remain ambivalent about ECT. In these cases, it may be useful to offer video educational tapes. The analogy of electroconvulsive therapy as an outpatient surgical procedure alleviates fears by placing ECT within a context of medical interventions. Especially helpful are vignettes of famous individuals who have shared publicly their psychiatric conditions and experiences with ECT.

Although inpatient ECT treatments can be monitored, compliance with outpatient continuation ECT or maintenance ECT provides additional challenges. Implementation of continuation or maintenance ECT may be constrained by multiple factors affecting compliance including distance, lack of family support, cost, fear of anesthesia or ECT, concern about memory loss, and unsubstantiated optimism regarding the remission of depressive symptomatology. Nonetheless, continuation or maintenance ECT is indicated for many situations: patients with severe recurrent illness, patients who are poorly responsive, nontolerant, at risk, or noncompliant on psychotropics; patients with a history of impulsive suicide attempts using psychotropics, and patients with a good response to ECT. (Clarke et al., 1991). Any noncompliance with ECT or missed ECT should be thought of as possibly a result or cause of relapse; low motivation leading to a missed ECT treatment may be an early indicator of relapse rather than the cause of relapse. The need for ECT should be reassessed every three months (Dubin et al., 1992). Whether inpatient or outpatient continuation or maintenance ECT, compliance assessment should be a standard element.

DAY HOSPITAL TREATMENT

Partial hospitalization, day treatment, and day hospitalization are similar terms used to describe day programs with individualized goals for patients. These programs are helpful for those patients who have little social or limited family supports, and who are not able to adequately function at home alone. The treatment is designed and tailored to achieve goals usually having to do with resocialization, rehabilitation and improved adjustment. The goals are to ease the stressful transition from the hospital back into the community and to insure continual treatment compliance. Day programs offer a range of therapies, and provide social and recreational activities designed to help individuals live more adequately in the community. Partial hospitalization decreases length of stay when admission is necessary. Day treatment set up requires low outlay of funds for staffing rather than for construction or equipment.

Thienhaus and Greschel (1988) noted that the transition of elderly psychiatric patients from inpatient to outpatient is frequently complicated for the patient and has a high potential for breakdown in follow-up. They recommend a program of interim care to reduce noncompliance during this critical transition. Partial hospitalization programs can affect compliance by working more intensely with individuals in preventing relapse by the omission or overuse of medicine.

For older adults, partial hospitalization requires the same programming and goals as for younger individuals although employment may not be a primary objective. Older adults may benefit from the involvement in transitional psychiatric treatment to prevent rehospitalization and to further assess self-care abilities. For frail elderly, intensive structured treatment may provide support when there are few resources available.

Earlier studies such as those of Meltzhoff and Blumenthal (1969), Guy, et al. (1969), and Belyaeva and Kabanov (1972), document the efficacy of partial hospital programs as significantly reducing rehospitalization. More recent studies have noted the social and financial benefits of day programs (Marishita, et al., 1989); Culhane & Culhane, 1993).

Despite the benefits noted, partial hospitalization is greatly under utilized compared with inpatient care. Since 1991, Medicare reimbursement has provided for day hospital treatment. This would argue for the development of more intensive outpatient treatment for a high risk special needs elderly population.

CONSULTATION AND LIAISON

Hospitalization is particularly stressful for the elderly patient. It frequently creates emotional problems or exacerbates existing psychiatric disorders (Ruskin, 1985). Accurate diagnosis often implies the difficult task of distinguishing dementia from depression which mimics a dementia-like syndrome with somatic symptoms stemming from physical illness. Adequate management includes the appropriate choice and use of psychotropic drugs, the assessment of competency, contacts with the patient's family and with various social agencies, and liaison work with the staff. In many cases, the consultation and liaison psychiatrist has to insist on additional medical work-up to determine the cause of delirium, to determine a potentially reversible cause of dementia, or to look for an occult malignancy in a depressed patient. The liaison psychiatrist at times has to take the role of patient advocate, and at other times acts as a mediator between the patient and the medical/surgical staff, as well as an educator for the latter, since most of the elderly, especially the cognitively impaired, are frequently viewed as difficult to manage. It makes the task of geriatric psychiatrists even more challenging when assistance is requested for problematic noncompliant elderly patients. The geriatric psychiatry consultant is required to assess and evaluate the patient as a whole, and to identify the relative contributions of the medical, psychodynamic, social, and behavioral factors contributing to noncompliance by the patient (Waller & Altshuler 1986). Noncompliant patients do tend to create a negative emotional climate from the treatment team. This is when the geriatric psychiatry consultant with good liaison skills can be most beneficial from the viewpoint of both understanding the problem behavior, as well as dealing with the burdensome environment that the behavior has produced (Waller & Altshuler 1986). The goal is to understand what makes a particular patient's behavior seem reasonable given the specific situation, since no behavior is random and even pathological behavior is an indication of something crucial. This enables the geriatric psychiatrist to view the patient separately from the self-defeating aspects of his/her behavior which may frustrate the physician and the treatment team. The most important issue is to see the patient as a "human being." The development of a therapeutic alliance with the patient is only feasible if all aspects of the patient's problems are considered. Howanitz and Freedman (1992) revealed interesting results from a study regarding patients' refusal to be treated. In this study, 70 percent of patients refusing treatment changed their minds within 24 hours of psychiatric consultation. It also showed the most common reason was that the patient did not believe that treatment was necessary. The second most common reason was the patient's fear of treatment. In this case, consultation is recommended to explore previous medical experiences with the patient and through this discussion the patient may realize that the current situation is less threatening than previous admissions. Patients who refuse treatment because of anger toward their doctor or hospital, if enabled to vent their anger, may agree with treatment. Overall, the study resulted in recommending that psychiatric consultants who deal with noncompliant patients in the hospital address particular reasons for refusing treatment and deal with them accordingly. Lipowski (1983) stated that the challenge for a geriatric psychiatry consultant is not only to develop an alliance with the patient for treatment compliance but also with the medical and surgical colleagues. Many negative attitudes may be encountered in the general hospital setting. The consultant's advice may be acknowledged but not acted upon, patients may be referred without adequate preparation, or they may be abruptly discharged before a psychiatric evaluation is completed. Close liaison work needs to be done with the treatment team to gain acceptability using sound clinical judgment, offering useful advice for patient management, and working as a team player.

REFERENCES

American Association of Retired Persons (1989). *Elder suicide: A national survey of prevention and intervention programs,* Washington D.C.

Atkinson, R. M., Tolson, R. L., & Turner, J. A., (1993). Factors affecting outpatient treatment compliance of older male problem drinkers *Journal of Studies on Alcohol, 54,* 102–106.

Atkinson, V., & Stuck, B. (1991). Mental Health Services for the Rural Elderly: The SAGE Experience, *The Gerontologist 31,* 548–551

Ayd, F. J. (1972). Once-A-Day Neuroleptic and Tricyclic Antidepressant Therapy *International Drug Therapy Newsletter, 7,* 33–40.

Blackwell, B. (1972). Drug therapy: Patient compliance *New England Journal of Medicine, 289,* 249–252.

Belyaeva, T., & Kabanov, M. (1972). Partial Hospitalization in a Psychiatric Clinic *Soviet Neurology and Psychiatry, 5,* 71–80.

Benbow, S. M. ECT in Late Life. (1991). *International Journal of Geriatric Psychiatry, 6,* 401–406.

Bergmann, K., & Eastham, E. J. (1974). Psychogeriatric ascertainment and assessment for treatment in an acute medical ward setting *Age Aging, 3,* 174–188.

Blackwell, B. (1992). *Compliance. Psychotherapy and psychosomatics, 58,* 161–169.

Blaschke, T. F. (1981). Potential drug interactions in aging patients In A. A., Raskin (Ed.) *Age and the Pharmacology of Psychoactive Drugs.* New York, Elsevier.

Campion, F. X. (1993). *Informed consent Resident & Staff Physician, 39,* 101–106.

Clarke, T. B., Coffey, C. E., Hoffman, G. W., & Weiner, R. D. (1991). Continuation therapy for depression using outpatient electroconvulsive therapy. *Convulsive therapy, 7,* 330–337.

Cohen-Mansfield, J. (1988). Agitated Behavior and Cognitive Functioning in Nursing Home Residents: Preliminary Results. *Clinical Gerontologist,* 7(3/4), 11–22.

Culhane, D., & Culhane, J. (1993). The Elderly's Underutilization of Partial Hospitalization for Mental Disorders and the History of Medicare Reimbursement Policies, *Journal Of Geriatric Psychiatry,* 26(1), 95–112.

Dubin, W. R., Jaffe, R., Roemer, R., & Siegel, L. (1992). The efficacy and safety of maintenance ECT in geriatric patients. *Journal of the American Geriatric Society, 7,* 706–709.

Feldman, E. B. (1983). *Nutrition in the middle and later years,* Boston: John Wright-PSG.

Finlayson, R. E., & Davis L. J. (1994). Prescription drug dependence in the elderly population: Demographic and clinical features of 100 inpatients. *Mayo Clinical Proceedings, 69,* 1137–1145.

Folstein, M. F, Folstein, S., & McHugh, P. R. (1975). Mini Mental State: A practical method of grading the cognitive state of patients for the clinician, *Journal of Psychiatric Research, 12,* 189–198.

Fox, H. (1993). Patients' fear of and objection to electroconvulsive therapy. *Hospital and Community Psychiatry, 44,* 357–360.

Golinger, R. C., & Federoff, J. P. (1989). Characteristics of patients referred to psychiatrists for competency evaluation. *Psychosomatics, 30,* 296–299.

Grunhaus, L., Pande, A. D., & Haskett, R. F. (1990). Full and abbreviated courses of maintenance electroconvulsive therapy. *Convulsive Therapy, 6,* 130–138.

Guy, W., Gross, M., Hogarty, G., & Dennis, H. (1969). A Controlled Evaluation of Day Hospital Effectiveness, *Archives of General Psychiatry,* 20(3), 329–338.

Halaris, A. (1986–87), Antidepressant Drug Therapy in the Elderly: Enhancing Safety and Compliance *International Journal of Psychiatry in Medicine, 16,* 1–19.

Hay, D. P. (1984). Physician Resistance to Treating the Elderly — Facing Our Own Future. *Wisconsin Medical Journal, 83,* 33–37.

Howanitz, E. M., & Freedman, J. B. (1992). Reasons for refusal of medical treatment by patients seen by a consultation and liaison service. *Hospital and Community Psychiatry,* 43(3):278–279.

Jarvik, L. F., & Perl, M. (1981). Overview of physiologic dysfunctions related to psychiatric problems in the elderly. In A. S. Levison, R. C. W. Hall, (Ed.), *Neuropsychiatric Manifestations of Physical Disease in the elderly.* New York: Raven Press.

Klein, L. E. et al. (1982). Aging and Its Relationship to Health Knowledge and Medication Compliance. *Journal of The Gerontologist, 22,* 384–387.

Kramer, B. (1987). Maintenance ECT: A survey of practice. *Convulsive Therapy, 3,* 260–268.

Lipowski, Z., & Wolston, E. J. (1981). Liaison psychiatry: Referral patterns and their stability over time. *American Journal of Psychiatry, 138,* 1608–1611.

Lipowski, Z. J. (1983). The need to integrate liaison psychiatry and geropsychiatry *American Journal of Psychiatry, 140*(8), 1003–1005.

Lipton, H. L., & Bird, J. A. (1994). The Impact of Clinical Pharmacists' Consultations on Geriatric Patients' Compliance and Medical Care Use: A Randomized Controlled Trial *Journal of The Gerontologist, 34,*(3), 307–315.

Liptzin, B. (1982). The geriatric psychiatrist's role as consultant. *Journal of Geriatric Psychiatry and Neurology, 16*(1), 103–112.

Lundin, D. V. et al. (1980). Education of Independent Elderly in the Responsible Use of Prescription Medications. *Journal of Drug Intelligence and Clinical Pharmacy, 14*, 335–342.

Mainprize, E., & Rodin, G. (1987) Geriatric referrals to a psychiatric consultation and liaison service. *Canadian Journal of Psychiatry, 32*(1), 5–8.

Marishita, L., Siu, A., Wang, R., Oken, C., Cadogen, M., & Schwartzman, L. (1989). Comprehensive Geriatric Care in a Day Hospital: A demonstration of the British Model in the United States. *The Gerontologist, 29*(3), 336–340.

McCartney, J. R., & Palmateer, L. M. (1985). Assessment of cognitive deficits in geriatric patients: A study of physician behavior *Journal of American Geriatric Society, 33*, 467–471.

McMullen, P., Ross, A. J., & Rees, J. A. (1991). Problems experienced with medicines by psychogeriatric patients in the community *The Pharmaceutical Journal, 247*, 182–184.

Meltzhoff, J., & Blumenthal, R. (1969). *The Day Treatment Center,* Springfield, Illinois: Charles C. Thomas.

Monroe, R. R. (1991). Maintenance electroconvulsive therapy. *Psychiatric Clinics of North America, 14*, 940–961.

Orsulak, P. J., & Kolodner, R. M. (1989). Improving antidepressant therapy: Role of drug level monitoring *Drug Therapy, 19*, 25–32.

Peterson, L. (1986). Rx Anger [special Issue: The Elderly Uncooperative Patient]. *Journal of Clinical-Gerotolotist, 6* (2), 19–21.

Pitt, B., & Silver, C. P. (1980). The combined approach in geriatrics and psychiatry: Evaluation of a joint unit in a teaching hospital district. *Age and Aging, 9*, 33–37.

Popkin, M. K., Mackenzie, T. B., & Callies, A. L. (1984). Psychiatric consultations to geriatric medically ill inpatients in a university hospital, *Archives of General Psychiatry, 41*, 703–707.

Reisberg, B., Borenstein, J., Salob, S. P., Ferris, S. H., Franssen, S. H., & Georgotas, A. (1987). Behavioral Symptoms in Alzheimer's Disease; Phenomenology and Treatment. *J Clin Psychiatry, 48* (5), 95–155.

Ruskin, P. E. (1985). Geropsychiatry consultation in a university hospital: A report on 67 referrals. *American Journal of Psychiatry, 142*(3), 333–335.

Salzman, C. N. (1982), Basic principles of psychotropic drug prescription for the elderly. *Hospital Community Psychiatry, 33*, 133–136.

Salzman, C., & Van Der Kolk, B. A. (1979). Management of the geriatric patient in a general hospital: Psychotropic drugs and polypharmacy in elderly patients in a general hospital. *Journal of Geriatric Psychiatry, 12*, 167–176.

Shute, G. E. (1986). Psychotherapy of reluctant, depressed elders *Clinical Gerontologist, 6*, 81–83.

Stoudemire, A., Hill, C. D., Morris, R., & Lewison, B. J. (1993). Long-term Outcome of Treatment-Resistant Depression in Older Adults. *American Journal of Psychiatry, 150*, 1539–1540.

Thienhaus, O. J., & Greschel, J. (1988). Nursing Interim Care: A novel practice concept, *Journal of Clinical-Gerontologist, 8* (1), pp. 27–35.

Thienhaus, O. J., Margletta, S., & Bennett, J. A. (1990). A study of the clinical efficacy of maintenance ECT. *Journal of Clinical Psychiatry, 51*, 141–144.

Thorton, J. E., Mulsant, B. H., Dealy R., & Reynolds, C. F., M.D. (1990). A retrospective study of maintenance electroconvulsive therapy in a university-based psychiatric practice. *Convulsive Therapy. 6*, 121–129.

Tonkin, A. L., & Bochner, F. (1994). Therapeutic drug monitoring and patient outcome. *Clinical Pharmacokinetics, 3*, 169–174.

Urquhart, J. (1994). Role of Patient Compliance in clinical Pharmacokinetics: A Review of Recent Research. *Clin Pharmacokinet, 27* (3), 202–215.

Waller, D. A., & Altshuler, K. Z. (1986). Perspectives on patient noncompliance. *Hospital and Community Psychiatry, 37*(5), 490–492.

Wantanabe, M., & Davis, J. M. (1990). Overview: Pharmacotherapeutic considerations in the elderly psychiatric patient *Psychiatric Annals, 8,* pp 423–432.

Wood, A. (1986). Uncooperative Behavior in Unipolar Depression: Managing Medication Non-compliance. *Journal of Clinical-Gerontologist,* [Special Issue: The Elderly Uncooperative Patient], *6* (2), pp. 109–112.

Yesavage, J. A., & Brink, T. L. (1983). Development and validation of geriatric depression screening scale: A preliminary report. *J Psychiat Res, 17* (1), 37–49.

20

Memory Disorders in Older Adults

ROBERT HIRSCHMAN

Alice Grant is a 76 year old depressed married woman with history of hypertension referred for a neuropsychological evaluation to determine if she was suffering actual memory loss (reflective of a neurodegenerative condition) or simply memory complaints related to depression (so called pseudo-dementia or depression related cognitive dysfunction). Ms. Grant complained of forgetfulness and associated feelings of agitation, anxiety, and stress. She was polite and spoke articulately although she displayed occasional word finding difficulties. She performed well on most cognitive tests (WAIS-R: Verbal IQ = 118, Performance IQ = 112, Full Scale IQ = 119) and very short term memory (WMS-R Verbal: 52nd %tile; Nonverbal: 40th %tile) but weak in delayed memory (Verbal: 18 %tile; Nonverbal: 20 %tile). Face-name learning (RBMT) was mildly impaired but she responded well to cueing. When asked to learn a route (RBMT), she recalled the key elements of the route but out of sequence. She generated a score of 30 on the Beck Depression Inventory. Contributing to her dysfunction was the burden of attempting to care for her severely ill, dependent, demanding, and agitated husband. We concluded that she was suffering from major depression with associated mild memory impairment and recommended that she receive assistance in placing her husband as well as treatment for her memory problems and continued treatment for depression. We suggested a number of specific memory strategies and worked closely with her therapist and her daughter to implement this plan. The memory techniques included writing down appointments and important information in a memory book, setting an hourly watch alarm to cue her to check her book, posting a schedule and calendar in her kitchen, and paraphrasing information she is told in conversation. Given her sequencing difficulties, we recommended providing a written series of steps to complete complex tasks. We also recommended providing a combination of maps and directions that refer to landmarks to help her find her way about.

A ten month follow-up evaluation revealed significantly improved affect (Beck Depression Inventory = 5) and concentration as well as stable cognitive functioning (VIQ = 121; PIQ = 121, FSIQ = 122) but continuing weaknesses in delayed memory. She increased her activities by attending 2 hour exercise classes, socializing, participating in church and community organizations, and going out to dinners at least twice a week. Her daughter reported that she sometimes stubbornly refused to follow some suggestions but for the most part responded well to cues and offers of assistance. The therapist continues to see Ms. Grant, maintain contact with her family, and collaborate with her internist and psychiatrist.

AGING AND MEMORY

At an age where one is expected to integrate a near lifetime of knowledge and experiences to achieve developmental tasks involving integrity, acceptance, wisdom, and guidance, the specter of forgetfulness lays heavily on people's minds. It is not death but cognitive deterioration that poses dire threats to the older adult's self-perceptions and social relationships, and near phobic reactions. Health practitioners and researchers have scrambled to meet the epidemic of memory complaints. Where Alzheimer's disease and related neurodegenerative dementias are concerned, more reliable assessments for making accurate diagnoses earlier in the disease process are emphasized, as are experimental drug treatments, alternative living and community support arrangements, and support groups or more formal interventions for family caregiver stress. Where "age associated memory impairment" and "depression related cognitive dysfunction" are suspected, psychopharmacologic, cognitive-behavioral, and memory enhancing interventions are often prescribed.

The social consequences of memory impairment may be devastating. Social relationships depend on joint shared memories of past experiences. Forgetting of shared experiences, personal commitments, social obligations, and rules for specific social activities, roles, or encounters frequently result in exclusion or withdrawal. Family turmoil and isolation frequently result. The distress caused by this isolation, conflict, forgetfulness, or psychiatric symptoms often leads to increased visits to a physician, although the reasons for these visits are often unclear. To the extent that problems involving distress and memory problems can be identified, interventions may be designed and implemented. Unfortunately, little is known about the effectiveness of these various interventions and even less about how to foster motivation, commitment, follow-through, and generalization of these interventions.

TYPES OF MEMORY LOSS AND INTERVENTIONS

Interventions and associated compliance issues differ as a function of the nature and cause of the memory deficit. Memory complaints are common with 50% over age 60 reporting serious problems (Lowenthal, et al., 1967). These problems range in severity, cause, type of memory affected, and discrepancy between self-perceived memory and performance on standardized memory tests. The assessment of these problems requires measures of different types of memory (California Verbal Learning Test, Wechsler Memory Scale-Revised, Rivermead Behavioural Memory Test), perceived memory (Memory Functioning Questionnaire, Metamemory in Adulthood Questionnaire) and associated or contributing factors such as depression (Beck Depression Inventory, Geriatric Depression Scale) or other psychiatric symptoms (SCL-90R).

Milder deficits are typically viewed as being more amenable to direct cognitive interventions. Deficits related to psychiatric distress or depression are typically amenable to cognitive-behavioral, relaxation, and/or psychopharmacologic interventions. Using meta-analysis, Scogin and McElreath (1994) found psychotherapy in general (effect size = .78) and cognitive therapy in particular (effect size = .85) to be highly effective treatments for geriatric depression. Such interventions also sometimes produce beneficial effects on memory functions, although such benefits may be temporary because in many cases a progressive dementia becomes evident over the subsequent three to five years (Alexopoulous, et al., 1993, Kral & Emery, 1989).

Discrepancies between self-perceived memory functions and performance on tests may be related either to overestimation or underestimation of memory problems. These discrepancies may be partially amenable to psychoeducational approaches. Discrepancies between memory perception and function in the direction of overestimation of deficits may be related to affect. Zarit, Gallagher, and Kramer (1981) found that subjective memory complaints show a greater decline as a result of cognitive-memory interventions than does actual memory performance. The improvements in perceived memory were correlated with improvements in affect.

In cases where there is low discrepancy between memory perception and function, memory interventions may both reduce complaints and improve performance without there being a corresponding change in affect (Zarit, Cole, & Guider, 1981). Alternatively, in cases where individuals are highly anxious about their memory problems, combining psychotherapeutic and memory enhancing interventions may be necessary to produce positive results. For example, Yesavage (1984) found that relaxation training improved the ability of older adults to use mnemonic techniques and thereby resulted in improved recall. This combined approach was also helpful in the case of Ms. Grant discussed above whose anxiety extended to attempting some new, unfamiliar strategy to improve memory.

In cases where there is underestimation of deficits, these individuals are unlikely to request help for memory problems. To the extent that family members or health professionals identify potentially remediable or compensatable memory deficits, the major focus will need to be on the initial stages of the behavior change process, i.e., motivation enhancing interventions (Miller & Rollnick, 1991; Prochaska & DiClemente, 1982).

In cases where the memory deficit is more pronounced or where an initially self-aware person with memory problems starts to forget that they forget, environmental modifications become the treatment of choice. Therapists assist family members in structuring the home environment so that objects needed for everyday living are always returned to the same place and external cues such as alarms and schedules are provided to prompt initiating a functional or recreational activity. Organizing and color coding objects needed for activities of daily living and placing them in the areas where they will be needed helps to create a prosthetic environment for the memory impaired person (Fowler, Hart, & Sheehan, 1972; Skinner & Vaughan, 1983). These approaches also capitalize on implicit memory or procedural learning (Eslinger & Damasio, 1986); memory disordered individuals can often re-learn how to complete everyday functions without being able to recall or declare verbally how they complete these activities.

Memory enhancing interventions typically involve components of organization, imagery, and compensatory aids (Scogin & Prohaska, 1993). Organization includes categorizing items such as a grocery list into several sets such as paper goods, spices, and fruits, and chunking a large number of individual items into a smaller number of groups of items (such as telephone numbers in the form xxx–xxxx). This strategy facilitates both encoding and retrieval of learned information. Imagery includes the method of loci where elements of a familiar image (e.g., one's bedroom) are linked to different items on a list (such as a set of errands). Imagery also includes novel interacting images such as linking a person's facial feature with that person's name. These strategies facilitate improved encoding of the information to be remembered. Compensatory aids include external methods or physical reminders such as writing down lists, appointments in a calendar, or notes of things needing to be done and placing these notes in a conspicuous place such as the bathroom mirror.

THE ROLE OF PERCEIVED CONTROL

In geropsychological research, a widely accepted principle involves the maximizing of a sense of internal control over one's environment, relationships, and health in order to maximize quality of life and produce significant decreases in morbidity and mortality. For example, high perceived controllability and predictability of an impending relocation was associated with significantly reduced post-relocation mortality (Schulz & Brenner, 1977) as well as subsequent placement in a nursing home (Rodin, 1986). Incorporating self-instructional and control enhancing methods in a psychological intervention produced stable reductions in urinary free cortisol over an 18 month period of time (Rodin, 1983). The psychological intervention without the control enhancing component produced only a transitory reduction, and the no treatment control showed no reduction. Perceived control is also associated with reduced preoccupation with symptoms and more positive appraisals of health (Levkoff, Cleary, & Wetle, 1987). Generally, increased perceived control ameliorates the impact of negative life events and optimizes health and adaptive outcomes in older adults.

Following this line of research, it is plausible that memory enhancing interventions that maximize perceived control may be particularly effective. One means to accomplish this goal is to develop self-taught memory training programs. In one such program, Scogin, Storandt, and Lott (1985) developed a manual that described memory changes associated with aging, discussed strategies to improve memory in the face of these changes, and presented memory exercises to be completed daily. It took sixteen participants between 16 days and 4 weeks to complete this program. These participants showed improvement on some but not all measures of memory functions relative to a delayed training control group. Scogin and Prohaska (1992) found beneficial effects of a similar program on memory performance relative to a no treatment control, but they found no superiority for this program relative to an attention-placebo intervention. With regard to memory complaints and ratings by family members, they found significant reductions in subjects administered the self-instruction program relative to the attention-placebo participants.

While it is relatively easy to monitor compliance with treatment during a structured, therapist administered intervention, it is more difficult to do so for a self-administered program and for periods of time following the formal administration of a program. In a three year follow-up study, Scogin and Bienias (1988) found that only 28% of participants reported using mnemonic strategies. Scogin and Prohaska (1993) suggest that providing ongoing booster sessions and increased opportunities to generalize or apply what they have learned may result in better long-term effects although there is as yet no data supporting this suggestion.

The context of medical care and specifically the lack of perceived patient control inherent in this system may be partly responsible for the lack of compliance with memory programs in older adults. Health professionals typically prefer patients to be deferential (Wills, 1978) and are less likely to give information and support to older adults than to younger adults (Greene, et al., 1987).

In their overall approach to medical problems, older adults are more likely than younger adults to adopt a traditional medical model view where the responsibility for both the cause and solution to problems are attributed to external agents. The older adult adopting this model feels impotent to diagnose, solve, and appraise changes in their problems and rely on health professionals to complete these tasks for them (J. Karuza, et al., 1990). Self-help approaches are inconsistent with this model and are also more generally not a familiar means of controlling health in this cohort. Further, memory enhancing interventions in general and self-administered ones in particular require a high degree of active participation and effort (Scogin & Prohaska, 1993), inconsistent with the socialization of a passive medical model role in this cohort.

POTHOLES AND PITFALLS

The road to improvement of memory function and/or complaints is hazardous at best. We lack even a road map informing us what the exact nature of the problem is. Without a clear definition of the problem, all the good intentions and zeal in the world may take us in the wrong direction at a cost of precious health care dollars, unmet expectations, disappointment, and suffering. We need to identify the anticipated terrain and lay of the land before we can negotiate these problems more effectively.

The issues of discriminating memory complaints versus dysfunction and identifying the type and severity of dysfunction have been discussed above. The memory enhancing interventions and the role of increasing perceived control have been reviewed. However, even with these issues sorted out, there is no reason to expect higher rates of compliance and success with these problems than we have for controlling addictive behavior, hypertension, weight loss, or high risk sexual behaviors. We need to sort out how the biopsychosocial factors resulting in noncompliance generally may produce noncompliance in the population of older adults with memory complaints or dysfunction.

There are many reasons for noncompliance with memory enhancing interventions. First, some individuals may be unaware that there is a problem or forget what the problem is, thereby producing reluctance to seek help or follow recommendations. Others may appear rebellious if not hostile, perceiving messages about their problem and suggested solutions as usurping what is left of their waning sense of control. Still others may be resigned and lack the energy to invest in a memory rehabilitative program. Yet others may rationalize their difficulties as being the result of normal aging, retirement, losses, family stressors, or environmental changes, and further perceive no potential benefit to addressing adjustment to these changes.

There are also individuals who are ambivalent; they are either very aware of their difficulties or emphatic with their complaints but need additional positive incentives to participate in a suitable program. Retrieving memories of past successful learning or self-improvement activities may be of benefit. Alternatively, some individuals may have difficulty visualizing how seemingly tedious mnemonics will help them with their everyday life. Concrete examples and monitoring with feedback may help address these concerns.

Despite their apparently respectful stance toward the medical profession, older adults show no increase in compliance rates and express many reasons for noncompliance. Atwood, et al. (1992) found that non-adherence among older adults in 3 community based clinical studies was related to forgetting, side effects, unrelated illness, and competing outside stressors. Further, mild cognitive impairment may result in medication non-compliance which in some conditions worsens the cognitive impairment. Computer assisted medication recall training has been shown to be effective in increasing medication adherence (Leirer, et al., 1988).

Finally, there exists controversy on whether individuals with more severe memory impairment can benefit from memory enhancing interventions. Zarit, Cole, and Guider (1981) suggest screening these individuals out to avoid failure experiences and to reassure the remaining participants that their memory loss is mild, normal, and not the beginning of incipient decline and dementia. Some dementia care units in nursing homes are now experimenting with simplified cognitive interventions that promote some experience of success, focus, and optimal level of stimulation that is neither too intense to be overwhelming nor so limited as to produce a state of sensory deprivation and confusion.

THE THREE R'S: RELATIONSHIP, REPRESENTATIONAL MEANING, AND REMOVING BARRIERS

While likely not sufficient, necessary elements to improve compliance with memory enhancing interventions must address issues of relationship, meaning, and obstacles. Health care professionals must work to establish and maintain a collaborative partnership with both the patient and family members. Key ingredients to this process include respect, warmth, empathy, and open communication. All steps of the communication process need to be attended to, including reception, comprehension, memory, personal acceptance, and behavior (Leventhal and Hirschman, 1982). Communicating the nature of the problem, the need for intervention, and the precise steps involved in intervention so that these messages are heard, understood, remembered, and personally accepted are essential to compliance. Structuring the relationship so that it invites participation and activity on the part of the patient will also likely combat the passivity barrier and foster both improved compliance and perceived control.

Impaired concentration, memory, abstract reasoning, and organization as well as depression and anxiety interfere with the communication process. Because messages may not be received by the patient, there may remain a lack of accurate awareness of the problem, lack of motivation to change, and/or lack of commitment to persist through the change process. Therefore, special attention needs to be paid to each step in the communication process in a manner that reduces anxiety and increases confidence. The practitioner and patient need to develop collaboratively a memory plan which addresses issues of motivation, strategy selection, and strategy use (Duke, Haley, & Bergquist, 1991). Once these issues are effectively negotiated, specific messages need to be provided to facilitate implementation of the agreed upon plan. For example, identification of external cues may be necessary for an individual to apply newly learned mnemonic strategies to everyday situations (Robertson-Tchabo, Hausman, & Arenberg, 1976).

In addition to addressing relationship issues with the patient, these same issues frequently need to be addressed with family members. Caregivers for Alzheimer's patients clearly show prominent psychiatric distress and depression (Cohen, et al., 1990) and these symptoms have been associated with violent family interactions (Paveza, et al., 1992). While the stress in family members of older adults with more mild memory problems or complaints may be less severe, family members will still likely need the same type of supportive and communicative relationship that their relatives need in order to address their needs and be more effective in facilitating compliance with a treatment regimen. Further, cultural variations in family beliefs and caregiving practices need to be incorporated in these approaches (Segall and Wykle, 1988). Family members are frequently a vital but unheralded part of the treatment alliance.

Patients attempt to understand and regulate their treatment through the formation of schemata or representations (H. Leventhal, Diefenbach, & E. Leventhal, 1992). Currently, we sorely lack data on how individuals represent memory problems and treatments. We have not identified the rules patients follow in appraising themselves as experiencing symptoms of a memory disorder, nor have we described what factors these symptoms might be attributed to. Individuals' theories of how memory works, what symptoms of forgetfulness indicate, and how interventions for memory problems and complaints work may greatly influence both compliance and the success of the treatment. One intervention may involve helping patients interpret their symptoms and treatment in a more adaptive manner.

Once we know how individuals' theories of memory function change as a result of experience, we may be able to facilitate adaptive changes in representations. For example, an individual may experience success using physical reminders and may be more amenable to working to develop new habits to compensate for memory loss and maintain social involvement. As treatment progresses, an examination of how the patient represents social relationships may provide a key to maintaining or rebuilding these vitally important relationships. Given that most patients think of health problems in terms of acute diseases, some attention may need to be directed to presenting the issue of memory limits as a chronic one needing ongoing coping and use of compensatory strategies.

The ability to link information and experiences with specific models (e.g., parents or grandparents) may either impede or facilitate the treatment process. To the extent that an adaptive representation is formed and concrete goals agreed to, constructive problem-focused as well as emotion-focused coping may be facilitated. Furthermore, this process may facilitate realistic and positive appraisals of outcome.

The role of barriers cannot be overstated. Whether it is money, transportation, weather, family conflict, or illness, any factor may impede treatment. Neurobehavioral limits in ability to process information, solve problems, or initiate behavior may pose additional barriers to compliance. Attempts to "conserve energy" may pose yet another barrier (E. Leventhal, et al., 1993). These barriers may change over time particularly if one has a progressive dementia or suffers a stroke. Frequent boosters and guided practice in applying techniques to everyday situations may be required. Involving all members of the health care team as well as the family is frequently necessary to initiate and maintain change, as was evident with the case of Alice Grant discussed above.

A particularly worrisome barrier is the tendency of health professionals to forget the strategies that promote an effective treatment alliance for the treatment of patients' memory problems (Meichenbaum & Turk, 1987). Checklists placed in one's office or in patients' charts may serve as reminders. Taking the time to listen to patients' ideas, attend to the communication process, and enlist the collaboration of family members are necessary if memory enhancing interventions are to be successful. As the younger generations age, they may be able to look confidently toward a user friendly future where they are functioning independently, socially active, and confident in their abilities to cope with change, to integrate memories, and to continue getting the most out of life.

REFERENCES

Alexopoulos, G. S., Meyers, B. S., Young, R. C., Mattis, S., & Kakuma, T. (1993). The course of geriatric depression with "reversible dementia": A controlled study. *American Journal of Psychiatry, 150,* 1693-1699.

Atwood, J. R., Haase, J., Rees-McGee, S., Blackwell, G., et al. (1992). Reasons related to adherence in community-based field studies. *Patient Education and Counseling, 19,* 251-259.

Cohen, D., Luchins, D., Eisdorfer, C., Paveza, G., Ashford, J. W., Gorelick, P., Hirschman, R., Freels, S., Levy, P., and Shaw, H. (1990). Caring for relatives with Alzheimer's disease: The mental health risks to spouses, adult children, and other family ccaregivers. *Behavior, Health, and Aging, 1,* 171-182.

Duke, L. W., Haley, W. E., & Bergquist, T. F. (1991). Cognitive-behavioral interventions for age-related memory impairments. In P. A. Wisocki (Ed.), *Handbook of clinical behavior therapy with the elderly client.* New York: Plenum Press.

Eslinger, P. J., & Damasio, A. R. (1986). Preserved motor learning in Alzheimer's disease: Implications for anatomy and behavior. *Journal of Neuroscience, 6,* 3006-3009.

Fowler, R., Hart, J., & Sheehan, M. (1972). A prosthetic memory: An application of the prosthetic memory concept. *Rehabilitation Counseling Bulletin, 16,* 80-85.

Greene, M. G., Hoffman, S., Charon, R., & Adelman, R. (1987). Psychosocial concerns in the medical encounter: A comparison of the interactions of doctors with their old and young patients. *The Gerontologist, 27,* 164-168.

Karuza, J., Zevon, M. A., Gleason, T. A., Karuza, C. M., & Nash, L. (1990). Models of helping and coping, responsibility attributions, and well-being in community elderly and their helpers. *Psychology and Aging, 5,* 194-208.

Kral, V. A., & Emery, O. B. (1989). Long-term follow-up of depressive pseudodementia of the aged. *Canadian Psychiatry, 34,* 445-446.

Leirer, V. O., Morrow, D. G., Pariante, G. M., & Sheikh, J. I. (1988). Elders' nonadherence, its assessment, and computer assisted instruction for medication recall training. *Journal of the American Geriatrics Society, 36,* 877–884.

Leventhal, E. A., Leventhal, H., Schaeefer, P., & Easterling, D. (1993). Conservation of energy, uncertainty reduction, and swift utilization of medical care among the elderly. *Journal of Gerontology, 48,* 78P–86P.

Leventhal, H., Diefenbach, M., & Leventhal, E. A. (1992). Using common sense to understand treatment adherence and affect cognitive interactions. *Cognitive Therapy and Research, 16,* 143–163.

Leventhal, H., and Hirschman, R. S. (1982). Social psychology and prevention. In G. Sanders and J. Suls (Eds.), *Social psychology of health and illness*. Hillsdale, NJ: Lawrence Erlbaum Associates.

Levkoff, S. E., Cleary, P. D., & Wetle, T. (1987). Differences in the appraisal of health between aged and middle-aged adults. *Journal of Gerontology, 42,* 114–120.

Lowenthal, M. F., Berkman, P. L., Buehler, J. A., Pierce, R. C., Robinson, B. C., & Trier, M. L. (1967). *Aging and mental disorder in San Francisco*. San Francisco: Jossey Bass.

Meichenbaum, D., & Turk, D. C. (1987). *Facilitating treatment adherence*. New York: Plenum.

Miller, W. R., & Rollnick, S. (1991). *Motivational interviewing: Preparing people to change addictive behavior*. New York: The Guilford Press.

Paveza, G. J., Cohen, D., Eisdorfer, C., Freels, S., Semla, T., Ashford, J. W., Gorelick, P., Hirschman, R., Luchins, D., and Levy, P. (1992). Severe family violence and Alzheimer's disease: Prevalence and risk factors. *The Gerontologist, 32,* 493–497.

Prochaska, J. O., & DiClemente, C. C. (1982). Transtheoretical therapy: Toward a more integrative model of change. *Psychotherapy: Theory, Research, and Practice, 19,* 276–288.

Robertson-Tcabo, E. A., Hausman, C. P., & Arenberg, D. (1976). A classical mnemonic for older learners: A trip that works! *Educational Gerontology, 1,* 215–226.

Rodin, J. (1986). Health, control, and aging. In M. M. Baltes & P. B. Baltes (Eds.), *Aging and the psychology of control*. Hillsdale, NJ: Lawrence Erlbaum Associates.

Rodin, J. (1983). Behavioral medicine: Beneficial effects of self-control training in aging. *International Review of Applied Psychology, 32,* 153–181.

Schulz, R., & Brenner, G. (1977). Relocation of the aged: A review and theoretical analysis. *Journal of Gerontology, 32,* 323–333.

Scogin, F., & Bienias, J. L. (1988). A three-year follow-up of older adult participants in a memory-skills training program. *Psychology and Aging, 3,* 334–337.

Scogin, F., & McElreath, L. (1994). Efficacy of psychosocial treatments for geriatric depression: A quantitative review. *Journal of Consulting and Clinical Psychology, 62,* 69–74.

Scogin, F., & Prohaska, M. (1992). The efficacy of self-taught memory training for community dwelling older adults. *Educational Gerontology, 18,* 751–766.

Scogin, F., & Prohaska, M. (1993). *Aiding older adults with memory complaints*. Sarasota, Florida: Professional Resource Press.

Scogin, F., Storandt, M., & Lott, L. (1985). Memory skills training, memory complaints, and depression in older adults. *Journal of Gerontology, 40,* 562–568.

Segall, M., & Wykle, M. (1988). The black family's experience with dementia. *The Journal of Applied Social Sciences, 13,* 170–191.
Skinner, B. F., & Vaughan, M. E. (1983). *Enjoy old age: A program of self-
   management.* New York: W. W. Norton.
Wills, T. H. (1978). Perceptions of clients by professional helpers. *Psychological Bulletin, 85,* 968–1000.
Yesavage, J. A. (1984). Relaxation and memory training in 39 elderly
   patients. *American Journal of Psychiatry, 141,* 778–781.
Zarit, S. H., Cole, K. D., & Guider, R. L. (1981). Memory training strategies
   ands subjective complaints of memory in the aged. *The Gerontologist,
   21,* 158–165.
Zarit, S. H., Gallagher, D., & Kramer, N. (1981). Memory training in
   the community aged: Effects of depression, memory complaint, and
   memory performance. *Educational Gerontologist, 6,* 11–27.

Index